Safe and Effective Medication Use in the Emergency Department

Safe and Effective Medication Use in the Emergency Department

Victor Cohen BS, PharmD, BCPS, CGP
Assistant Professor of Pharmacy Practice
Arnold & Marie Schwartz College of Pharmacy and
Health Sciences
Long Island University
Clinical Pharmacy Manager for the
Department of Emergency Medicine

and

Director of Emergency Medicine and Pharmacy
Practice Residency Programs
Maimonides Medical Center

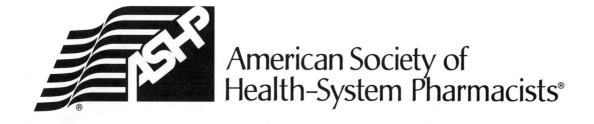

American Society of
Health-System Pharmacists®

Any correspondence regarding this publication should be sent to the publisher, American Society of Health-System Pharmacists, 7272 Wisconsin Avenue, Bethesda, MD 20814, attention: Special Publishing.

Director, Special Publishing: Jack Bruggeman
Acquiring Editor, Special Publishing: Hal Pollard
Senior Editorial Project Manager: Dana Battaglia

Library of Congress Cataloging-in-Publication Data

Cohen, Victor. Safe and effective medication use in the emergency department / Victor Cohen. p. ; cm.
  Includes bibliographical references and index.
  ISBN 978-1-58528-233-3
  1. Hospital pharmacies. 2. Emergency medicine—Safety measures. 3. Drug interactions. I. American Society of Health-System Pharmacists. II. Title.
  [DNLM: 1. Pharmacy Service, Hospital—organization & administration. 2. Emergency Service, Hospital—organization & administration. 3. Interdepartmental Relations. 4. Medication Systems, Hospital. 5. Safety Management. WX 179 C678s 2009]
  RA975.5.P5C64 2009
  362.17'82—dc22

                                                                                    2009019314

ISBN: 978-1-58528-233-3

Dedication

To my wife, Samantha, who has provided me with insurmountable love, support, and confidence to complete this work.

To my father Jacobo, mother Esther and sister Diane, who have always encouraged me.

To my brother Henry, a mentor and role model, who proved to me that I can overcome all barriers.

To Grandpa Max, who in his dying days still asked, "Did you finish the book yet?"

To pharmacists, emergency medicine physicians, nurses, patient care technicians, and all other emergency department staff who work as a team to sacrifice their lives to save others without daily acknowledgements, you are all blessed.

CONTENTS

Reviewers   ix

Preface   xi

PART I Crossroads Between Emergency Medicine and Pharmacy Practice 1

1   Emergency Medicine: An Overview   3

2   Challenges Facing Emergency Medicine Quality and Safety: Medication Management   9

3   Aligning the Principles of Pharmacotherapy with Emergency Medicine   15

4   Emergency Clinical Pharmacy Services: Historical Perspective and Systematic Review   21

5   Unique Characteristics of the Emergency Department and the Emergency Department Pharmacist   31

6   Academic-Based Emergency Department Clinical Pharmacy Services and the PharmER Pyramid   35

PART II Anatomy of a Safe Medication Use System: Operational Considerations . . . 43

7   Defining a Safe Medication Use System in the Emergency Department   45

8   Establishing Relationships in the Emergency Department: A Pharmacy Leadership and Advocacy Role   49

9   Improving the Drug Order and Delivery Process in the Emergency Department with Information Systems   57

10   Emergency Department Unit of Use Formulary and Drug Distribution System   69

11   Reviewing Medications for Appropriateness in the Emergency Department   77

PART III Assuring Quality of Emergency Care Pharmacotherapy: Focus on Quality Measures, High-Risk, High-Cost Medication, and Response to Medical Emergencies 87

12   Antimicrobial Stewardship in the Emergency Department   89

13   Significance of Drug Interactions in the Emergency Department   103

14   Responding to Toxicologic and Public Health Emergencies   111

15   Emergency Care Pharmacotherapy of the Critically Ill: Tools to Expedite Care   133

16   Clinical Decisions and Instructional Support System: Clinical Pharmacy Service and Informatics   149

17   Target Medication Reconciliation in the Emergency Department   161

18   Emergency Care Pharmacotherapy Considerations in Special Populations: Geriatric, Pediatric, and Obstetric   167

PART IV Fostering Interest in Emergency Care Pharmacotherapy 181

19   Education for Emergency Medicine Pharmacotherapy: A Blueprint for PGY2 Specialty Residency   183

20   Designing an Undergraduate PharmD Intern Practice Model in the Emergency Department   189

21   Role of the Pharmacy Technician: Use of Board-Certified Support Personnel to Facilitate Clinical Pharmacy Services in the Emergency Department   201

22   Future of Clinical Pharmacy Services in the Emergency Department   205

PART V **Appendices** **211**

Appendix A: Policies and Procedures   213

    Policy and Procedure for Monitoring
    Medications and Supplies for
    Emergency Response   213

    Policy and Procedure for Code Team
    and PharmD Role   214

    Policy and Procedure for Acute Stroke   216

    Policy and Procedure for the Treatment
    of Thrombolytic for Acute Myocardial
    Infarction (AMI)   218

Appendix B: Dosing Guides and Tables   221

    Adult ED Acute Area Medication Floor
    Stock Par Level List   222

    Acute Care Area Medication Floor Stock
    List for Refrigerated Medications   223

    Acute Care Area Controlled Drug Floor
    Stock List   224

    Resuscitation Care Area Medication
    Floor Stock List   224

    Resuscitation Care Area Controlled
    Drug Floor Stock List   226

    Pediatric ED Controlled Drug Floor
    Stock List   227

    Clinical Steps for Safe Antidote Ordering
    and Delivery Process in the ED   228

    Bioterrorism Monthly Inventory List   233

    Antidotes for Chemical Agents   234

    Radiologic and Nuclear Antidotes Monthly
    Inventory List   235

    Pandemic Influenza Preparedness   237

    Chronic Care Medications for Natural
    Disasters   239

    Emergency Medicine Pharmacotherapist
    General Principles and Guide to Managing
    Critical Care Infusions   242

Appendix C: Educational Outcomes, Goals,
and Objectives for Emergency Medicine   246

    Educational Outcomes, Goals, and
    Objectives for Postgraduate Year
    Two (PGY2) Pharmacy Residencies
    in Emergency Medicine   246

Index   255

REVIEWERS

Roberta Aguglia, BSPharm, RPh
Associate Director of Operations
Department of Pharmaceutical Services
Maimonides Medical Center
Brooklyn, New York

Patricia Caruso, MSPharm, PharmD
Clinical Pharmacy Manager of Antibiotics and Infectious
    Diseases
Department of Pharmaceutical Services
Maimonides Medical Center
Brooklyn, New York

Fredrick B. Cassera, BS, MS, MBA
Director
Department of Pharmaceutical Services
Maimonides Medical Center
Brooklyn, New York

Tanya Clairborne, PharmD
Clinical Pharmacy Specialist
Emergency Medicine
SENTARA
Hampton, Virginia

Hillary Cohen, MD, MPH
Attending Physician
Department of Emergency Medicine
Maimonides Medical Center
Brooklyn, New York

Steven J. Davidson, MD, MBA, FACEP
Chairman
Department of Emergency Medicine
Maimonides Medical Center
Brooklyn, New York

Lydia B. Fancher, PharmD, BCPS
Emergency Medicine Pharmacy Practice Resident
Department of Pharmaceutical Services
Maimonides Medical Center
Brooklyn, New York0

Christian Fromm, MD
Director, Division of Research
Emergency Medicine
Maimonides Medical Center
Brooklyn, New York

Estevan Garcia, MD
Vice Chairman, Pediatric
Emergency Medicine
Maimonides Medical Center
Brooklyn, New York

William M. Goldman, BS, PharmD
Associate Director for Clinical Services
Department of Pharmaceutical Services
Maimonides Medical Center
Brooklyn, New York

Connie Grande, RN, BSN
Project Implementation Support Nurse
Department of Emergency Medicine
Maimonides Medical Center
Brooklyn, New York

Amie Jo Hatch, PharmD
Pharmacy Practice Resident
Department of Pharmaceutical Services
Maimonides Medical Center
Brooklyn, New York

Samantha P. Jellinek, PharmD, BCPS, CGP
Clinical Pharmacy Manager, Medication Reconciliation
    & Safety
and the Acute Care for Elders (ACE) Unit
Clinical Coordinator, Pharmacy Practice (PGY-1) and
Emergency Medicine Specialty (PGY-2) Residencies
Department of Pharmaceutical Services
Maimonides Medical Center
Brooklyn, New York

Kelly R. Klein, MD
Department of Emergency Medicine
Maimonides Medical Center
Brooklyn, New York

Antonios Likourezos, MA, MPH
Research Associate
Department of Emergency Medicine
Maimonides Medical Center
Brooklyn, New York

Michael Lapatto
Maimonides Medical Center
Department of Emergency Medicine
Brooklyn, New York

Eustace Lashley, MD, FACEP
Director, Adult Emergency Medicine
Maimonides Medical Center
Department of Emergency Medicine
Brooklyn, New York

John Marshall, MD, FACEP
Vice Chairman for Academics
Department of Emergency Medicine
Maimonides Medical Center
Brooklyn, New York

Domenic Martinello, MD
Chief Resident
Department of Emergency Medicine
Maimonides Medical Center
Brooklyn, New York

Brad Miller, PharmD
Clinical Pharmacy Specialist
Emergency Medicine
Spectrum Health Butterworth Hospital
Pharmacy Department
Grand Rapids, Michigan

Sergey M. Motov, MD
Assistant Residency Program Director
Department of Emergency Medicine
Maimonides Medical Center
Brooklyn, New York

Kathy Peterson, RN
Director of Nursing
Emergency Medicine
Maimonides Medical Center
Brooklyn, New York

Kenneth N. Sable, MD, FACEP
Director, Division of Medical Informatics
Associate Vice Chairman for Operations
Department of Emergency Medicine
Maimonides Medical Center
Brooklyn, New York

Linda Salem, RN, BS
Director of Clinical Systems
MIS Department
Maimonides Medical Center
Brooklyn, New York

Lindsay Stansfield, PharmD
Pharmacy Practice Resident
Department of Pharmaceutical Services
Maimonides Medical Center
Brooklyn, New York

Gloria Tsang, MD
Emergency Medicine Resident
Department of Emergency Medicine
Maimonides Medical Center
Brooklyn, New York

Angela Torres, PharmD
Emergency Medicine Pharmacy Practice Resident
Department of Pharmaceutical Services
Maimonides Medical Center
Brooklyn, New York

Janet Williams RN, CNS
Director of Nursing
Emergency Medicine
Maimonides Medical Center
Brooklyn, New York

PREFACE

As a pharmacy intern at Northeastern University during my undergraduate years of pharmacy school, I recall the day I was on Coronary Care Unit rounds at Massachusetts General Hospital, not sure of my role and wishing at the time that there was someone to tell me what to do. The pharmacy preceptor visited and showed me all the problems that the team had just created and that I failed to fix. During my endocrine rotation at St. Johns University, I witnessed an endocrinology specialist, an expert I hoped to resemble, who helped couples become pregnant with hormone therapy through an understanding of pharmacology. It was during my Toxicology rotations of my post-baccalaureate PharmD (at that time PharmD was a two-year post graduate requirement) when I discovered my interest—toxicology. It was so fascinating and the practitioners at the New York City Poison Control Center were great mentors with this relentless pursuit for knowledge of pharmacology and toxicology. Despite this, I still felt peripheral to the care of the patient. One day, during my rotation at Mary Imogene Bassett Hospital in Cooperstown, I witnessed a code and saw everyone running toward the bedside; I was excited and intensely focused but was upset that I did not have the skills to respond or assist in saving the patient's life. I remember requesting to initiate an emergency medicine rotation at Miami VA Healthcare System where I was completing my first year of residency training. I recall running with the medical team toward the front of the medical center where a patient was just dropped off by his friend; the patient appeared unresponsive and in respiratory distress after injecting heroin. The nurses were not sure what to do; I suggested to the physician to try naloxone. Even with the chaos that this event created, I knew I was hooked.

Despite having a good knowledge base in toxicology, I needed more knowledge on how to respond during an emergency, and it was not until I began my second year of postgraduate training at Robert Wood Johnson University Hospital where I witnessed what the expectation for a pharmacist is within an emergency department. I recall my first days responding to a Trauma code, gowning up, assisting with delivery of a patient to the CT scanner, or being paged for a pediatric code that the ICU physician would not start until the pharmacy team was present to dispense medications.

These experiences developed my passion for emergency medicine and the perseverance to understand the role of a pharmacist. At that time, there were few clinical pharmacy jobs available within the ED setting so I compromised and took an academic position with the intent to establish and foster an emergency medicine pharmacy practice service.

Since then, I have worked over ten years with numerous physicians and nurses in a multidisciplinary manner to ensure optimal use of medications. First, we used a paper system, and then we transformed the system into an electronic one. Over the years, as a result of these experiences, I have been asked "what do you do as a pharmacist in the emergency department?" or "what value do you bring?" I have been questioned how to solve this problem clinically and operationally. Furthermore, when pharmacy issues arise, I am a catalyst for change and implementation through education and communication, which are often lacking within healthcare institutions due to politics and economics. With this journey in mind and the current exposure given to the ED due to the recent Institute of Medicine report, it was time to shed light on what I have experienced.

Safe and Effective Medication Use in the Emergency Department is intended to serve several purposes. First, this book is an introductory text for allied health care professional students, residents, and practitioners of all disciplines because it serves as a resource to explaining the emergency department, its history, its essential role in healthcare, circumstances that have overwhelmed this resource, and the inherent risks associated with an overloaded system. Second, this book is intended for undergraduate and postgraduate PharmD students, first-year pharmacy practice residents who may be doing an elective clerkship in emergency medicine as part of their advanced practice pharmacy experiences, and second-year postgraduate pharmacy residents who have developed an interest for this area of specialization. This text provides instruction on the role of pharmacists, pharmacist activities in the emergency department, and how to blend into the chaos of the department. Most importantly, this book instructs on how to respond during emergency care.

Safe and Effective Medication Use in the Emergency Department can serve as a primer to pharmacist practitioners who either want to establish a clinical pharmacy services in the ED, plan to establish one, or have been re-deployed and are tasked to provide services to the ED. This text provides practitioners with answers to what are the contextual elements of emergency medicine clinical pharmacy services, and how to implement sustainable services. Fourth, this text can serve as a primer to administrators, quality assurance experts, and regulatory groups as a means to understanding the impact on various regulations and the strides that healthcare systems have to go through to achieve these goals. This text may also be used by educators in all fields of medicine to illustrate patient safety issues and the interconnectedness of all disciplines and their processes;

communication is the most essential component to ensure a safe medication use system.

Safe and Effective Medication Use in the Emergency Department serves as an entry into the world of emergency medicine pharmacotherapy; the fusion of experience of current practice and evidence-based pharmacotherapy can foster a research agenda in emergency medicine pharmacotherapy. There is no current text that describes the specific issues associated with emergency medicine pharmacotherapy within the ED. This text may help improve deployment of technology into the ED or show how to modify technology to achieve regulatory goals and assure better continuity. This text was also intended for the medical director and nursing director of emergency departments to identify how they may deploy pharmacy to be advantageous to the overall clinical operations of the ED. We describe pharmacy leadership and management and introduce the PharmER pyramid model as a means to establishing a sustainable clinical pharmacy service that achieves The Joint Commission's Medication Management Standards. The PharmER pyramid acts as building blocks or the establishment of structure within the ED, which if implemented, can help evaluate processes or measure outcomes. This text also covers how best to respond to public health emergencies and explains current issues associated with care of specific patient populations (geriatric, obstetric, and pediatric).

This book is a fusion of evidence from the literature, and when there was no evidence, we provided our experience or that of those who have successfully implemented activities and wrote of their observations. Published peer-reviewed data from pharmacy, pharmacotherapy, emergency medicine, public health, toxicology, critical care, infectious diseases, quality assurance, and medication safety were used to compile this book. We visited other EDs, and my research included observing the needs of pharmacists by attending numerous ED-pharmacy conferences.

I acknowledge those days at Robert Wood Johnson University hospital where I participated in trauma codes on a daily basis. I acknowledge the healthcare staff of the pharmacy department and ED at Maimonides who provided me with countless opportunities to improve the process of care; the pharmacy interns, some would complain about not knowing what to do, some cried over what they saw in the ED, and some excelled in the ED; and the PGY-1 and PGY-2 residents who have helped me sustain this service. The physicians, nurses, and research teams of the ED who request my assistance at times, guided me, and accepted my specialty skills as an advantage to use and apply for the better good of the patient. Ultimately, this book was written to improve direct patient care in the ED, and I acknowledge each patient who I see suffering and who I seek to help quickly and efficiently.

Victor Cohen
BS, PharmD, BCPS, CGP,
Assistant Professor of Pharmacy Practice
Arnold & Marie Schwartz College of
Pharmacy and Health Sciences
Long Island University

Clinical Pharmacy Manager
Department of Emergency Medicine
Residency Program Director
Emergency Medicine and Pharmacy Practice
Maimonides Medical Center

Part I

Crossroads Between Emergency Medicine and Pharmacy Practice

Part I provides a discussion of the emergency medicine specialty and its current challenges to assuring quality of care. It introduces a model that aligns pharmacy practice and emergency medicine to ensure a safe medication use system.

1

Emergency Medicine: An Overview

The emergency department is a natural laboratory for the study of error.

Dr. Patrick Croskerry

Objectives

- Define emergency medicine specialty
- Trace the history of the emergency medicine specialty
- Describe the physicians approach to the emergency department patient
- Describe how emergency medicine physicians think
- Describe how to reduce cognitive errors
- Review system causes of medication errors and methods for prevention

Most pharmacists gain their awareness of pharmacy's role in the emergency department (ED) through undergraduate Pharmacy elective clerkships or during their pharmacy practice residency rotations. Based on this limited experience, pharmacy students assess whether they want to pursue this area as a career. Despite the television depiction of the ED, the cold reality is that the ED is a place where many sick people go to get help.

To be able to improve the patient's experience and ensure safety and quality, one must have an understanding of what emergency medicine is, its historical place in medicine, its parallel to the growth of hospital pharmacy, the distinct approach that the emergency medicine specialist takes toward the patient, how the emergency clinicians thinks, and how this thought process to the novice physician can produce error. Furthermore, it is essential to understand the current ED crisis of overcrowding due to the public's enhanced demand for emergency care services while there is a shrinking supply of these services. The result of this crisis is the public demand for quality care and safety. Pharmacists must ensure the provision of safe medication use to achieve definite outcomes into practice.

WHAT IS EMERGENCY MEDICINE?

Emergency medicine involves the immediate care of urgent and life-threatening conditions found in critically ill and injured patients. Emergency Physicians are really specialists in breadth because their training encompasses acute problems that span several clinical disciplines.[1] No other specialty can match the astounding variety of patients found in the ED. The Australian College of Emergency Medicine defines emergency medicine as the field of practice based on the knowledge and skills required for the prevention, diagnosis, and management of acute and urgent aspects of illness and injury affecting patients of all age groups with a full spectrum of episodic undifferentiated physical and behavioral disorders. Furthermore, emergency medicine encompasses an understanding of the development of pre-hospital and in-hospital emergency medical systems and the skills necessary for this development.[2]

HISTORY OF EMERGENCY MEDICINE

The specialty of emergency medicine can be traced back 30 years ago. In the 1960s, any physician board-certified in other specialties, such as internal medicine, surgery, and even psychiatry, would care for acute, emergent, and traumatic illnesses. However, in the early 1960s, the United States public began to demand improved quality of care in hospital EDs. In response to this demand, hospitals developed full-time emergency services dedicated to providing quality medical care to patients with life- or limb-threatening conditions. These events led to the establishment of emergency medicine as the twenty-third recognized medical specialty in the United States and are intimately tied to changes in the healthcare delivery system.[3]

Interestingly, Theodore Taniguchi, Director of Hospital Pharmacy Services at University Hospital, University of Washington, Seattle, presented to the pharmacy section of the American Association for the advancement of science in Denver in 1961 a program that provided efficient prescription services to the ED despite the pharmacy being closed.[4] Taniguchi, in this report, forecast that the number of ambulatory patients who use the hospital ED for medical care will increase, forcing a similar growth in hospital pharmacists in the US. Thus, Taniguchi, from the University of Washington, was the first to describe a pharmacy and ED collaboration, albeit omitting any discussion of the clinical presence of the ED pharmacist.

EMERGENCY PHYSICIANS APPROACH TO THE PATIENT

The approach to the ED patient is usually scripted and well orchestrated because the same questions are repeated: Do I need to resuscitate?, How great is the threat?, and How quick must I act?[5] The first question takes seconds and is usually based on a clinician's gestalt.

In true resuscitative emergencies, the usual sequence of history, physical examination, laboratory data, and testing is modified because of the need to take rapid action. In the most extreme cases, management begins with treatment, physical examination, laboratory testing, and history. This action must be taken unhesitatingly with a well-prepared planned approach, and there may be no time for the assessment of risk to benefit of treatment option.

Emergency physicians work with a "bias toward action," that is action before all information needed is available, with the rationale that this method can save lives. Part of the art of emergency medicine is the ability to reliably discriminate between cases requiring emergency action and those allowing the traditional sequence approach. This tool is what the emergency physician uses so effectively; however, this bias to action approach can lead to an indiscriminate approach to the patient and can result in less than optimal care.[5]

MANAGEMENT CONCURRENT WITH DIAGNOSIS

Traditionally, medicine has focused on diagnosis as the central important task of the clinician. Emergency medicine makes it clear that this is erroneous. In medicine in general, especially emergency medicine, the central task is not diagnosis; it is management.[5] In fact, a diagnosis cannot be made under the constraints of an ED evaluation, and emergency medicine supports the notion that there may not be a diagnosis. A diagnosis is helpful, but even without it, decisions must be made and actions taken.

Those in emergency medicine understand that patients want more than simply a diagnosis. They want explanation and reassurances. Simply providing the diagnosis, however correct, dismisses the patient's concerns and will leave them unsatisfied. By empathizing with patient fears, the physician can strengthen rapport with the family and take a position as their friend and ally, rather than a remote authority. Thus, the intellectual tasks are to come up with a reasonable plan of management, which may include but not be limited to, making a diagnosis.

HOW DO EMERGENCY PHYSICIANS THINK?

Medicine is essentially about making decisions; in emergency medicine, this general property of medicine is intensified.[5] The emergency physician is forced to act in the face of great uncertainty and within tight time constraints. How emergency physicians make decisions is essential to how well they perform.

The ED is the third most likely site for significant errors to occur, second only to the operating room and the patient's hospital room.[6] Compared with the total time spent in each arena, the risk of harm in the ED is disproportionate to the other settings. Croskerry et al. has suggested that thinking about how the emergency physician thinks and assessing how this thinking could err can impact quality of care and help to devise strategies to prevent error.[7] Cosby et al. further describes how knowing how emergency physicians think can help in preventing cognitive error.[8] This may have direct implications to the practice of pharmaceutical care in the ED or to any clinical pharmacy services that attempt to promote safety and improve quality.

Many models for medical decision making exist, such as the Hypothetico-deductive method that goes through a sequence of steps including generating a hypothesis, refining and testing it, undergoing causal reasoning, and subsequent diagnostic verification. Another method of medical decision making is based on the normative principles and basic statistics. For example, first the disease prevalence is known and then sensitivity, specificity, negative and positive predictive values are calculated using 2×2 tables, and then the pretest probability, post test probability and Bayes theorem is used to update or revise beliefs in light of new evidence.[9] Evidence-based medicine is another skill used to apply best possible information to a unique patient situation.[9]

All of these methods are time consuming and laborious and not ideal for the emergency medicine practitioner. Furthermore, the intention is to achieve a diagnosis; the emergency physician is interested in management of the patient as opposed to a diagnostic endpoint. According to Cosby et al. emergency physicians use a specialty bias, which is a distinct approach applied in emergency medicine, to rule out the worst rather than accept the most likely.[8] The advantage of this method is one avoids the can't-miss diagnosis; the disadvantage is potential for overuse of resources.

Cosby et al. described that the emergency physician uses the concept of **decision threshold**, including "**threshold to threat**," "**threshold to test**," and "**threshold to admit**." This is in contrast to the traditional internist who uses the concept of **index of suspicion.** An emergency physician will have a threshold of probabilities to determine if they should treat a patient or not treat a patient. In simplistic form, consider one disease; a patient either has the disease or does not have it; this creates four probabilities; the patient has the disease and is treated or not treated or the patient does not have the disease and is treated or not treated.[5]

If the patient is almost certain to not have a disease, then the probability is zero, and he or she will not be treated; in contrast, if a patient almost definitely has a disease, with a probability of 1, the correct decision is to treat the patient since the cost and risks of treatment outweigh the negative consequences not to treat. Thus, the emergency physician's task is not to make a diagnosis but instead to discover whether the probability of disease is over or under the treatment threshold and then act accordingly. Diagnostic and laboratory tests aid in elucidating the decision threshold. However, when the probability of disease is very low, these tests are not routinely ordered because of a large number of false positives, which can outweigh the occasional detection of a patient with disease. Similarly, when the probability of disease is very high, it is better to treat everyone, rather than test everyone, because the consequence of a large number of false negatives erroneously denied treatment outweigh the occasional patient without disease who is spared unnecessary therapy. With intermediate probabilities, testing and treating only those patients with positive tests provides the best overall outcome. Thus, the clinician's task is to decide whether the patient falls above or below the treat–test threshold. Therefore, testing is only useful in changing management decisions between the two thresholds. This threshold approach provides rationale for understanding physician's varying choices when faced with what seems to be similar clinical scenarios. Anything that helps the emergency physician revise their probability assessment is considered a test. A therapeutic trial or a period of observation or a clinical scoring system can help sort out probabilities.[5]

Emergency physicians also use naturalistic[10] or event-driven decision making to identify when action thresholds have been crossed. First, the emergency physician will classify a current situation as typical or atypical, based on matching clinical presentations to stored patterns or schemata. If the situation is typical, then stored patterns evoke a customary set of responses. If the situation is not typical, variations of customary responses are considered first, and then novel one-of-a-kind responses are considered. Experience is critical in developing a sufficiently rich set of stored schemata; the vast majority of clinical problems can be recognized and dealt with by a preplanned response. The emergency physician will then engage in a serial evaluation of the available courses of action, beginning with the most typical response, and evaluating each mentally by simulating the expected outcomes.

Thus, it is not the best of all possible responses that is sought in the ED, but instead one that is good enough. The payoff for accepting a good, but not necessarily, best response is that decisions are quick and effortless. Most of the expertise of physicians lies in their ability to constructively perceive the problem, which leads to a solution without much conscious effort. This is in sharp contrast to laboriously identifying all responses and painstakingly identifying the best option.

Learning this method of decision making is not easy. It can be gained with experience and is communicated by narratives of meaningful cases. It does not appear attainable through a formal decision analysis.[8]

Emergency physicians may also use *heuristics thinking* to simplify clinical decision-making operations.[11–12] Heuristics are shortcuts, rules of thumb, maxims, or any strategy that achieves abbreviation and avoids the laborious working through of all known options in the course of problem solving. Croskerry, describes Sutton's law, or "going for where

the money is" as a classic example of heuristic thinking. These shortcuts considerably reduce the cost of search, and in a vast majority of cases, will be correct. However, inevitably heuristic thinking will be associated with error, and a price will be paid for cutting corners. Reason has termed this type of thinking "flesh and blood" decision making.[13] However, heuristic decision making, if good, leads to expedient patient disposition and optimal utilization of resources.

ERRORS IN DECISION MAKING

Based on the unique decision-making processes of emergency medicine, a number of errors may arise. First, misdiagnosis can occur due to knowledge gaps, inexperience, faulty information gathering, faulty patterns of recognition, or misuse or misinterpretation of tests.[8]

Other errors in decision making have been described by Elstein's error classification[11] and includes inaccurate estimates of pretest probability, inaccurate estimate of disease prevalence, and an inaccurate estimate of the strength of the evidence.

Cosby and Croskerry describe other cognitive biases that may cause errors in emergency medicine decision making. For example, *anchoring* is the tendency to be unduly persuaded by features encountered early in the presentation of illness, thereby committing to a premature diagnosis; attaching a diagnostic label to patients early in their presentations allows the clinician to fall prey to anchoring.[14] An example is an emergency clinician "anchors" to an initial presenting sign of a patient, such as having an abnormal heart rate. The clinician treats the patient for atrial fibrillation with diltiazem, which would otherwise be appropriate. However, the clinician does not see underlying acute hyperglycemia hyperosmolar state as the underlying etiology.

Management of hyperglycemic hyperosmolar state requires rapid and copious fluid resuscitation and insulin therapy for improved glucose utilization to support cardiac function. The elevated heart rate is only a symptom of the more ominous underlying metabolic problem of hyperglycemia and insulin resistance. Use of diltiazem in this emergent condition will certainly lower the heart rate as it has potent negative chronotropic and inotropic effects; however, it also may inhibit insulin release and further reduce glucose uptake into the heart cells, resulting in cardiogenic shock and potential for subsequent death.

Another common source of error is *confirmation bias,* which is attention that is directed disproportionately toward observations that appear to confirm a hypothesis instead of seeking evidence that may disprove it.[11]

The *conjunction fallacy* is another source of error in which the likelihood of two or more independent instances occurring is overestimated by mistakenly linking them in a cause–effect relationship.[8]

Another cognitive error is *bounded rationality*, which suggests a restrictive "keyhole" view of the problem. Another term used to describe this is *search satisficing*, where the physician calls off the search for further abnormalities, because of satisfaction in finding the first.[8]

Prevalence bias, or the tendency to misjudge the true base rate of disease, is another source of cognitive error. This is an example of how we can be misled by the representative heuristic. For example, this error can be made by having the mistaken belief that circumstantial factors represent the event that we are anxious to not miss. For example, the assumption that a patient who comes to the ED must be sicker than if he visited a clinic is an example of prevalence bias. Erring on the side of caution can lead to an overuse of resources; safe and prudent decision making may sometimes be costly.

Hindsight bias is another cognitive phenomenon that may be a source of error. This is the "knew it all along" effect. This is the second guessing that can occur and creeps into our decision process.

Representative bias is another problem whereby we emphasize the relatively rare and esoteric cases, which although interesting, contribute little to the learning process. Similarly a phenomenon that occurs in medical journals that leads to errors associated with the *availability heuristic*. This is when we tend to overestimate the prevalence of a disease if we have recently seen a case or read about one because we are more conscious and it is easily recalled; therefore, it may be overrepresented. In contrast to the availability heuristic, Reason describes the *"out of sight, out of mind" failure mode* that occurs when we have not seen a problem or disease and miss it completely when it comes along.[13] Other influences of human performance associated with decision making are the affective errors, and personal impairment, such as fatigue, stress, and interpersonal conflicts.

PREVENTING ERRORS IN DECISION MAKING

Preventing cognitive errors can be done by reducing the cognitive load. For example, development and simplification of diagnostic and treatment protocols, the implementation of clinical decision rules, and practice guidelines.[8] Examples of these approaches are the Advance Cardiac Life Support, Advance Trauma Life Support, and Pediatric Advance Life Support algorithms that provide a shared approach to management. Electronic prompts aid in obtaining the desired response. Memory devices may be useful in addition to resources such as online consultations and electronic or online textbooks. Furthermore, shared responsibility and accountability, using teamwork principles, reduce cognitive error. Cognitive forcing strategies, such as locking functions, may assist with error prevention. Also, human performance improves when sleep deprivation is minimized and impaired team members are recognized.

The speed–accuracy trade off SATO phenomenon is well described as the trade-off that occurs when accuracy is sacrificed for speed. There is an inverse relationship between speed and accuracy in the field of industrial psychology. Thus, the faster the production line goes, the more errors are likely to occur.[15] Similar problems occur when limitations in resource availability (RA), such as available beds, staffing, fatigue, task overload, and time constraints compromise the continuous quality improvement (CQI) of care and decision making, leading to trade-offs (RACQITO).[16] The vital signs of the ED may sometimes become unstable. Errors of RACQITO occur in other medical settings such as ICUs and operating rooms and have received widespread coverage in the US

media.[17] Errors are not sole responsibility of physicians and nurses; they are forced by the operating characteristics of the system in which they practice.

SYSTEM-RELATED CAUSES FOR MEDICATION ERRORS IN THE EMERGENCY DEPARTMENT: RACQITO

Howard A. Peth described that the specialty of emergency medicine is characterized by unique systems challenges that place patients at increased risk for medication errors. First, patients present to the emergency physician as strangers. Unlike physicians in pediatrics or internal medicine, emergency physicians are rarely familiar with their patients' medical histories, medication lists, allergy history, renal function, and so on, and emergency physicians rarely have immediate access to the medical records of patients who present to the ED. In addition, off-hours contact with physicians who may be familiar with ED patients' medical histories is often not possible. Second, emergency physicians provide service every day and night of the year. They are often required to dispense drugs directly from the ED at hours when pharmacists may not be available to serve as a crucial safety check in the drug-ordering and delivery scheme. Third, emergency physicians often administer potentially dangerous medications on an emergency basis to critically ill or injured patients, increasing the risk that critical safety checks may be omitted. In addition, the route of administration used in an emergency can lead to a greater risk of an adverse event. When a medication is given intravenously or via a central line, the risk of an adverse event rises dramatically. Finally, a reliance on verbal orders, which is inherent in emergency medicine, increases the risk that a potentially ambiguous medication order is misinterpreted or misunderstood.[18]

A team approach is strongly recommended for the successful outcome with each stage of drug ordering and delivery.[18] There are five stages of drug ordering and delivery: 1) prescribing, 2) transcribing, 3) dispensing, 4) administrating, and 5) monitoring, as depicted in Figure 1-1.

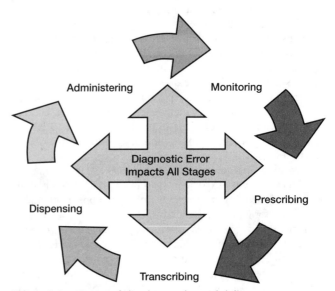

Figure 1–1. Stages of the drug order and delivery process are contingent on the correct diagnosis.

Each of these stages represents a vulnerable link in a chain along which any variety of errors can occur—explaining the complexity involved in preventing adverse drug events. A breach along any one of the links in the chain can lead to an adverse drug event. A diagnostic error, the most common medical error in the ED may adversely impact all links of the chain. Thus preventing medication errors is inherently dependent on accurate diagnosis, suggesting a team approach is needed. Although it appears that certain individuals may have greater responsibility along certain links in the chain, and other individuals may have a greater role elsewhere, a cohesive team can synergistically impact risk of error.[18]

SUMMARY

Pharmacists interested in emergency medicine practice must be aware of the unique nature of emergency medicine, the practice setting, the approach taken, the risks associated with this approach, methods to prevent risk, and current system demands. Pharmacists interested in improving safety and enhancing patient quality may need innovative, nontraditional approaches to implementing a safe medication use system within the ED.

References

1. Graf J. Emergency Medicine. In: Freeman B. *The Ultimate Guide to Choosing A Medical Specialty, Second Edition.* New York: McGraw Hill, 2007;181–198.
2. Australasian College for Emergency Medicine [homepage on the Internet]. West Melbourne, Australia [1999 December]. Definition of Emergency Medicine. Available from: http://www.medeserv.com.au/acem/open/documents/definition.htm.
3. American Board of Emergency Medicine [homepage on the Internet]. East Lansing, MI [revised 2008 Jun 23]. ABEM History. Available from: http://www.abem.org/PUBLIC/portal/alias__Rainbow/lang__en-US/tabID__3573/DesktopDefault.aspx.
4. Taniguchi T. Providing An Emergency Department Dispensing Service. Hospitals, 1962;36:126–130.
5. Wears R. The Approach to the Emergency Department Patient. In Harwood-Nuss A. *The Clinical Practice of Emergency Medicine, Third Edition.* New York: Lippincott Williams & Wilkins, 2001;1–4.
6. Leape LL, Brennan TA, Laird N, et al. The nature of adverse events in hospitalized patients: Results of the Harvard Medical Practice Study II. *N Engl J Med* 1991; 324:377–84.
7. Croskerry P. The cognitive imperative: Thinking about how we think. *Acad Emerg Med* 2000; 7:1223–1231
8. Cosby KS, Croskerry P. Patient safety: A curriculum for teaching patient safety in emergency medicine. *Acad Emerg Med* 2003;10(1):69–78.
9. Kovacs G, Croskerry P. Clinical decision making: An emergency medicine perspective. *Acad Emerg Med* 1999;6:947–952.
10. Klein GA, Orasanu J, Calderwood R, Zsambok CE. *Decision Making in Action: Models and Methods.* Norwood, NJ: Ablex Publishing Corp., 1995.
11. Elstein AS, Heuristics and biases: Selected errors in clinical reasoning. *Acad Med* 1999;74:791–794.
12. Redlemier DA, Ferris LE, Tu JV, Hux JE, Schull MJ. Problems for clinical judgment: Introducing cognitive psychology as one more basic science. *Can Med Assoc J* 2001;164:358–60.
13. Reason J. *Human Error.* New York: Cambridge University Press, 1990.
14. Tversky A, Kahneman D. Judgment under uncertainty: Heuristics and biases. *Science* 1974;185:1124–1131.
15. Foley P, Murray N. Sensation, perception and systems design. In: Salvendy G (ed) *Handbook of Human Factors.* New York: John Wiley and Sons, 1987.
16. Vincent C, Taylor-Adams S, Stanhope N. Framework for analyzing risk and safety in clinical medicine. *Br Med J* 1998;316:1154–1157.
17. Donchin Y, Gopher D, Olin M, et al. A look into the nature and causes of human errors in the intensive care unit. *Crit Care Med* 1995; 23:294–300.
18. Peth HA. Medication errors in the emergency department: A system approach to minimizing risk. *Emerg Clin North Am* 2003;21:141–158.

2

Challenges Facing Emergency Medicine Quality and Safety: Medication Management

Objectives
- Review public concern for patient safety
- Discuss incidence cost of medical injury and the "tip of the iceberg"
- Review the emergency department: Safe haven or serious threat to quality of care
- Describe etiology of emergency departments in crisis
- Discuss the quality chasm: Another challenge facing emergency departments
- Describe Institute of Medicine (IOM) goals IOMs for healthcare improvement to medication use in the emergency department (ED)

PUBLIC CONCERN OF PATIENT SAFETY

There is a significant public concern associated with patient safety as indicated in one survey in which 47% of people reported they were very concerned with a medical error happening to them or their family when getting hospital care, compared with 40% when going to the doctor's office for care, or 34% when getting a prescription filled. In addition 6% of respondents reported they personally suffered harm due to medical injury in the preceding year.[1-2]

INCIDENCE COST OF MEDICAL INJURY

There is a rationale for this concern; according to the Institute of Medicine *To Err is Human: Building Safer Health-System,* medical injury causes an estimated 44,000–98,000 deaths per year. This ranks medical errors as the 8th leading cause of death. Medical errors result in $17–29 billion in excess cost.[1] It is also important to remember that we discover only those

errors that result in significant harm to patients—"the tip of the iceberg." In the iceberg model, the submerged errors include those that occurred, but did not result in injury and the near misses, those errors that almost happened and could have had dire consequences.[3] The "tip of the iceberg" model can also be used to illustrate how a medical error can manifest and result in medical injury. Figure 2-1 depicts an iceberg model of the case described in Chapter 1 of a hyperglycemic hyperosmolar state. The tip of the iceberg represents the initial presenting tachycardia; what is not seen to the clinician is the submerged part of the iceberg that represents the hyperglycemic hyperosmolar state that may not be managed and result in a diagnostic and medical error and potential for injury.

In another case, a patient was prescribed a caffeine citrate infusion for a lumbar puncture-induced headache. Central pharmacy instructed the night shift nurse to administer the infusion over 90 minutes. The night nurse never administered the infusion, and the morning shift nurse requested the injectable to be sent so she could administer it. The morning shift nurse administered the dose of caffeine citrate over 2 minutes. Although this occurred without incident, various process-related issues within the system broke down to permit this near miss to occur. Correction of these processes is a challenge and must be part of a system of continuous quality improvement.

As reported by the Institute of medicine in *Crossing the Quality Chasm,* there are serious problems in the quality of care in the United States.[4]

ED: SAFE HAVEN OR SERIOUS THREAT TO QUALITY OF CARE

The emergency department (ED) is an important portal in the healthcare system, especially for those patients who are most vulnerable. Despite a decline in number of EDs, the use of

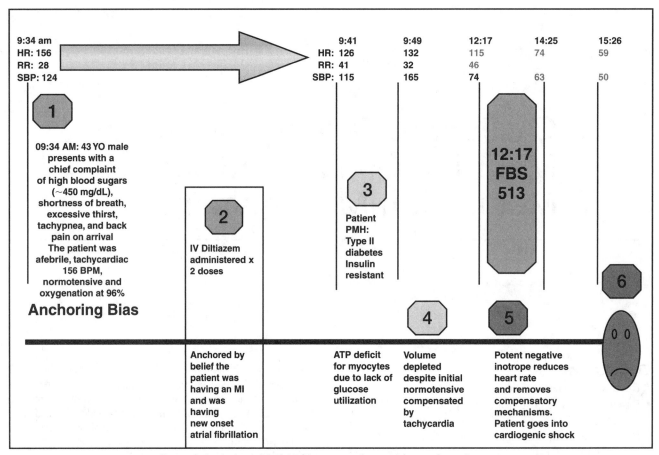

Figure 2–1. Iceberg Model of hyperosmolar state hyperglycemic state.

emergency medical services has increased, which has led to concerns about the capacity of those EDs that continue to operate. Annual number of ED visits increased 18% in the United States between 1994 and 2004 from 93 million to 110 million, yet the number of EDs decreased by 12% during this same period.[5] This increased volume together with the high complexity of emergency practice and shrinking resources, according to the Institute of Medicine, is what creates an environment that sacrifices quality and is prone to errors.

Furthermore, the lack of continuity with patients, coupled with inadequate information infrastructure for care across the continuum, often forces emergency providers to see patients without all the information needed to make cost effective, high-quality decisions.[1] These factors rationalize why over the past decade, National Emergency Department's ability of assuring the provision of quality of care and patient safety has been scrutinized. These factors have also lead to The Committee on the Future of Emergency Care in the United States Health-Systems to conclude that the ED is a high-risk, high-stress environment that is fraught with opportunities for error.[1] Leape and colleagues have demonstrated in a landmark study of hospitalized patients that although the ED was a site for only 3% of adverse events, it was the site of 70% of those events attributed to negligence.[6–7] Studies of hospital admissions and malpractice claims have also found the ED to be the site of a significant number of errors resulting in adverse events. Two of the most common types of errors in the ED are failures to diag-

nose a patient properly and medication errors.[7] To reduce these threats to quality of care and assure that EDs continue to be regarded as safe havens to the public, novel and transparent system-based strategies to ensure quality of care are needed.

CAUSES OF EMERGENCY DEPARTMENT CRISIS: A SUPPLY AND DEMAND PHENOMENON

Emergency departments are in crisis; this crisis can be attributed to various phenomena that have occurred simultaneously. First, the demand for ED services has increased. This increase is due to constraints on where a patient may go for their care by HMOs, stricter enforcement of the Federal Emergency Medical Treatment and Active Labor Act (EMTALA), and more patients without insurance seeking care in the ED.[8]

There are also supply-side constraints. In many communities, the number of EDs decreased because of hospital-closures and mergers, leaving fewer facilities to respond to the growing demand. An 8% decline in EDs has been observed from 1994 to 1999. Downsizing and reconfiguration of hospital inpatient capacity has led to delays in admitting patients from the ED. Furthermore, there are fewer

---

TABLE 2-1

Medication Management Standard and Related Task

MM1.10 Patient-specific information standards and related actions.

MM2.10 The hospital has defined criteria to create a formulary.

MM2.20 Medications are properly and safely stored throughout the hospital.

MM2.30 Develop a policy for identification of medications and procedures for safe use of medications brought from home.

MM2.40 Develop a system that identifies the drugs available in response to a medical emergency and ensure that the drugs are secured to guarantee their availability.

MM3.10 The hospital procedure for writing "as needed" medication orders for drugs that have multiple indications is specified.

MM3.20 Medication orders are written clearly and interpreted/transcribed accurately.

MM4.10 All medication orders are reviewed for appropriateness.

MM4.20 Medications are prepared safely.

MM4.30 Medications are appropriately labeled.

MM4.40 Medications are dispensed safely to the patient.

MM4.50 A safe practice for providing medications when the pharmacy is closed is developed by the organization.

MM4.70 Recalled or discontinued medications are retrieved and disposed.

MM4.80 Medications returned to the pharmacy are appropriately managed.

MM5.10 Medications are administered safely and accurately.

MM6.10 Effects of medications are monitored to ensure effectiveness and to reduce adverse events.

MM6.20 Hospital has a process to evaluate and learn from adverse drug reactions and medication errors.

MM7.10 High-risk/high-alert medications

MM7.40 Organization institutes safe practices to protect patients who participate in investigational studies involving medication. Monitors patients' responses to investigational drugs to evaluate safety.

MM8.10 Hospital evaluates its medication management system.

Adapted from Hoying MR. *The Compliance Guide to JCAHO's Medication Management Standards, 2nd Ed.* Massachusetts: HCPro.

---

discharge options because of reduced investment in skilled nursing facilities and home healthcare services, adding to the bottleneck in inpatient units and the ED overload. Nursing shortages have also contributed to hospital capacity constraints.[8]

Overcrowded EDs have collateral damage and result in hospitals under stress: diversion of ambulances to other facilities delays treatment, and other serious threats to patient care emerge. Patients face longer waits in the ED for needed services. Overcrowding in EDs has been associated with an inability to ensure quality of care standards; patients may not receive life-saving antimicrobials in time to be most beneficial to survival. Thus, global ED issues have a direct impact on patient care in the field, and safeguards within the field are needed to protect against these uncontrollable factors.[8]

REGULATORY CHALLENGES FACING THE ED

In addition to the human toll exacted by medication errors, preventable drug-related morbidity and mortality represent an enormous economic burden on society. For example, cost-averaging statistics place the drug-related morbidity and mor-

tality financial tab at $76.6 billion in the ambulatory setting, the largest component of this total going toward drug-related hospitalizations.[9–11] The number of deaths from medication errors is increasing: deaths attributed to medication mistakes more than doubled between 1983 and 1993,[12] and there are signs that this trend will continue. The Joint Commission for the Accreditation of Healthcare Organization (TJC) now requires its 17,000 member organizations to have specific procedures in place that target the prevention of medication errors with medication management standards.[13] Thus Emergency Departments are challenged to comply with The Joint Commission standards that include medication management as listed in Table 2-1.[14]

CROSSING THE QUALITY CHASM: ANOTHER CHALLENGE FACING EMERGENCY DEPARTMENTS

According to the IOM, the gap between current healthcare and the healthcare we could have has been termed the

---

TABLE 2-2

National Aims for Healthcare Quality

- Safety: achieves the same level of "being safe" as we have in our homes
- Effectiveness: avoids overuse of ineffective care and under-use of effective care
- Patient-Centered: honors the patient and respects choice
- Timeliness: reduces waiting time for both patients and those who give care
- Efficiency: reduces waste
- Equity: closes racial and ethnic gaps

Adapted from Institute of Medicine. *To Err is Human: Building a Safer Health-System*. Washington, DC: National Academy Press, 2001.

"chasm." To fill the chasm, major system changes in healthcare will be required, and as a result, national aims for improvement have been set as seen in Table 2-2.[1,15]

NATIONAL AIMS FOR HEALTHCARE IMPROVEMENT TO MEDICATION USE IN THE ED

If we examine each of the national aims for improvement as it pertains to medications in the ED, an emergency medicine/health service research agenda and quality improvement strategy begin to emerge.

To improve patient *safety*, we could develop effective reporting systems that could reduce sentinel events in EDs, including medical errors and near misses, such as ADR reporting and medication error reporting, irrespective if the event caused harm, so we can take action to avoid risk in the future. We can examine high risk medication use in the ED, and target active surveillance systems or create automated guidance to reduce risk with high risk medications. Furthermore, when events do occur, we can use tools, such as root cause analysis or failure mode effect analysis (FMEA) to learn from our errors.

In the area of *effectiveness*, we could focus on underuse and overuse of diagnostic and therapeutic approaches in emergency medicine. For example, we could improve the use of thrombolytics therapy for acute myocardial infarction and stroke. We would reduce the risk of overuse of antibiotics through the collaborative development of protocols for optimal antimicrobial therapies.

To make emergency care pharmacotherapy *patient centered*, we would assure that the patient was aware of the medications being administered. We would inquire if the patient had any problems in the past with this type of medication, and we would make every effort to educate, counsel, and reassure the patient as it pertains to the medication needs of the patient in the emergency department. Greater involvement of families to assist with identifying medication issues will also be attempted. We will assure that the desired endpoint of therapy is reached, or at minimum, followed and addressed to ensure the goal of therapy is attained.

To improve *timeliness,* we need to determine the key time limits needed for vital drug therapies and work to achieve and improve them. This may include all medications placed in easily accessible locations to expedite care. We would develop and implement automated systems that simplify medication ordering, transcribing, and administering.

To improve *efficiency,* we need a better understanding of how delays in therapy may affect the throughput in EDs, and how pharmacists can facilitate and expedite therapy to prevent these delays and reduce overcrowding in the ED.

To improve *equity* of healthcare services in the ED, the pharmacist will consider the cultural, ethnic, pharmacogenomic considerations that affect the emergency care pharmacotherapy provided to the patients and identify areas of disparity. Furthermore, as we consider emerging healthcare issues, we will further identify the role that pharmacy plays in healthcare preparedness for bioterrorism and natural disasters.

SUMMARY

The public is concerned over safety and quality of healthcare. Incidence and cost of injury due to medical errors (medication and diagnostic) are significant. The EDs reputation as a safe haven for the sick is being challenged due to the current threats to quality of care, such as reduced emergency care resources; yet, the demand for these resources has increased. Evidence supports that medical error occurs disproportionately for the time spent in the ED and that these errors are largely preventable. Contributing to lack of quality are factors associated with ED overcrowding that eventually make their way down to the patient. Novel strategies are needed to protect against these risks. To improve safety and quality of emergency care and prevent diagnostic and medication error, EDs also face the external regulatory forces such as TJC and IOM national aims that are demanding that the "chasm" of healthcare quality be filled by assuring full compliance with quality standards. Needless to say, EDs are facing significant challenges.

References

1. Institute of Medicine. *To Err is Human: Building a Safer Health-System*. Washington, DC: National Academy Press, 2001.
2. Kaiser Family Foundation/Agency for Healthcare Research and Quality. *National Survey on Americans as Health Consumers: An Update on the Role of Quality Information*. Rockville, MD: AHQR, Dec 2000.
3. Heinrich HW. *Industrial Accident Prevention-A Scientific Approach*. New York: McGraw Hill,1941.
4. Committee on Quality Health Care in America. Institute of Medicine. *Crossing the Quality Chasm*. Washington, DC: National Academy Press, 2001.
5. United States Department of Health and Human Services Centers for Disease Control and Prevention National Center for Health Statistics. Advance Data from Vital and Health Statistics. 2006;376:1–24.
6. Leape LL, Brennan TA, Laird N, et al. The nature of adverse events in hospitalized patients. Results of the Harvard Medical Practice Study II. *N Engl J Med* 199 ;324(6):377–384.
7. Brennan TA, Leape LL, Laird N, et al. Incidence of adverse events and negligence in hospitalized patients. Results of the Harvard Medical Practice Study I. *N Engl J Med* 1991;324(6): 370–76.

8. Brewster LR, Rudell LS, Lesser CS. Center for Studying Health System Change: The ER in Crisis. 2001;38:1–4.

9. Bootman JL, Harrison DL, Cox E. The health care cost of drug-related morbidity and mortality in nursing facilities. *Arch Intern Med* 1997;157:2089–96.

10. Johnson JA, Bootman JL. Drug-related morbidity and mortality: A cost-of-illness model. *Arch Intern Med* 1995;155: 1949–56.

11. Schneider PJ, Gift MG, Lee YP, et al. Cost of medication-related problems at a university hospital. *Am J Health-Syst Pharm* 1995;52:2415–8.

12. Phillips DP, Christenfeld N, Glynn LM. Increase in US medication-error deaths between 1983 and 1993. *Lancet* 1998; 351:643–4.

13. Peth HA Jr. Medication errors in the emergency department: A systems approach to minimizing risk. *Emerg Med Clin North Am* 2003;21:141–158.

14. Hoying MR. *The Compliance Guide to JCAHO's Medication Management Standards.* 2nd Ed. Massachusetts: HCPro, 2005

15. Burstin H. Crossing the Quality Chasm in Emergency Medicine. *Acad Emerg Med* 2002;9(11):1074–1077.

3

Aligning the Principles of Pharmacotherapy with Emergency Medicine

Objectives
- Discuss divergent principles
- Review aligned principles
- Describe the ED pharmacist role in assuring alignment

As drug use is an essential part of emergency care, pharmacotherapeutic principles should align with the principles associated with the practice of emergency medicine. However, this is not always the case, and the emergency care pharmacotherapist is an essential team member who can ensure these principles align for safe and cost effective, yet expedient, use of drug therapy in the ED.

Guiding principles of pharmacotherapy (PTH) have been described and are listed in Table 3-1.[1]

PTH PRINCIPLES IN CONTRAST TO EMERGENCY MEDICINE

The first PTH principle requires that there should be a justifiable and documented indication for every medication that is used. This corresponds with the traditional practice of medicine that has focused on diagnosis as the central important task of the clinician. Emergency medicine makes it clear that this may not be fully necessary for acute stabilization. In emergency medicine, the central task is not diagnosis; it is management. Often a diagnosis cannot be made under the constraints of an ED evaluation; this is the insight that the emergency medicine specialty has given to their colleagues—the notion that there is not always a diagnosis. If one is made, it is helpful; but if not, decisions must still be made and actions are taken.[2]

The emergency care pharmacotherapist needs to practice under this merged paradigm as opposed to the traditional pharmacist, who if no indication is present will not validate or verify the appropriateness of the medication prescribed. This traditional pharmacotherapy principle if applied to the ED may delay therapy.[3] An emergency care pharmacotherapist rationalizes the indication based on the management paradigm and uses his or her risk-to-benefit threshold or event-driven assessment for risk of use of the medication to avoid delay and expedite administration.

The emergency care pharmacotherapist is present at the bedside and sees the patient. Witnessing the patient allows the pharmacotherapist to develop a rich set of experiences that can relate to and rationalize the treatment and management of the patient. There is no substitute for practical experience. No current pharmacotherapy textbook addresses the experiences witnessed in this arena because unique presentations occur frequently, and only astute clinicians can detect, using his gestalt, whether the threshold for treatment has been crossed and if risk exists with treatment. The emergency care pharmacotherapist with extensive experience in the ED is valuable to the novel resident or attending and can aid in informing the common schemata in the community, locality, or region.

Another PTH principle that is in contrast to emergency medicine principles is that medications should be used at the lowest dosage and for the shortest duration that is likely to achieve the desired outcome. Circumstances in the ED, often at the height of the patient's acute illness, require that higher than normal doses be used. For example, based on PTH principles, intravenous nitroglycerin are recommended to begin at a rate of 5–10 mcg/min and titrated every 15 minutes to desired endpoint.[4] This is in contrast to what is practiced during emergency care and the need for expedient care and acute stabilization. Nitroglycerin is started at a dose rate of 30–50 mcg/min in patients with acute pulmonary edema or patients with acute coronary syndrome with unrelenting chest pain refractory to sublingual nitroglycerin. This increased initial dosing allows for more rapid resolution and can result in avoidance of

TABLE 3-1

Alignment of Pharmacotherapy Principles with Practice of Emergency Medicine

Pharmacotherapy Principles	Aligns	Counters
1. There should be justifiable and documented indication for every medication used.		X
2. A medication should be used at the lowest dosage and for the shortest duration that is likely to achieve the desired outcome.		X
3. When a patient is adequately treated with a single drug, monotherapy is preferred.		X
4. Newly approved medications should be used only if there are clear advantages over older medications.		X
5. Whenever possible, the selection of medication regimen should be based upon evidence obtained from controlled clinical trials.		X
6. The timing of drug administration should be considered as a possible influence on drug efficacy, adverse effects, and interactions with other drugs and food.	X	
7. A medication regimen should be simplified as much as possible to enhance patient adherence.	X	
8. A patient's perception of illness or the risks and benefits of therapy may affect adherence.	X	
9. Careful observation of a patient's response to treatment is necessary to confirm efficacy, prevent, detect, or manage adverse effect, assess compliance and determine the need for dosage adjustment or discontinuation of drug therapy.	X	
10. A medication should not be given by injection when giving it by mouth would be just as effective and safe.		X
11. Before medications are used, lifestyle modifications, should be made, when indicated, to obviate the need for drug therapy or to enhance pharmacotherapy outcomes.	X	
12. Initiation of a drug regimen should be done with full recognition that a medication may cause a disease, signs, symptoms, syndrome, or abnormal lab tests.	X	
13. When a variety of drugs are equally efficacious and equally safe, the drug that results in the lowest healthcare cost or is most convenient for the patient should be chosen.		X
14. When making a decision about drug therapy for individual patients, societal effects should be considered.		X
15. The possible reason for failure of medication regimens include inappropriate drug selection, poor adherence, improper drug dose, or interval, misdiagnosis, concurrent illness, interactions with foods or drugs, environmental factors, or genetic factors.	X	

Adapted from Dipiro JT, Talbert R, Yee GC, et al. Guiding principles of pharmacotherapy. *Pharmacotherapy: A Pathophysiological Approach, Sixth Edition*. New York: McGraw Hill, 2005.

intubation as opposed to the slower more deliberate titration that actually may worsen the potential for resolution. Because time is limited for titration in an overcrowded ED, the clinician will probably choose the path of least resistance, which is immediate intubation as opposed to slow titration. Intubations in patients with respiratory compromise are frequently prevented with diligent and rapid respiratory and pharmacotherapy interventions.

Initiating analgesic therapy is another example. Doses of morphine need to be at high levels in most patients who present with pain to the ED and have a pain score of 10/10. Without optimal dosing, the patient will experience significant pain throughout the stay within the ED, which is made worse by the fact that a timely re-evaluation may not occur for some time.[5]

Another example is the titration of a labetalol drip in the case of a dissecting aorta; it is essential to reduce the blood pressure as expeditiously as possible to prevent further dissection. Using the initial bolus doses of 20 mg IV push over 2 minutes with repeat doses of 40–80 mg at 10-minute intervals up to 300 mg is likely to delay achieving the preferred outcome of hemodynamic stability while ceasing further aortic dissection.[4] Based on this dosing regimen, the 300-mg dose can take up to 1 hour, and at that point may be excessive or the patient may have ruptured the aorta and gone into a cardiogenic shock. Thus, often the endpoint of a

hypertensive emergency of 25% reduction in mean arterial pressure is not achieved appropriately. As Brooks and colleagues reported in a retrospective chart review of patients treated for hypertensive emergency in the ED or ICU for at least 30 minutes, only 32% of patient were treated appropriately, 57% were excessively treated, and 13% had failed a 2-hour acute phase treatment window for achieving the intended endpoint.[6]

The emergency care pharmacotherapy team assists with titration of a labetalol drip at 2 mg/min with precision-guided bolus doses; minute-to-minute monitoring is conducted to allow the nurse and physicians to maintain normal operations and handle the incoming surges with the security of a trained specialist in pharmacotherapy and pharmaceutical care to assist in safely achieving the specifically desired endpoint.

When a variety of drugs are equally efficacious and equally safe, the drug that results in the lowest healthcare cost or is most convenient for the patient should be chosen. This is another example of contrasting principles between pharmacotherapy and emergency medicine as seen with the use of enoxaparin, a low–molecular-weight heparin administered as a subcutaneous dose every 12 hours for acute coronary syndrome instead of heparin administered by intravenous infusion. Enoxaparin is preferred over heparin requiring a bolus and a continuous infusion, which requires titration and monitoring of the aPTT. The prolonged duration of action of enoxaparin makes it a favorite among emergency physicians, and ease of administration makes it extremely desirable to nursing staff. Despite the risk with the use of enoxaparin, such as the risk of bleed, or the less than full reversal with protamine, as well as lack of efficacy data that show early use reduces mortality, the convenience makes it the drug of choice despite its high acquisition cost. The emergency care pharmacotherapist intervenes and expedites the procurement, administration, and monitoring of heparin as a way to avoid use of the more expensive enoxaparin.

The use of a newly approved medication only if there is a clear advantage over the older medications is in contrast to what may occur in the ED setting. An example of this problem is the marketing of fosphenytoin as a new and improved antiepileptic that can be administered quicker than phenytoin and results in less vascular necrosis when given intravenously. Prematurely but often at the advice of the neurology specialist the emergency medicine physicians will follow the recommendations. Recent reports have confirmed that use of fosphenytoin in the ED is no safer and no more effective than use of phenytoin; furthermore, it is excessively more costly than phenytoin.[7]

Another example of this misaligned principle is the initial marketing of intravenous ketorolac for pain management as a preferred nonsteroidal anti-inflammatory drug over oral ibuprofen because it was suggested that the parental dosage form provided more rapid and enhanced pain relief. Published reports have refuted the superiority of ketorolac over oral ibuprofen; furthermore, oral ibuprofen has been associated with similar onset, but improved pain relief than that of intramuscular ketorolac.[8–10] This coincides with yet another principle of pharmacotherapeutics—a medication should not be given by injection when giving it by mouth would be just as effective.

PTH PRINCIPLES ALIGNED WITH EMERGENCY MEDICINE

Timing of drug administration should be considered as a possible influence on drug efficacy, adverse effects, and interactions with other drugs and food. Emergency medicine principles of practice stress the importance of initial immediate emergency care as the most essential component to positive outcomes. For example, protocols have been developed and workflow operations have been modified to assure efficacy of thrombolytics, with timely administration, to the patient presenting with a brain or heart attack. Emergency department process changes were made to assure antibiotic time within 4 hours for community-acquired pneumonia and goal-directed therapy for sepsis within 1 hour.

Although timing of administration of pharmacotherapy as an influence on drug efficacy and toxicity while providing emergency care is an aligned principle in certain circumstances, it may not be taken into consideration. For example, because emergency physicians are biased to action, they may not take timing of administration of a medication in the ED as an important consideration to reduce risk for toxicity. Risk assessments for drug interactions are not extensively done. This may lead to drug–drug interactions involving the recent administration of an emergency care medication with that of a medication recently taken from home. This may result in permanent and major disability.

An illustration of this occurred when the timing of the administration of subcutaneous sumatriptan and its impact of drug toxicity was not considered in a patient with migraine presenting to the ED within 24 hours of use of a selective serotonin-reuptake inhibitor. Furthermore there was no thorough knowledge of the patient's past medical history, and this can further predispose patients to an adverse event, as seen in the case study and the accompanying ECGs.

A proposed set of emergency care pharmacotherapy principles that align the goals of pharmacotherapy with those of emergency medicine is listed in Table 3-2.

■ Case Study

Timing of Drug Administration of Sumatriptan: Possible Influence in Sudden Coronary Vasospasm

A 44-year-old woman presented to the ED with multiple complaints including non-productive cough, diarrhea, and headache that started the day before. Numbness of both hands developed 3 hours prior to coming to the ED. She also complained of generalized weakness that had been ongoing "for a while," which prevented her from going to work. She saw her primary medical doctor who prescribed sumatriptan for her presumed migraine headache for the first time. She denied recent fevers, chest pain, shortness of breath, abdominal pain, vomiting, or urinary symptoms.

The patient reported having a medical history only significant for type II diabetes mellitus. Specifically, there was no history of a seizure disorder. However, she was taking multiple medications including topiramate, escitalopram, and zolpidem. She denied any significant family history or any use of alcohol, tobacco, or illicit drugs.

On physical examination, she was a well-appearing female, alert, and in no apparent distress. She had a temperature of 36.8°C (98.2° F), a heart rate of 70 beat/min, a respiratory rate of 20 breath/min, a blood pressure of 143/74 mmHg, a pain score of 5/10, and an O_2 saturation of 99%. The rest of her physical examination was within normal limits. Specifically, there were no focal neurological deficits. Work up in the ED with laboratory tests, including a complete blood count, a prothrombin time, blood chemistry, lipid profile, liver functions, plasma lipase, and urinalysis, did not reveal any abnormalities. Her blood glucose level was 110 mg/dL.

With the above findings, the emergency physician's impression was that the patient was probably suffering from a viral syndrome. The patient received intravenous hydration with one liter of normal saline and reported feeling better. The patient was being prepared for discharge; however, because she had an unfilled prescription for sumatriptan, the emergency physician decided to give her the first dose in the ED. She was given a subcutaneous injection of 6 mg sumatriptan for her presumed migraine headache. Ten minutes later, she had foaming at the mouth, urinary incontinence, and

TABLE 3-2

Emergency Care Pharmacotherapy Principles

1. Most pharmacotherapy is a temporizing measure; thus, risk/benefits should be assessed because in most cases there is time.
2. The risks of drug therapy must be applied to the emergency care setting as this setting is able to manage drug reactions.
3. Protocols should guide medications that have proven to be time sensitive, and these protocols should be team developed and prac_ticed and contain the complete course of the ED visit.
4. ED pharmacotherapist should manage medications that require titration to assure endpoints are achieved and not exceeded and should be consulted when using medications that are not used frequently.
5. New pharmacotherapy should not be introduced unless it has proven outcome benefit within the ED setting and no risk of harm.
6. Oral pharmacotherapy is preferred over parenteral; however, if rapid attainment of levels or resolution is needed, parenteral administration is preferred if justified by evidence-based medicine.
7. The pharmacotherapist should procure all emergent drugs and record their use during medical emergencies.
8. Medications should be available in the ED for the pharmacist to prepare immediately during an emergency.
9. Drug-induced disease assessments and recording should be conducted by the ED pharmacist in suspected cases as a mechanism of pharmacovigilance and to improve drug use within the community.

reduced responsiveness. It was suspected that the patient might have had a seizure, as she appeared postictal. She was moved to a more critical area of the ED for cardiac monitoring. Her vital signs remained stable. A neurological examination revealed that her left pupil was 4 mm in diameter and unreactive to light, while the right pupil was 3 mm in diameter and sluggishly reactive. A non-contrast computed tomography (CT) of the head

was ordered. An electrocardiogram (EKG) was performed at 1:30:39 PM. The EKG revealed normal sinus rhythm with a greater than 1 mm ST segment depression in the inferior leads and greater than 1 mm ST segment elevation in the anteroseptal and lateral leads (Fig. 3-1A).

A second EKG performed at 1:32:57 PM revealed that the ST segment depression in the inferior leads and the

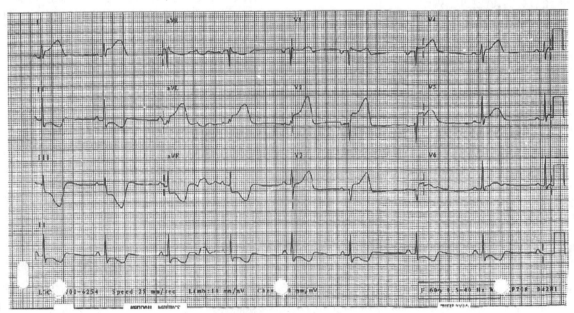

A

Figure 3–1. Case study EKG.

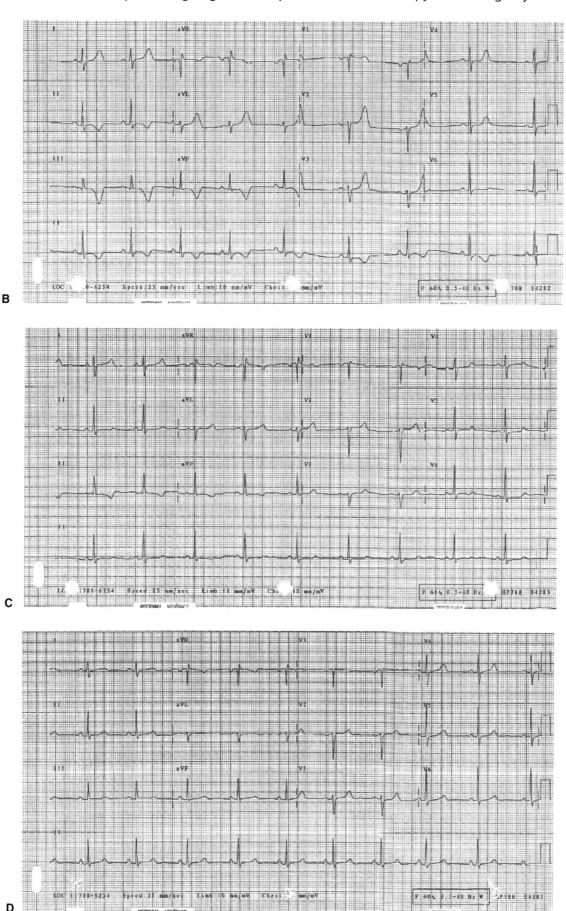

Figure 3–1. Case study EKG. *(continued)*

ST segment elevation in the anteroseptal and lateral leads had resolved. However, there was a new T wave inversion in the inferior leads (Fig. 3-1B). On re-examination, the patient was aroused and was able to follow commands. Her pupils were both equal and reactive to light. A third EKG performed at 1:36:19 PM showed further resolution of the ST-T wave changes (Fig. 3-1C). A fourth EKG performed at 3:03:29 PM showed complete resolution of the ST-T wave changes (Fig. 3-1D).

The patient's CT scan of the head was normal. Repeat laboratory tests were sent including cardiac enzymes and a urine toxicology screen. After regaining her baseline mental status, the patient indicated that a tightness of her chest developed shortly after the sumatriptan injection. She was admitted for further monitoring with telemetry. Two sets of cardiac enzymes, including myoglobin, creatine kinase (MB fraction), and troponin I, were normal. Although the patient denied any use of illicit drugs, her urine toxicology screen was positive for cocaine. A cardiac catheterization and coronary angiography were performed the next day, and she was found to have normal coronary arteries. She was discharged from the hospital to home the next day with a follow-up appointment with her primary medical doctor.

SUMMARY

As the need to assure patient safety and quality has increased and because complexities of pharmacotherapy continue to grow, it is essential to examine the similarities and differences in approaches to pharmacotherapy taken by emergency medicine clinicians and those that govern the principles of pharmacotherapy. Once understood, a mutual understanding will be developed that can foster a partnership to achieve the goal of safe, but efficient, quality emergency care pharmacotherapy.

References

1. Dipiro JT, Talbert R, Yee GC, et al. Guiding principles of pharmacotherapy. In Dipiro JT. *Pharmacotherapy: A Pathophysiological Approach, Sixth Edition*. New York: McGraw Hill, 2005.
2. Wears R. The approach to the emergency department patient. In: Harwood-Nuss. *Clinical Practice of Emergency Medicine, 3rd ed*. Philadelphia: Lippincott Williams & Wilkins. Philadelphia, 2001.
3. No Authors Listed. Organizations join forces against Joint Commission medication rules. *ED Manage* 2006(8):85–87.
4. Rynn KO, Hughes F, Faley B. An emergency department approach to drug treatment of hypertensive urgency and emergency. *J Pharm Pract* 2005;18(5):363–376.
5. Thompson C. Pain persists among emergency department patients. *Am J Health-Syst Pharm* 2004;61(23): 2480, 2483, 2489.
6. Brooks TW, Finch CK, Lobo BL, et al. Blood pressure management in acute hypertensive emergency. *Am J Health-Syst Pharm* 2007;64(24):2579–2582.
7. Coplin WM, Rhoney DH, Rebuck JA, et al. Randomized evaluation of adverse events and length of stay with routine emergency department use of phenytoin or fosphenytoin. *Neurol Res* 2002;24(8); 842–848(7)
8. Neighbor ML, Puntillo KA. Intramuscular Ketorolac versus oral ibuprofen in emergency department patients with acute pain. *Acad Emerg Med* 1998;5(2):118–122.
9. Turturro MA, Paris PM, Seaberg DC. Intramuscular ketorolac versus oral ibuprofen. *Ann Emerg Med* 1995;26(2):117–120.
10. Wright JM, Price SD, Watson WA. NSAIDS use and efficacy in the emergency department: Single doses of oral ibuprofen versus intramuscular ketorolac. *Ann Pharmacother* 1994; 28(3):309–312.

4

Emergency Clinical Pharmacy Services: Historical Perspective and Systematic Review

Objectives
- Rationalize the role of the pharmacist in the ED
- Review historical perspective of published reports of the pharmacist role in the ED
- Introduce ED clinical pharmacy services: A systematic review
- Explain fostering a research agenda

RATIONALIZING THE ROLE OF THE PHARMACIST IN THE ED

Strategies for improving safe and effective use of medications have included integration of clinical pharmacy services in the inpatient and outpatient setting. There is evidence that including pharmacists on the care team improves the quality and safety of patient care in both settings.[1-2] This strategy has been sporadically adopted for the ED setting.

There are several reasons for including a clinical pharmacy service on the ED care team. With the ever-increasing number of drugs available and the increased complexity of drug selection, administration, and monitoring, there is justification for having a clinically trained doctor of pharmacy on the care team.[3] The ED pharmacist can ensure that patients' medication needs are met while in the ED.

Participation of a pharmacist on the care team is in line with guidelines of the Joint Commission on Accreditation of Healthcare Organizations (JCAHO) standards for promoting a multidisciplinary approach to patient care. Because medication errors are a serious problem in EDs, as recommended by the IOM, pharmacists may be able to lead system changes that can reduce or eliminate errors.[3] Furthermore, pharmacists are in a good position to evaluate which medication is most cost-effective for patients and the hospital.

HISTORICAL PERSPECTIVE OF THE PHARMACIST IN THE ED

Emergency clinical pharmacy services is not a new concept. As far back as the 1970s, hospitals began to integrate pharmacists into the ED. Initially, their roles involved improving medication billing and inventory, and in some cases, pharmacists were integrated on "Code" teams.[4-5] In 1961, Theodore Taniguchi, Director of Hospital Pharmacy Services, University Hospital, University of Washington, Seattle, made a presentation to the pharmacy section of the American Association for the Advancement of Science in Denver. Taniguchi was the first to forecast that ambulatory patients using hospital emergency departments for medical care would increase and would be one of the growth factors of hospital pharmacists in the United States. He reported a program that provided efficient prescription services to the emergency department despite the pharmacy being closed.[6] Decades later, numerous descriptive reports have been published describing the role and activities of clinical pharmacy services in the ED. In 1976, Elenbaas et al. was first to report on the general pharmacotherapeutic role of the clinical pharmacist in the ED.[4-5] Czajka et al. in 1979 described ED clinical toxicology consult services provided by a pharmacist, without being present full time in the ED.[7] In 1981 and 1985, Whalen and Powell et al. in two distinct reports justified costs for a decentralized pharmaceutical service in the emergency room and described 24-hour emergency pharmaceutical services with a pharmacist in the ED.[8-9] In 1986, Kasuya et al. published a pharmacist-conducted on-call consultation service that supported the primary care of patients who were admitted to the University of Illinois Chicago ED, and this paper was followed by a report on a follow-up observation of this 24-hour pharmacotherapy services in the ED published by

Berry et al. in 1992.[10–11] Levy in 1987 illustrated and informed on services provided in the ED by a clinical pharmacist and explained how to document these activities.[12] Duke et al. in 1991 published a report on the impact of a pharmacist-physician designed asthma protocol to improve quality of care for patients visiting the ED.[13] In 2003, Cohen et al. published a qualitative description of the ED pharmacist role and rationalized the role of the pharmacist as provider with potential liability if the national pharmacist scope of pharmacy practice is not modified to fit actual needs of patients and role of pharmacists in the emergency care system.[14] In 2006, Carter et al. reported pharmacists conducting medication histories and improving safety in hospital emergency departments.[15] In 2006, Idrees et al. published a call to action for hospital pharmacists in response to the IOM report on the future of emergency care in the U.S. health system to improve emergency care in the United States.[16] Subsequently, in 2007, Lada et al. published a report on pharmacist intervention and the resulting significant cost avoidance.[17]

Despite this historical account and what appears to be a significant body of literature on the role of the pharmacist in the ED, the cost benefit and role in error reduction of a pharmacist in the ED is still in question by select emergency medicine and nursing societies, as well as hospital administrators. Even within the pharmacy departments, the employment of a clinical pharmacist assigned to the ED is not common. Despite more than four decades of literature on the role of the ED pharmacist, this role is still perceived as a new addition to the healthcare team and to the pharmacy world in general.

On this basis, we ascertain the scope of involvement of pharmacy practice or services provided in the ED (What is emergency medicine clinical pharmacy services?), to summarize the economic, humanistic, and clinical outcome data associated with ED pharmacists (What is the impact of the ED pharmacist?), and identify areas in need of future research. Thus, we conducted a systematic review of the published literature.

ED CLINICAL PHARMACY SERVICES: A SYSTEMATIC REVIEW

A search of MEDLINE (1966 through May 23, 2008), The Cochrane Library (1993-January 1st 2008), International Pharmaceutical Abstracts (1964 to January 1st 2008) and CINAHL Plus (1982 to January 1st 2008) databases was conducted using the keywords "ED or emergency department," and "clinical pharmacist or clinical pharmacy services." Manual searches of the bibliographies of included articles were performed. Articles were excluded if the pharmacist providing services to ED patients did not routinely practice in the ED, but rather provided consultations for ED patients. A single pharmacist performed the initial systematic search as described, with subsequent review by a second pharmacist of all included and excluded studies. The primary author reviewed the final selection of articles for completeness.

DATA ANALYSIS

Qualitative analyses were conducted to characterize pharmacists' activities and impact in the ED. The articles were categorized using several characteristics such as description of the services, various activities of the ED pharmacists, interventions reported, analysis of cost savings and cost avoidance, analysis of medication error reduction and involvement in conducting medication histories, and outcome measures or satisfaction data associated with the ED pharmacist or pharmacy service. The search returned 533 citations; however, only 17 citations met the inclusion criteria. Each of these reports provided a description of clinical pharmacy services at a total of 12 different institutions.[4–5,9–12,15,17, 19–25] The specifications of these institutions are depicted in Table 4-1.

EPIDEMIOLOGY OF CLINICAL PHARMACY SERVICES IN THE ED

Reports of clinical pharmacy services in the ED began to emerge in 1977.[4] Teaching hospitals are the predominant type of institutions reported in 11 of 12 articles (92%) that have deployed pharmacists to the ED with a mean rate of 61,000 annual admissions (21,000 to over 120,000) servicing what appear to be large metropolitan areas.

Hours of operation did not appear to be correlated with annual admission rates.[4–5,9–12,15,17, 19–25] Only 3 of the 12 institutions (25%) described having a satellite pharmacy.[9,18,21]

WHAT DO PHARMACISTS DO IN THE ED?

Table 4-2 lists over 30 job responsibilities or tasks reported among the 17 articles, with various articles reporting multiple tasks that the ED clinical pharmacist assumes. The scope of involvement varied between institution due to the various needs of the ED, the training of the pharmacist, and the allocation of resources. The time spent on each activity also varied and depended on the presence of an ED satellite, availability of pharmacy technicians, and technology of the ED (automated dispensing machines, computer physician order entry, etc).

The most common role for the ED pharmacist, reported in 73.3% of the articles, was to perform consultations.[4–5,10–12,17–21,24]

Sixty-seven percent report each of the following activities, including answering drug information questions[9–12,17–19,21–23] and providing staff education.[4–5,12,17–22,24] Fifty-three percent of articles report each of the following activities, including precepting students,[4–5,9,12,18–20,23] providing pharmacokinetic monitoring,[10–12,17–20,22] aiding in poison/toxicology cases,[10–12,17–20,22] participating in drug distribution activities,[9,12,17–21,23] and counseling patients on inpatient and outpatient therapy.[4–5,18–22,24] Forty-seven percent of articles report each of the following activities including obtaining medication histories,[11,15,18–20,22–23] precepting residents,[4–5,9–10,19–20,23] and documenting interventions.[12,15,18–22] Forty percent of articles report conducting research,[4–5,12,17,19,23] participating on rounds,[9,12,18–20,23] participating on code/trauma teams,[9,11–12,19–20,23] and recommending dose adjust-

TABLE 4-1

Description of ED and Pharmacy Services at Time of Study Publication

Ref.	Hospital	Pharmacy Services	Type of Hospital	Annual ED Admissions	No. of ED Beds	CPS implementation
4	Truman Medical Center (Kansas City, MO)	NR	Teaching	30,000	NR	1974
5	Truman Medical Center (Kansas City, MO)	NR	Teaching	40,000	NR	1974
9	Detroit Receiving Hospital (Detroit, MI)	Satellite pharmacy, 24/7 coverage	Teaching	72,000	NR	1980 (hospital opening)
10	University of Illinois at Chicago (Illinois, Chicago)	24/7 coverage; Pharmacist, Weekdays 7 am to 5 PM; Pharmacy residents, remainder	Teaching	21,000	NR	1979
18	Toronto East General and Orthopaedic Hospital (Toronto, Ontario)	Day shifts Monday-Friday and as requested during satellite pharmacy hours of 7:30 am–7:30 PM.	Community with teaching affiliation	New ED built with capacity for 65,000	NR	1989
12	Detroit Receiving Hospital (Detroit, MI)	Satellite pharmacy, 24/7 coverage	Teaching	75,782	NR	1980 (hospital opening)
19	Children's Medical Center (Dallas, TX)	Pharmacist, 24/7 coverage	Teaching	Over 120,000	NR	2002
20	University of Rochester (Rochester, NY)	Pharmacist, Weekdays 10 am–6 PM	Teaching	90,000	120	Initiated at study onset. (2000)
21	Grady Health System (Atlanta, GA)	Satellite pharmacy, 3 pm–11pm daily; Pharmacist, 10 am–7 PM Weekdays	Teaching	Over 100,000	120*	2001*
22	University of Kentucky, Chandler Medical Center (Louisville, KY)	Critical Care Pharmacy residents Monday-Saturday 4 pm–12 am	Teaching	NR	NR	NR
17	Detroit Receiving Hospital (Detroit, MI)	Satellite pharmacy, 24/7 coverage	Teaching	Over 84,000	100	1980 (hospital opening)
11	University of Illinois at Chicago (Chicago, IL)	24/7 coverage; Pharmacist, Weekdays 7 am to 5 PM; Pharmacy residents, remainder	Teaching	NR	NR	1979
15	University of Kansas Hospital (Olathe, KS)	Pharmacist completed ED medication histories for 3 months during the hours of 9 am–11 PM.	Teaching	Over 40,000	NR	NR
23	Saint Joseph Medical Center (Tacoma, WA)	Pharmacist, 10 am–8:30 pm daily	Tertiary Care	50,000	35	2005*
24	Cape Fear Valley Medical Center (Durham, NC)	For 3 months in 2005, a pharmacist was assigned to take medication histories between 9 am and 11 PM.	Community	Over 91,000	44 adult beds 13 pediatric beds	2006*
27	University of Rochester (Rochester, NY)	NR	Teaching	93,000	NR	NR

* Results from personal correspondence.
ED = Emergency Department, CPS = Clinical Pharmacy Services.

TABLE 4-2

Percent Frequency (%) of Reported Activities by ED Pharmacist from 1976-Present in Published Literature

Obtain medication histories (47)[11,15,18–20,22–23], allergy histories (33)[12,15,17,19,21] and immunization histories (7)[15]

Conduct drug use evaluations (20)[12,18–19] and conduct quality assurance (13)[12,19]

Monitor and report adverse drug reactions (20)[12,18–19]

Conduct research (40)[4–5,12,17,19,23]

Provide staff education (67)[4–5,12,17–22,24]

Precept students (53)[4–5,9,12,18–20,23] and residents (47)[4–5,9–10,19,20,23] and fellows (7)[19]

Provide pharmacokinetic monitoring (53)[10–12,17–20,22]

Follow-up microbiology culture data (7)[23]

Participate on rounds (40)[9,12,18–20,23], conduct chart reviews (27)[12,18,20,23], and perform consultations (73)[4–5,10–12,18–21,24]

Participate in code and/or trauma teams (40)[9,11–12,19–20,23]

Participate in drug distribution activities (53)[9, 12,17,19,21,23]

Answer drug information questions (67)[9,10,12,17–19,21–23]

Recommend appropriate pharmacotherapy (27)[17,19,20,22], monitor clinical outcomes (20)[12,19,23], and document interventions (47)[12,15,18–22]

Aid in poisoning/toxicology cases (53)[10–12,17–20,22]

Counsel patients on in-patient and out-patient therapy (53)[4–5,18–22,24]

Drug identification (27)[12,18–19,23]

Coordinate ambulatory health services (7)[5]; provision of 24/7 pharmacy services (13)[17,19]

Facilitate patient transfer to the floor and assure continuity of care once patient is transferred (27)[18–20,23]

Prepare medications trays and CPR kits for ambulance units (7)[9]

Maintains inventory of all drug supplies in ED (20)[9,18,20]

Assists nurses with calculating drip rates (20)[9,19,23], preparing IVs (27)[9,17,21,23], and recommending drug compatibility (33)[12,17,19,20,23]

Prospective review of medication orders (20)[9,20,23]

Participation in emergency preparedness (13)[20,24]

Disease state/drug therapy management (20)[4,5,23]

Participation on hospital committees (20)[4,5,23]

Recommend/monitor serum drug concentrations (33)[5,10–11,18–19] and perform emergency serum drug levels (13)[10,11]

Participate in the acute MI and STEMI team (7)[23]

Monitor and inform providers about medication side effects and interactions (13)[12,19]

Recommend alternative drugs if there is a shortage (7)[19]

Discuss patient compliance with provider (13)[12,19]

Recommend dosage adjustments (40)[12,17,19–21,23] and alternate routes of administration (20)[12,17,19]

Assure compliance with CMS and JC standards (7)[23]

Screen patients/order pneumococcal and influenza vaccinations (7)[23]

Indigent care/Outpatient prescription management (13)[17,19]

Compounding (7)[22]

Anticoagulation services (7)[17]

Transcription of orders (27)[17,19,21,23]

Fill emergency room outpatient prescriptions for difficult to find, after hours, emergent prescriptions (7)[19]

Maintain formulary compliance of medications in the ED (33)[4–5,9,17,21]

Maintain ED compliance with pharmacy procedures (20)[4,5,9]

CPR=Cardiopulmonary Resuscitation; ED=Emergency Department; IV=Intravenous; MI=Myocardial Infarction; STEMI=ST Segment Elevation Myocardial Infarction

ments.[12,17,19–21,23] Thirty-three percent of articles report obtaining allergy histories,[12,15,17,19,21] recommending drug compatibility,[12,15,17,19] recommending and monitoring serum drug concentrations,[5,10–11,18–19] and maintaining formulary compliance of medications in the ED.[4–5,9,17,21] Twenty-seven percent report conducting chart reviews,[12,17,19,20,23] recommending appropriate pharmacotherapy,[17,19,20,22] identifying drugs,[12,18,19,23] facilitating patient transfer to the floor and assuring continuity of care once patient is transferred,[18–20,23] preparing intravenous admixtures,[9,17,21,23] and transcribing orders.[17,19,21,23]

Several institutions reported unique pharmacists' activities or job responsibilities in their ED. Kasuya et al. described the emergency services provided by pharmacy residents at the University of Illinois at Chicago. These services included providing emergency drug levels for select drugs using an enzyme-mediated immunoassay technique (EMIT system) located in a pharmacy lab within the ED. Residents would interpret results and provide a written pharmacotherapeutic consultation including interpretation of level and appropriate patient management. Pharmacy residents provided clinical pharmacy services to the ED between the hours of 5 PM and

7 AM on weekdays, and 7 AM to 7 AM the following days on weekends and holidays, through use of an on-call pager.[10]

Mialon et al. described ED clinical pharmacy services provided at the Children's Medical Center in Dallas, Texas. One of the main focuses of their ED Pharmacy Program was to decrease the potential for medication errors. This is done in a number of ways including tracking "due times" for repeat medications, completing medication histories, and documenting all weights, heights, and allergies. They reported an 80% reduction in medication errors after implementation of clinical pharmacy services, and a projected cost savings of more than $800,000 per year. Pharmacists also provided discharge counseling for all newly diagnosed epileptics, diabetics, asthmatics, and patients with other disease states, as appropriate. They also provided these patients with a website link for more information if they have questions once they are discharged.[19]

Wymore et al. described culture and susceptibility report follow-up by the ED pharmacist. The pharmacist reviews a report of the culture and susceptibility results of patients seen in the ED daily and de-escalates or discontinues therapy as needed. If the patient has been discharged, and the results would change therapy, the patient is contacted and necessary arrangements are made for the patient to receive an appropriate antibiotic prescription. These extra measures prevent patient re-admission to the ED.[24]

WHAT IS THE IMPACT OF THE PHARMACIST IN THE ED?

Various studies report outcome data including intervention analysis, cost analysis, medication error prevention, and medication histories and survey data.

Six studies reported information about pharmacist interventions including number and types of interventions, time per intervention, and acceptance rate. Results are described in Table 4-3.

The mean duration of observation for these studies was 11 months (1–30 months). The mean number of interventions was 1500 (183–3787) with a mean acceptance rate of 93% (89–98.6%).[10–11,17,21,22,25] Five of 6 (83%) of the reports were retrospective with a mean duration of observation of 12 months (1–30 months). The mean number of interventions was 1371 (173 to 3787) with a mean acceptance rate of 93% (89–98.6%).[10–11,21–22,25] Categories of interventions reported were within the normal scope of a generalist-trained clinical pharmacist suggesting process and quality improvements with interventions conducted similar to pharmacists in other settings. However, intervention categories differed between institutions suggesting a need for standardization. Documentation methods differed between institutions and included paper cards, personal digital assistant, and computer programs. Four studies reported cost-related outcomes, as seen in Table 4–4.

The mean duration of observation for these articles was 11 months (0.5–36 months). Average reported cost avoidance was $355,021 over this time frame.[12,17,20,21] A retrospective study design was used in three of four studies. The mean duration of observation for these articles was 14 months (0.5 to 36 months) with a reported average cost avoidance of $130,103.[12,20,21]

As illustrated in Table 4-5, three studies reviewed medication error reduction when a clinical pharmacist is present

in the ED, and one study reported total number of medication histories recorded by a clinical pharmacist.

This data suggest that a pharmacist in the ED can reduce medication errors.[15,22,25] It also contributes to the achievement of various ASHP 2015 Health-System Pharmacist initiatives such as increasing the number of hospitals that will have pharmacists involved in obtaining medication histories upon admission and will be involved in medication safety within the institution.[28]

Lastly, two studies reported results of surveys. Both of these studies administered internal surveys to assess staff perception of clinical pharmacy services in the ED.[4,254] These results are listed in Table 4-6.

FOSTERING A RESEARCH AGENDA

Bearing limitations of the published literature, ED clinical pharmacy services have been established for over 30 years now and are predominantly deployed in teaching institutions and in larger metropolitan areas where dense populations are served. Pharmacy hours of operation vary significantly, and only few hospitals have satellites suggesting that pharmacists and pharmacy services within the ED are patient-care focused and require presence and visibility to provide services.

The summary of the data implies that ED pharmacists are already conducting a form of prospective review of medication orders in various institutions as needed. Standards for methods for prospective review based on models used by these organizations should be described, made transferable to other institutions, and be used as best practices to meet the Joint Commission's standards for MM4.10 prospective review of medication orders. Variations in the standard should be internally based on the unique characteristics of the ED setting, and as long as they are rational, acceptance of these unique entities should be permitted.[26]

This data suggests voluntary demand for pharmacy services in the ED derived not from regulatory requirements but instead from acknowledgement of a unique core of skills best suited and delivered by a pharmacist. Essentially, EDs need clinical pharmacy services as part of good operating procedure. The ED is a healthcare setting fertile for novel programs and unique practices developed based on the demand and need of the patients and the community using this resource.

This cost avoidance data lacks formal structured pharmacoeconomics analysis. Despite this limitation, the implications of this data are that hiring a pharmacist deployed to the ED pays for itself through cost avoidance data. Whether this is sufficient for hospital administrators to support funding is still in question. However, this data suggests that at minimum an ED pharmacist may improve process, reduce error, and improve quality of services demanded by ED healthcare staff at no additional cost to the institution. The summarization of this data may be limited because each institution used a different method to calculate cost savings and cost avoidance; however, each method was consistent within the institution. In most cases, these figures were calculated to justify ED services and pharmacy service expansion.

TABLE 4-3

Analysis of Interventions

Ref.	Study Design	Duration	Number of Interventions	Type of Intervention	Time Per Intervention	Acceptance Rate
10	Retrospective	2 years	2283*	Therapeutic consultation: 90% Drug information: 10%	68 minutes: 1st year 134 minutes: 2nd year	91.5%
21+	Retrospective	5 months	401	Dose/frequency adjustments: 29% Formulary interchange: 16% Professional services: 13% Allergy documentation: 9%	Majority (52%) 21–30 minutes	89%
22	Retrospective	1 month	201	Pharmacotherapy: 36% Patient counseling: 23% Pharmacy to dose: 20% Pharmacy clarifications: 6% Pediatric questions: 5% Toxicology: 5% Codes: 2% Compounding: 1% Pharmaceutics: 1%		
17	Prospective	4 months	2,150	Drug information: 16.8% Dosage adjustment: 16.4% Nursing questions: 14.7% Formulary interchange: 8.4% Pharmacotherapy: 8.4% Order clarifications: 7.6% Change to alternative drug therapy: 7.3% Compatibility issues: 6.7% Patient information: 3.6% Change route of administration: 3.1% Discontinue drug therapy: 2.7% Toxicology: 2% Allergy notification: 1.9% Drug therapy duplication: 0.4% Drug interaction: 0.09%		
11	Retrospective	2.5 years	3,787	Asthma/COPD: 33% Toxicology: 22% Seizures: 17.5% Cardiology: 11% Miscellaneous: 9% Pharmacokinetic: 7.5%	100 minutes ± 83 minutes	
24	Retrospective	1 month	183	Dose calculation: 29% Inappropriate dosage, drug, route, or schedule: 26% Order clarification: 16% Allergy documentation: 12% Miscellaneous or unspecified: 8% Approval of nonformulary medication: 4% Identification of duplicate therapy: 4% Clarification of medication history: 1% Identification of drug interaction: 1%		98.6%

*Reported as number of consults

TABLE 4-4

Analysis of Cost Avoidance

Ref.	Study Design	Duration	Analysis	Outcome
12*	Retrospective	3 years	Analysis of clinical interventions. Cost savings primarily based on material cost-savings resulting from the costs of the drug plus necessary equipment. Pharmacist and nursing time for drug preparation not included.	**Annual cost avoidance/year = $41,571.20 in 1989 $54,007.09 in 1990 $93,561.22 in 1991**
20*	Retrospective	2 weeks	Informal cost analysis using 14 randomly selected days during the CPS phase-in period. Data from quality assurance logs, maintained using ASHP's CliniTrend software, were used to calculate cost savings based on changing medication, dosage, route of administration, and avoiding inappropriate choice of medications.	Reported Average cost avoidance/day = $589.00; **Projected Annual cost avoidance/year = $214,985**
21	Retrospective	5 months	Pharmacist interventions characterized into events avoided due to intervention; further divided by cost avoidance, based on an internally validated model.	Reported Total cost avoidance = $192,923; **Projected Annual cost avoidance/year = $385,846**
17	Prospective	4 months	Analysis of interventions based on cost and probability of harm if the intervention had not taken place. Interventions were reviewed by a physician and pharmacist. Pharmacist wage and supplies incorporated into calculation.	Reported Total cost avoidance = $1,029,776; **Projected Annual cost avoidance/year = $3,089,328**

*Report cost savings which are equivalent to cost avoidance

TABLE 4-5

Analysis of Medication Errors and Medication Histories

Ref.	Study Design	Duration	Medication Errors	No. of Medication Histories
22	Retrospective	1 month		93
23	Prospective	3 months	Sample size was 252 medication histories. Medication histories taken by ED providers were 78% incomplete and 18% contained immunization histories. Medication histories taken by pharmacist were 100% complete and 100% contained immunization histories. Pharmacists documented 7% more medication allergies than ED providers.	
24	Retrospective	1 month	Sample size was 490 medication errors for 198 patients. When a clinical pharmacist was present in the ED there was a 66% relative risk reduction in the number of medication errors (p=0.0001). The acceptance rate of pharmacist recommendations was 98.6%	

TABLE 4-6

Studies with Survey Results

Ref.	Study Design	Results
4	A 14-item questionnaire administered to determine staff attitudes toward the pharmacist and clinical pharmacy services in the ED. 54 questionnaires were distributed to 17 ED physicians (residents and attendings), 20 to all residents who had completed a one month or more rotation in the ED in the previous year, and 17 to the ED nursing staff. Medical students on rotation, and nonprofessional personnel in the ED were excluded.	Response rate: 72% 100% of respondents agreed that the pharmacist was a benefit to patient care and an important component of the department. 95% felt the pharmacy role was transferable to other emergency departments. 87% physicians agreed that the pharmacist is capable of providing primary care to select patients once a diagnosis has been made. 83% of physicians were willing to have their patients charged for these services.
25	A 26-item survey administered to medical and nursing staff to determine staff perceptions of the ED Pharmacy Services. 50% (91 of 182) ED staff members were randomly selected to receive an e-mail request to complete the web-based survey. Staff members included all attendings, fellows, residents, and midlevel providers (nurse practitioners and physicians assistants).	Response rate: 82% 99% of respondents agreed that the pharmacist improved quality of care. 96% felt the pharmacist was an integral part of the team 93% had contacted the pharmacist at least a few times during their last five shifts.

ED=Emergency Department, CPS=clinical pharmacy services

There are obvious limitations of applicability of internal surveys from one institution across to other institutions around the country; however, a common positive theme toward the role of the pharmacist in the ED was expressed by nursing and medical staff, again suggesting that the pharmacist does not intrude or disrupt the emergency care process.

Limitations to this systematic review include publication bias as those who have unsuccessfully implemented services within the ED setting may not have pursued full publication of their data. Furthermore, descriptive reviews have been written by pharmacists, suggesting a positive bias toward their efforts.

Selection bias may have occurred as our search strategy has selected articles that report on benefits of pharmacists in the ED. We did not include grey literature that may include anecdotal commentary from some in the emergency medicine and nursing societies that do not agree with the clinical impact of a pharmacist in the ED. For example, as quoted in the September 2007 issue of *Emergency Medicine News*,[28] Dr. Tom Scaletta, Director of the American Association of Emergency Medicine, stated "Prospective pharmacy review of ED prescriptions was likely unnecessary especially when a doctor-nurse team was capable of making a good decision about when to give a medication" and that "It would slow things down and force hospitals to use resources for something that wasn't necessary. That means something else wouldn't get the resources it needed." Despite this contention, medication errors are not uncommon in the ED, the majority of which are preventable and directly related to negligence.[29] Furthermore, there are no randomized, controlled trials supporting the contention that a pharmacist in the emergency care team would slow things down. As illus-

trated in Table 4-4, annual cost avoidance data suggest a return on investment, justifying the ED pharmacist position and avoiding the assumed opportunity cost suggested by Dr. Scaletta.

To reduce publication bias, multiple searches from various databases were conducted; however, no data suggesting a negative impact of the ED pharmacist was reported. However, a clinical pharmacist may miss errors and be involved in drug-related morbidity so this must be considered.

Most of the studies published were not of high quality compared to the gold standard, randomized controlled trials. As such, inference to the impact of a clinical pharmacist in the ED as a strategy for one specific element, such as reducing medication errors, improving quality, or cost avoidance may not be generalized to all ED settings. In fact, because of the broad mix of activities and patients, it is unlikely to accumulate effect size sufficient to show statistical significance of any individual element.

LIMITATIONS AND FUTURE DIRECTION

This systematic review describes the role of the clinical pharmacist in the ED as described in published literature. Seventeen articles were included for review; a description of services and an analysis of outcomes were reported. The level of evidence to this point is mostly the equivalent of level 4 data, which is similar to a heterogeneous group of case reports describing successful establishment and roles of pharmacists providing a heterogeneous group of services all within the general scope of the pharmacists and described throughout select geographical regions.

What would be of greatest interest would be descriptions of how organizations first decided upon deploying a pharmacist into the ED because this insight may provide an understanding of organizational gaps in care or processes that were resolved with deployment of a pharmacist in the ED. For example was it economic, humanistic, or clinical forces that incorporated the pharmacist within these ED settings? It would be of great value for those with ED clinical pharmacy services to describe the nature of origin of ED clinical pharmacy services and to describe problem resolution that this intervention provided.

Higher level data such as randomized controlled trials are required. Most notably, studies of institutions with and without pharmacists at varying seasonal and peak time activities and with explicit measurable outcomes that are standardized and accepted across disciplines would be the gold standard. However employing gold standard scientific methodology may be difficult because the variation in activity completed on a daily basis may not permit for consistent effects to be measured. Perhaps an index such as the Dow Jones industrial average, which takes a cumulative average of performance quality indicators, safety measures, and other varying tasks as an overall assessment of benefit would better support a national movement toward having pharmacists in the ED and could better delineate where, when, and how the ED pharmacist can be best utilized to improve quality.

There are other limitations to these studies. For example, the scope of involvement varied greatly between institutions. It may also be due to a lack of an established framework or guidelines pertaining to ED clinical pharmacy. While job responsibilities can be classified into similar categories across institutions, time allocation and resources vary greatly. This is necessary, to some degree, because the needs of each institution vary. However, more articles are needed to describe how to implement clinical pharmacy services and standard practice. This will occur naturally as more governing bodies, such as the Joint Commission, implement or clarify policies regarding ED practice. In the meantime, institutions with ED clinical pharmacy services should be encouraged to conduct studies and publish results of their efforts to provide a framework for institutions who seek to implement clinical pharmacy services and also as a means to justify these positions.

Also while 17 studies have been included in this review, they are mostly descriptive in nature. This review cites several studies that report cost avoidance and savings and decrease in medication errors associated with clinical pharmacy services. These outcomes are often not the primary outcome of the study. More data is needed that describes these outcomes in more detail, and institutions with clinical pharmacy services in the ED are encouraged to conduct and publish their research efforts. Clinical pharmacists should have formal, standardized documentation methods that incorporate types and number of interventions and associated cost savings.

Additionally, studies documenting ED pharmacist involvement on patient-specific outcomes are needed. An example of such outcome data has been reported by Zed et al. who conducted a prospective cohort study of Vancouver general hospital outpatient VTE treatment program over a 7-year period and measured recurrent rates of VTE at 3 and 6 months following discharge. Bleeding complications, throm-bocytopenia, and patient satisfaction were evaluated. The investigators reported that 305 patients were safely and effectively managed by ED based outpatient treatment program for VTE, and patient satisfaction was at a high level. [27]

Third, many institutions conduct internal pilot studies to determine cost savings and impact of clinical pharmacy services in the ED. These pilot programs are often completed by a pharmacy resident and are used as justification for implementing permanent services in the ED. Many such studies are presented as posters or presentations at local and national meetings. This review only included abstracts searchable in International Pharmaceutical Abstracts (IPA) or descriptions published in pharmacy journals (in the form of letters to the editor or an article written in a monthly column). Individuals performing such studies are also encouraged to publish the results of their pilot programs in emergency medicine or pharmacy journals.

SUMMARY

A review of the literature revealed that pharmacists have been involved in ED care for decades; they provide traditional clinical pharmacy services, respond to medical emergencies, provide consultation on medication issues, reduce medication errors, and conduct medication histories upon admission to the healthcare system and may be cost saving and or cost avoiding. The ED pharmacist does not disrupt the emergency care process or delay care. The level and standardization of evidence must improve to gain cross disciplinary acceptance. A research agenda has been implicated and proposed.

References

1. Kaboli PJ, Hoth AB, McClimon BJ, Schnipper JL. Clinical pharmacist and inpatient medical care: A systematic review. *Arch Intern Med* 2006;166:955–964.
2. Beney J, Bero LA, Bond C. Expanding the roles of outpatient pharmacists: effects on health services utilization, costs and patient outcomes. Cochrane database of systematic reviews. The Cochrane Library 2007;Issue 4.
3. Institute of Medicine. *To Err Is Human: Building a Safer Health System.* Kohn LT, Corrigan JM, Donaldson MS, eds. Washington, DC: National Academy Press, 2000.
4. Elenbaas RM, Waeckerle JF, Kendall WK. The clinical pharmacist in emergency medicine. *Am J Hosp Pharm* 1977;34: 843–846.
5. Elanbass RM. Role of the pharmacist in providing clinical pharmacy services in the emergency department. *Can J Hosp Pharm* 1978;123–125.
6. Taniguchi T. Providing an emergency department dispensing service. *Hospitals* 1962;36:126–130.
7. Czjaka PA, Skoutakis VA, Wood GC, Autian J. Clinical toxicology consultation by a pharmacist. *Am J Hosp Pharm* 1979; 36(8):1087–89.
8. Whalen FJ. Cost justification of decentralized pharmaceutical services for the emergency room. *Am J Hosp Pharm* 1981;38: 684–687.
9. Powell MF, Solomon DK, McEachen RA. Twenty-four hour emergency pharmaceutical services. *Am J Hop Pharm* 1985; 42:831–835.

10. Kasuya A, Bauman JL, Curtis RA, et al. Clinical pharmacy on-call program in the emergency department. *Am J Emerg Med* 1986;4(5):464–467.

11. Berry NS, Folstad JE, Bauman JL, Leikin JB. Follow-up observations on 24 hour pharmacotherapy services in the emergency department. *Ann Pharmacother* 1992;26;476–480.

12. Levy DN. Documentation of clinical and cost saving pharmacy interventions in the emergency room. *Hosp Pharm* 1993;28(7):624–627, 630–634, 653.

13. Duke T, Kellerman A, Ellis R, Self T. Asthma in the emergency department: Impact of a protocol on optimizing therapy. *Am J Emerg Med* 1991;9(5):432–435.

14. Cohen V. The Emergency Department Pharmacist. In: O'Donnell J, editor. *Drug Injury Liability, Analysis and Prevention.* Tucson, AZ: Lawyers & Judges Publishing Company, Inc., 2005;733–742.

15. Carter MK, Allin DM, Scott LA, et al. Pharmacist-acquired medication histories in a university hospital emergency department. *Am J Health-Syst Pharm* 2006;63:2500.

16. Idrees U, Clements E. The state of US emergency care: a call to action for hospital pharmacists. *Ann Pharmacother* 2006; 40:2251–2253.

17. Lada P, Delgado G. Documentation of pharmacists' interventions in an emergency department and associated cost avoidance. *Am J Health-Syst Pharm* 2007;64:63–8.

18. Laivenieks N, McCaul K. O'Brodovich. Clinical pharmacy services provided to an emergency department. *Can J Hosp Pharm* 1992;45:113–5.

19. Mialon PJ, Williams P, Wiebe RA. Clinical pharmacy services in a pediatric emergency room. *Hosp Pharm* 2004; 39:121–4.

20. Fairbanks RJ, Hays DP, Webster DF, et al. Clinical pharmacy services in an emergency department. *Am J Health-Syst Pharm* 2004;61:934–7.

21. Ling JM, Mike LA, Rubin J, et al. Documentation of pharmacist interventions in the emergency department. *Am J Health-Syst Pharm* 2005;62:1793–7.

22. Weant KA, Sterling E, Winstead PS, et al. Establishing a pharmacy presence in the ED. *Am J Emerg Med* 2006;24: 514–5.

23. Wymore ES, Casanova TJ, Broekemeier RL, et al. Clinical pharmacist's daily role in the emergency department of a community hospital. *Am J Health-Syst Pharm* 2008;65:395–9.

24. Brown JN, Barnes CL, Beasley B, et al. Effect of pharmacists on medication errors in an emergency department. *Am J Health-Syst Pharm* 2008;65:330–3.

25. Fairbanks RJ, Hildebrand JM, Kolstee KE, et al. Medical and nursing staff highly value clinical pharmacists in the emergency department. *Emerg Med J* 2007;24:716–9.

26. American Society of Health-System Pharmacists. 2015 initiative. http://www.ashp.org/s_ashp/cat1c.asp?CID=218&DID= 255. Accessed June 6, 2008.

27. Zed PJ, Filiatrault L. Clinical outcomes and patient satisfaction of a pharmacist-managed, emergency department-based outpatient treatment program for venous thromboembolic diseases. *CJEM* 2008;10:10–17.

28. SoRelle R. EM groups persuade Joint Commission to temper pharmacy review policy. *Emerg Med News* 2007;29:1–4.

29. Leape LL, Brennan TA, Laird N, et al. The nature of adverse events in hospitalized patients. Results of the Harvard Medical Practice Study II. *N Engl J Med* 1991;324:377–84.

5

Unique Characteristics of the Emergency Department and the Emergency Department Pharmacist

Objectives

- Review the unique role of the ED pharmacist in managing drug use
  - Physical Constraints
  - Time and Volume Pressures
  - Limited Therapeutic Options
  - Variety of Patients
  - Temporizing Measures
  - Team Approach
  - Paucity of Information
  - Discharge Counseling

UNIQUE ROLE OF ED PHARMACIST IN MANAGING DRUG USE

It is one thing to practice pharmacy in the hospital; it is quite another to practice emergency care clinical pharmacy. The effective practice of emergency care clinical pharmacy (ECCP) requires an approach, a way of thinking, and personality characteristics different from all other pharmacy specialty services. Factors that have led to this unique brand of pharmacy to the patient includes: physical constraints, the pressure of time and volume, variety of conditions to treat, the paucity of information, the limitation of therapeutic options, and the constraint of disposition.

PHYSICAL CONSTRAINTS

The physical limitations of the ED to most pharmacists would be an immediate deterrent to practicing pharmacy with the exception of those who thrive in this overcrowded frenetic area. Ninety-one percent of ED directors reported crowding to be a problem.[1] Nearly 40% reported crowding

on a "daily" basis.[1] Schneider et al. conducted a point prevalence study to assess the degree of overcrowding in hospitals EDs. At the index time, there was an average of 1.1 patients per treatment space, and 52% of EDs reported more than 1 patient per treatment space. There was also evidence of personnel shortage, with a mean of 4.2 patients per registered nurse, 49% of EDs having each registered nurse caring for more than 4 patients and a mean of 9.7 patients per physician.[2] Sixty-eight percent of EDs had each physician caring for more than 6 patients.[2] Crowding was present in all geographic areas and all hospital types (teaching/non-teaching status of the hospital). Consistent with the crowded conditions, 11% of institutions were on ambulance diversion, thus not accepting new acute patients. Delays in transfer of admitted patients out of the ED contributed to the physical crowding. Twenty-two percent of patients in the ED were already admitted and were awaiting transfer to an inpatient bed; 73% of EDs were boarding 2 or more inpatients.[2] Pharmacists who are *not* accustom to a large workspace, a quite environment, physical order and structure, and who enjoy running back and forth will thrive in the emergency department.

TIME AND VOLUME PRESSURES

More than any other specialty in pharmacy practice, emergency department pharmacists (EDP) deal with patients as a turbulent flow in a constricted channel. In a true emergency, seconds to minutes make the difference between life and death or serious disability as seen with thrombolytic use for acute MI or for stroke. In these situations, EDPs, contrary to much of their previous training, must be prepared to assist the team to "treat first and ask questions later." The ideal EDP has the knowledge and skill to ensure that the "treat first and ask questions later" approach is safe and secured. The EDP helps expedite and facilitate this emergent care.

31

The time available for an EDP to evaluate the management and think about any given patient is severely limited by the demands of other patients being managed concurrently.

Traditional medication order review is likely to delay treatment. Underwood et al. conducted a retrospective chart review using a convenience sample of 134 consecutive patients admitted from the ED to measure the delay associated with pharmacist review of prescribed antibiotics for community-acquired pneumonia, which currently required antibiotic therapy within 4 hours upon arrival. The investigators calculated the order time and administration time for antibiotics stocked in the ED versus those not stocked. The investigators reported an increase in time to administration of antibiotics in the ED of 32 ± 37.41 minutes (p=0.0001) with a total range of 0–195 minutes and an interquartile range of 35–153 minutes that required pharmacy review compared to those not subject to review by pharmacy.[3] The authors concluded that pharmacy review increases time to administration, and the net effect of pharmacist review may increase harm to patient safety. This study has multiple design flaws and has not undergone peer review, but makes the point that for medication review by a pharmacist to be effective, it must be efficient in the ED and new models for medication review are required to assure no delays.

In a study we conducted in elderly patients visiting the ED, a median time from ED entry to initial diagnostic intervention was 37 minutes, IQR of 19–57 minutes. The median time to initial therapeutic intervention was 81.5 minutes with an IQR of 53–129.5 minutes.[4] Thus there is ample time to generate information needed to review medication orders. However, the pharmacist must be present in the ED to take advantage of the time from arrival at triage to the initial management. It is likely that much of the time delay in reviewing medication orders for the ED is due to the pharmacist not being present in the ED, perhaps reviewing orders from a satellite in the critical care area or in central pharmacy and unable to obtain the information about the patient.

The experienced EDP will adopt an efficient process to ensure the pharmacotherapy is indicated, there are no contraindications, the selection is appropriate, and the dose is optimal, prepared, and administered appropriately. With a time efficient process, cost avoidance and reduction of medication errors associated with overuse may rationalize the time delay and enable the EDP to manage the volume. The development of medication use protocols, use of CPOE, and decision support will facilitate and streamline pharmacy review. But, incorporation of an EDP with this expertise is most essential to ensure safety and expedite care.

The combination of time and volume pressures forces the EDP to be much more aware of priorities among patients. The EDP must triage and prioritize the less significant risk (verify routine medication orders such as acetaminophen, check for inappropriate abbreviations) from those that pose the highest risk. The EDP assists in identifying and managing a drug overdose or must expedite and verify appropriate use of the high risk and high cost, often inappropriately used, medications (i.e. antidotes, Dantrolene, Octreotide, Glucagon, Digibind) or attend a cardiac arrest event (code) and provide code support where difficult procedures need to be completed immediately, and the emergency care team may need support during acute stabilization. The EDP must cognitively, but quickly, either support or refute the physician's pharmacotherapy decisions without delaying management. Case by case, the importance of the pharmacist interventions becomes realized and accepted by the emergency care team.

Pharmacists, who are efficient, can streamline care and multitask, and can move from patient to patient quickly will thrive in this arena. Their ratio, depending on the number of pharmacists deployed to the ED, of number of patients seen at any one time may be 40–50:1. During peak seasons, EDPs can see 250–300 patients per 24 hour-day and experience at any one time up to 50–60 patients boarded (admitted), each with 10–12 medications prescribed by the admitting team that require verification.

LIMITED THERAPEUTIC OPTIONS

Only a small subset of the vast therapeutic armamentarium is available to the EDP promptly because most medications are stored in centralized pharmacies or in automated dispensing machines, potentially delaying the most important life-saving intervention, but appropriately securing to avoid diversion and inappropriate use. The EDP must devise a strategy to assure safety and still deliver therapeutic recommendations and treatments in a timely manner to be of benefit to the emergency physicians. The EDP must master the vast number of urgent and emergent conditions and the pharmacotherapy for these conditions so the EDP can expand the potential therapeutic options for emergency physicians. Once the EDP is consulted and assumes responsibility then the physician can move on to another patient. Reducing the time associated with processing patients by having an EDP assume responsibility for the pharmacotherapeutic tasks is a major advantage to emergency physicians.

VARIETY OF PATIENTS

Because the diverse emergency care environment has expanded to manage far more than emergency patients, such as ophthalmological and oncological emergencies and transplant patients, specialist consultation may not be immediately available.[5-6] Recommendations made by on-call specialists may be complex and require high risk and high cost therapies that emergency physicians are not accustom to using. The EDP can aid the emergency care team in effectively executing the instructions for pharmacotherapy by the on-call specialist. Examples include the patient with acute angle closure glaucoma, where multiple ophthalmological agents must be considered to reduce risk of morbidity, or the oncological patient requiring colony-stimulating factors. The EDP can assess and validate appropriateness and then expedite the operations required to administer these agents. Thus the EDP is specialized in emergency care, but must have a flexibility to attend to a vast array of pharmacotherapeutic issues in the ED.

TEMPORIZING MEASURES

Often, emergency physicians can provide only temporizing or symptomatic treatment, while definitive therapy must be deferred to another specialist. These temporizing measures may include a potentially dangerous medication for use only on an emergency basis to a critically ill or injured patient, increasing the likelihood of an adverse event because critical safety checks may be omitted. In addition, the route of administration used in an emergency can lead to a greater risk of an adverse event (when a medication is given intravenously or via a central line, the risk of an adverse event rises dramatically).[7] Avoiding therapeutic error with temporizing measures is a paramount function to EDPs.

TEAM APPROACH

The essence of the EDP is to facilitate and expedite a safe approach at the bedside with therapy in-hand of temporizing measures; however, the EDP must also assist with life-preserving measures that are being conducted by the emergency team in a continuous non-disruptive flow. The continuity needed is analogous to a symphony orchestra, where the conductor (emergency physician) calls out instruction and the violinist (pharmacist) fine tunes and rapidly engages with other instruments (nursing and patient care technicians). A team approach is essential.

PAUCITY OF INFORMATION

An EDP assists in resolving many constraints associated with paucity of information. The EDP acquires more data, identifies important issues of concern, and recommends optimal pharmacotherapy and appropriate disposition based on expected resolution of diseases or pharmacokinetics and dynamics of medications.

DISCHARGE COUNSELING

An EDP specialist supports communications needed in the ED. Pharmacist are educators and counselors with the ability to translate the medical jargon into layman terminology to assist patients or caregivers of the need for the care being provided and to allay the fear of the patient. Traditionally pharmacists use a secluded counseling area to provide these services; the emergency department rarely provides for such a remote location. The savvy pharmacist finds ways to be the patient advocate and provides this information despite the noisy chaotic environment.

Distinct to the outpatient or ambulatory pharmacist who may alert or alarm the patient of risk, the ED pharmacist must allay the fear of the patient, empathize with caregivers, and support the ED team during a crisis.

SUMMARY

Unique characteristics are involved in providing pharmaceutical care and emergency care pharmacotherapy within an emergency care setting. Matching the characteristics of the Emergency Department with the personality traits of the pharmacist who has been assigned to the ED is an essential component to successfully establishing and sustaining clinical pharmacy service in the ED.

References

1. Derlet R, Richards J, Kravitz R. Frequent overcrowding in US emergency departments. *Acad Emerg Med* 2001;8:151–155.
2. Schneider S, Gallery ME, Schafermeyer R, Zwemer FL. Emergency department crowding: A point in time. *Ann Emerg Med* 2003;42(2):167–172.
3. Underwood M, Peter D, Lucas C, Jouriles N. Pharmacist review of emergency department medication orders: How long does it take? *Ann Emerg Med* 2007;50(3):S40–S41.
4. Cohen V, Jellinek SP, Likourezos A, et al. Variation in medication information for elderly patients during initial interventions by emergency department physicians. *Am J Health-Syst Pharm* 2006;65:60–4.
5. McConnel JK, Johnson LA, Arab N, et al. The on-call crisis: A statewide assessment of the costs of providing on-call specialist coverage. *Ann Emerg Med* 2007;49:727–733.
6. McConnell JK, Newgard CD, Lee R. Changes in the cost and management of emergency department on-call coverage: Evidence from a longitudinal statewide survey. *Ann Emerg Med* 2008;Apr 1.
7. Peth HA Jr. Medication errors in the emergency department: A systems approach to minimizing risk. *Emerg Med Clin North Am* 2003;21:141–158.

6

Academic-Based Emergency Department Clinical Pharmacy Services and the PharmER Pyramid

Objectives

- Describe the demographics and facilities of the ED at Maimonides Medical Center
- Discuss role of academic-based ED clinical pharmacist
- Introduce the PharmER Pyramid
- Illustrate the physical infrastructure for medication storage and delivery in the ED

MAIMONIDES MEDICAL CENTER

MODERN ED IS A HOSPITAL WITHIN A HOSPITAL

The Department of Emergency Medicine at Maimonides Medical Center is a primary teaching facility for the medical school of the State University of New York and serves the Boro-Park community of Brooklyn, New York. The Department of Emergency Medicine sees 90,000 patients annually, with an admission rate of 25%. The acute adult facility is divided into an existing ED and a new ED (South and North side). The south side consists of a triage area, 23 general beds with 1 quiet room, 1 obstetric and gynecological room, 1 ophthalmologic room, an isolation room, and an asthma treatment area. The north side ED consists of a large resuscitation area that can store up to eight beds, an acute area with 12 beds, and 1 isolation room. Adjacent to the new ED is the boarded unit where up to 12 patients who can be admitted but are awaiting beds. Each area is staffed with board-certified emergency medicine physicians and nurses. Nurse practitioners and physician assistants staff a fast track area. Board-certified pediatric emergency medicine physicians staff the pediatric emergency department. As part of a major modernization project and to manage the volume of patients visiting the ED within the community, the emergency department has undergone expansion and major renovations as depicted in Figure 6-1A. Two emergency medication rooms (EMR) are available on both the new and existing wings of the facility (Figs. 6-1B,C). These rooms were designed for medication storage, dispensing, and pharmacist verification as depicted in Figure 6-1B. Special features in the design of these medication rooms include a combination self-locking door for restricted access; two computer terminals for pharmacy use; and the central location allows the pharmacist to have easy access to patient care areas (Figs. 6-1D, E, F). The emergency medication room on the existing side (Fig. 6-1B) is scheduled to be expanded and converted into a fully operational pharmacy satellite. However, the EDPs uses "station 4659" as their post for supporting the emergency care team. Station 4659 is conveniently located in front of the resuscitation rooms, at the point of entry of the patient by ambulance and has a view of the entire ED (Figs. 6-1G, H).

DEPARTMENT OF PHARMACY

The Department of Pharmacy (DOP) provides a centralized 24-hour distributional support service to the Department of Emergency Medicine. Two self-locking medication rooms are located in the ED and store most of the emergency medications. Each room of the ED is outfitted with automated dispensing machines. The room is able to fit five persons for procurement of medications.

The central pharmacy refills the floor stock daily, delivers medications that are not floor stock at 1.5 hour scheduled rounds from 8 AM until 12 midnight, and sends medications through the Translogic CTF 30 pneumatic tube system. At all times, the tube system may be used for dispensing stat medications and any missing medications. The central pharmacy also provides drug and poison information as needed.

text continues on page 39

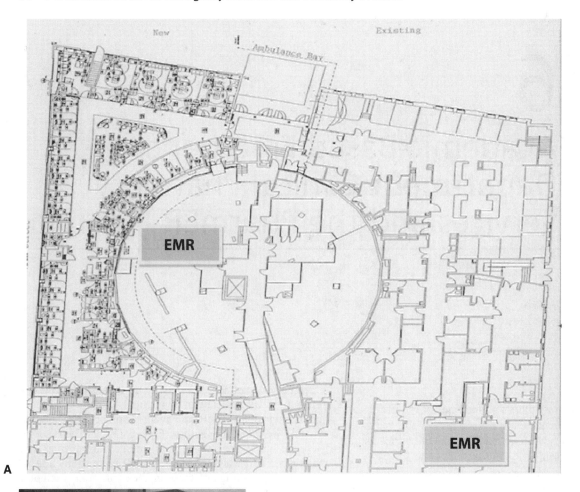

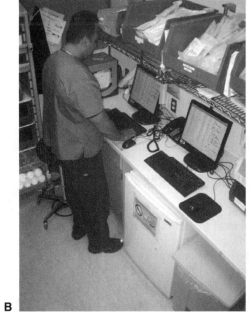

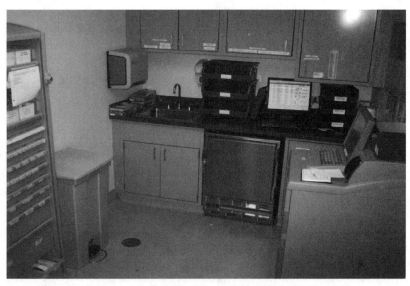

Figure 6–1. Emergency department expansion; (A) centrally located emergency medication rooms (EMR) for medication, storage, dispensing, and pharmacist verification; (B-C) space allocated for pharmacist verification and a source for drug information on new side.

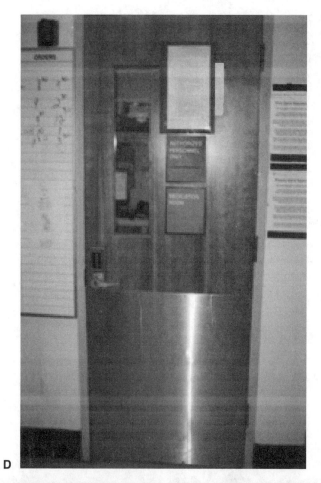

D

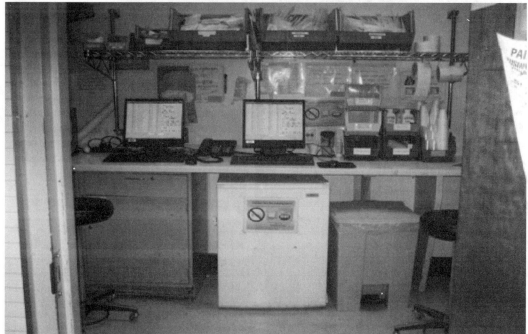

E

Figure 6–1. (D) Combination self-locking entry door for restricted access; (E) two computer terminals for pharmacy verification in the EMR.

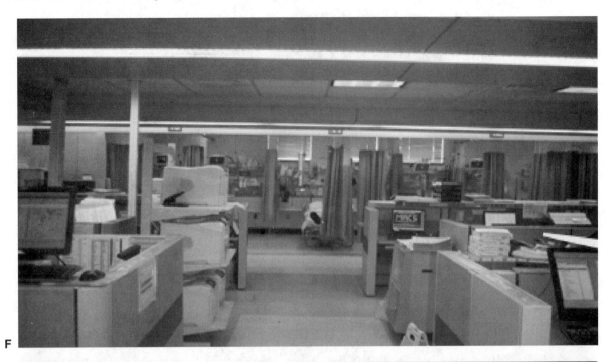

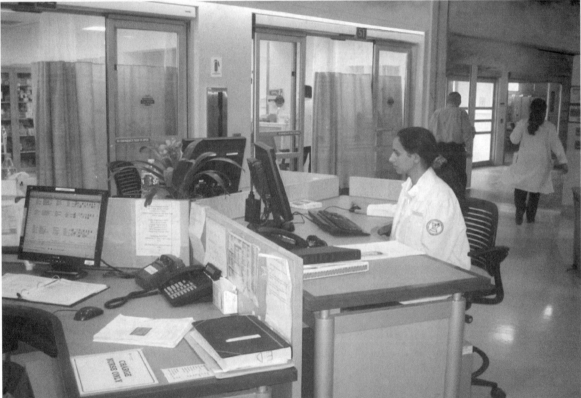

Figure 6–1. (F) Easy access to patient care areas in the ED; (G) Station 4659 used by the pharmacist for prospective review of medication orders and for active surveillance of resuscitation rooms.

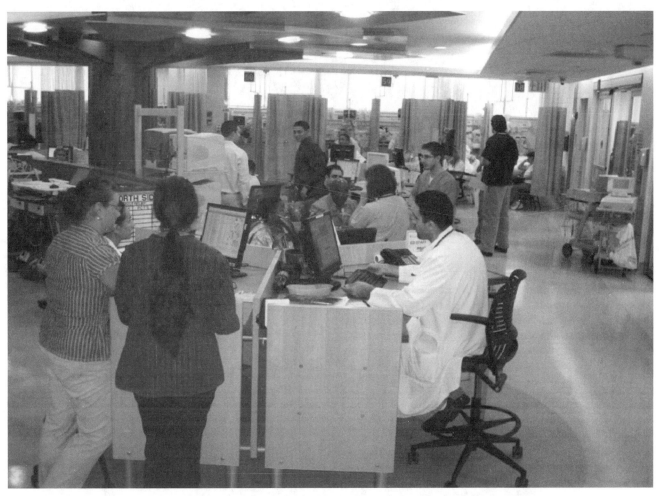

Figure 6–1. (H) Station 4659 enables interaction and surveillance of the new ED.

The Department of Emergency Medicine at Maimonides is busiest during the hours of 11 AM through 2 AM.

ROLE OF ACADEMIC-BASED ED CLINICAL PHARMACIST

Clinical pharmacy services were offered to the Department of Emergency Medicine by the Pharmaceutical Department at Maimonides Medical Center through an affiliation with the Arnold & Marie Schwartz College of Pharmacy & Health Sciences, Long Island University in July of 1998. Since the Department of Emergency Medicine supports a medical residency program, and a training program for Fiorello H. La Guardia Community College paramedic program, a clinical pharmacist specializing in emergency medicine seemed mutually beneficial. The ED would be used as a pharmacy practice-training site for entry level PharmD students. Ideal medication management within the ED had been a continued problem, overuse was well documented, and medication errors were not uncommon; therefore, the opportunity to improve these quality issues was mutually beneficial to the pharmacy department and the emergency department.

While present in the ED, the pharmacist provides a dual role that includes traditional and contemporary practice of pharmaceutical care.[1] The EDP specializes in acute stabilization of the urgent and emergent care pharmacotherapy to patients while also providing a generalist role with the goal of optimizing pharmaceutical care.

SUB-SPECIALIST IN EMERGENCY MEDICINE

Training and Education

The EDP is a post baccalaureate PharmD who completed two residencies, a pharmacy practice residency and a specialized residency in emergency medicine/toxicology. The EDP has been cross-trained to do resuscitative basic life support and common healthcare related procedures, i.e., phlebotomy, ECG, placing a patient on a cardiac monitor, assisting with intubation, and responding to trauma codes. These procedures are all important for the team approach to acute stabilization of the patient.

Certifications

The EDP is certified in Basic Life Support, Advanced Cardiac Life Support, Pediatric Advanced Life Support, and Advanced Hazardous Materials Life Support. The EDP

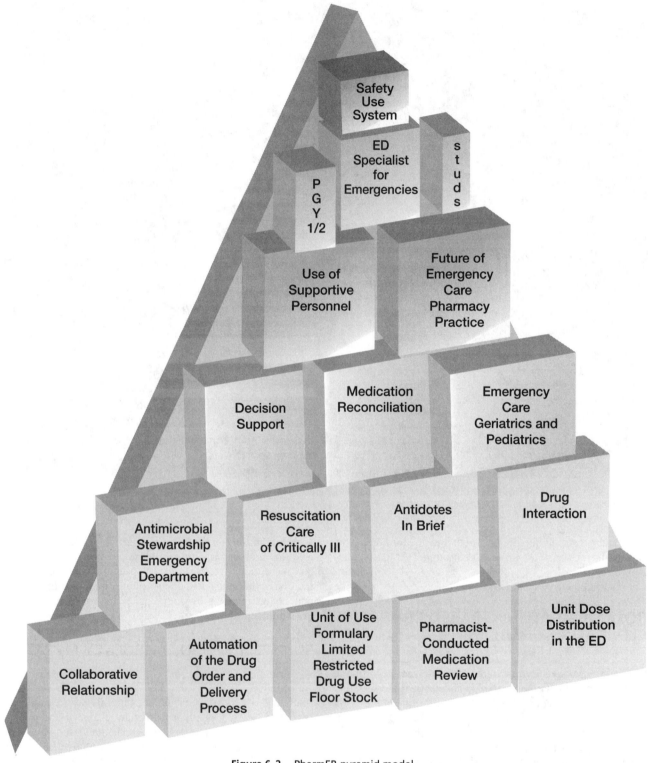

Figure 6–2. PharmER pyramid model.

is also a Certified Medical Investigator, important for detecting drug injury and providing expert testimony. Although these credentials attest to the ability to provide immediate life saving emergency care, they do not guarantee that the pharmacist will have the motivation or courage to participate meaningfully during a medical emergency. Furthermore, to become an authority is this area, pharmacist presence in the ED during the medical emergency is paramount.

Resuscitative Care

As described by Schwerman et al. in the 1970s, the involvement of a pharmacist during cardiac arrest permits the physician to focus on the diagnosis and immediate treatments, while the pharmacist focuses on the preparation and appropriateness of dosing of therapy needed. This collaborative team-oriented approach results in a high rate of success.[2]

At MMC, the EDP is a member of the Advanced Cardiac Life Support, the Disaster HazMat Decontamination, and Stroke Team and is a specialist in acute stabilization and resuscitation measures. Additionally, the EDP provides bedside consultation to assess for any potential drug-induced etiology associated with the clinical presentation.[3]

The EDP provides a rapid-approach, upon-anticipation, at the bedside pharmacotherapy consultation to support the medical staff procedures during stabilization of the patient. It is the proactive method that makes prospective review of medication orders unnecessary as medication regimens are recommended and facilitated by the responding emergency care pharmacist.

During a resuscitative event, the EDP monitors for life-threatening dysrhythmias and recommends immediate action and intervention. The EDP documents medications administered during a cardiac arrest. It is also not uncommon that the EDP, depending on the personnel available, may support the clinicians with procedures such as intubations, phlebotomy, and other nontraditional roles, such as manually ventilating a patient until he or she is placed on a respirator by the respiratory therapists.

Distinctively, the board-certified pharmacotherapist with a specialty in emergency medicine (EM pharmacotherapist) understands the uniqueness of the emergency medicine physician specialty and can relate to his or her needs. The EM pharmacotherapy specialist masters the symptoms associated with can't-miss diagnosis that emergency physicians are trained to rule out and masters the pharmacotherapy required for acute stabilization of these emergent conditions. The EM pharmacotherapist adds cognitive algorithmically based pharmacotherapeutic recommendations to assure safe but effective management of patients with multiple comorbid diseases states. The EM pharmacotherapist also distinguishes the importance of contraindications and precautions that in most cases would prevent the use of the drug therapy, but in the ED the intense monitoring and the risk-to-benefit consideration would permit its use.

PHARM-ER PYRAMID

The PharmER pyramid, as seen in Figure 6-2, is a leadership and management tool proposed to assist those interested in establishing clinical pharmacy services in the ED. The PharmER pyramid offers a stepwise approach to establishing a safe medication use system. The PharmER pyramid provides the structural elements for the pharmacist to imple-

ment in the ED; processes can be developed and measured and outcomes evaluated. As a whole, the pyramid is organized into services, which in turn, are divided into discrete subunits called "rubrics." Providing clinical pharmacy services to the ED entails making our way through each consecutive rubric. Each rubric differs in structure and process, intensity, and risk. Within each rubric are the tools the pharmacotherapist employs to assure safe and effective use of medications in the ED.

Based on a decade of service, we developed this model, the PharmER pyramid, for safe medication use (Fig. 6-2). The PharmER pyramid describes the elements of a safe medication use system within an emergency department. It illustrates steps needed to initiate a clinical pharmacy service in the ED that facilitates implementation of a safe medication use system within the ED. The PharmER pyramid is an emergency care pharmacotherapy multidisciplinary system that has developed processes to safeguard against medication errors, while assuring high quality pharmaceutical care and has enabled the pharmacist to remain an essential member of the medical emergency team.

Part II-IV includes a description of the PharmER pyramid model and its building blocks or steps that will help those that are challenged to comply with medication management standards. In addition, the PharmER pyramid will guide those interested in the emergency care setting to establish a sustainable academic-based ED clinical pharmacy service.

SUMMARY

To ensure safe medication use, day-to-day team surveillance of medication orders is needed to avert medication errors. At Maimonides Medical Center, we use the PharmER Pyramid model to safely manage emergency care pharmacotherapy needs. Through the integration of automation, clinical pharmacy, management, and the strong multidisciplinary team, including nursing, medicine, and information technology, a safe medication use process in the ED can lead to a system of quality healthcare.

References

1. Cohen V. Advance clinical pharmacy services: The emergency department pharmacists. In O'Donnel J, ed. *Drug Injury Liability and Analysis, 6th Edition.* Lawyers & Judges, 2004.
2. Schwerman E. The pharmacist as a member of the cardiopulmonary resuscitation team. *Drug Intell Clin Pharm* 1973; 7:299–308.
3. Ludwig DJ, Abramowitz PW. The pharmacist as a member of the CPR team: Evaluation by other healthcare professionals. *Drug Intell Clin Pharm* 1983;17:463–465.

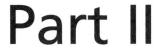

Part II

Anatomy of a Safe Medication Use System: Operational Considerations

In Part II, we continue to define the elements of a safe medication use system. However, in this section, we also provide in detail the "how to" of implementing clinical operations that have been sustainable in ensuring quality healthcare in the ED as it pertains to a safe drug ordering and delivery process.

7

Defining a Safe Medication Use System in the Emergency Department

Systems thinking is a discipline for seeing wholes. It is a framework for seeing interrelationships rather than things, for seeing patterns of change rather than static "snapshots." It is a set of general principles—distilled over the course of the twentieth century, spanning fields as diverse as the physical and social sciences, engineering, and management.... During the last thirty years, these tools have been applied to understand a wide range of corporate, urban, regional, economic, political, ecological, and even psychological systems. And systems thinking is a sensibility— for the subtle interconnectedness that gives living systems their unique character.

—Peter Senge

Objectives
- Introduce elements of the PharmER Pyramid model
- List the components of a safe medication use system in the ED
- Review how to define, characterize, ensure, and sustain safe medication systems in the ED

PHARMER PYRAMID MODEL

Over the past decade we have been constructing the building blocks to a safe medication use system in the ED. A safe medication use system can be defined and characterized using the PharmER pyramid, as depicted in Chapter 6 (see Fig. 6.2).

The PharmER pyramid includes multiple steps and blocks synonymous with building the foundation; it is a model that uses active surveillance by a pharmacist who triages and prioritizes optimization of care as it pertains to a whole system for use of pharmacotherapy in the ED. This model assures that the pharmacist is facilitating and assuring safety with emergency care, not creating unnecessary barriers to emergency care.

The PharmER pyramid acts to fill the day-to-day gaps within our traditional defenses against medication errors to assure a safe environment, as it pertains to medication use and improved quality. The PharmER pyramid fills the gaps in the Swiss cheese model of adverse outcomes. As depicted in Figure 7-1, gaps in defenses of safe medication use system exist. When gaps in defenses align, as seen in Figure 7-2, adverse outcomes occur and medical injury results. Active surveillance and implementation of the PharmER pyramid fills the gaps that arise in the safeguards used against medication errors, which are associated with the speed-over-accuracy trade off of the ED, as depicted in Figure 7-3.[1]

The PharmER pyramid is a response to the five stages of drug ordering and delivery. The five stages include prescribing, transcribing, dispensing, administration, and monitoring (Fig. 7-4). The PharmER pyramid strengthens each link of the chain so that when weaknesses arise they are detected and prevented.

The pyramid shape forms the backbone where each block (elements of emergency medicine pharmacy) sits. The pyramid shape represents the leadership and advocacy needed from pharmacy to remove barriers associated with creating safeguards to error in the emergency department. As Lucinda Maine, wrote "the time is right for pharmacy leadership" as

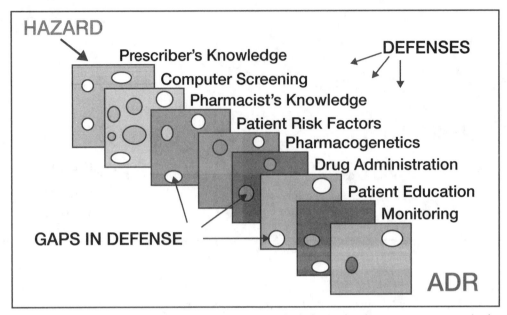

Figure 7–1. Swiss cheese model of adverse outcomes. The holes in the cheese represent gaps in the defenses.

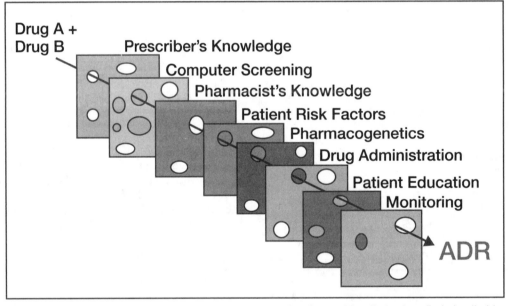

Figure 7–2. Swiss cheese model of adverse outcomes: each safeguard has limitations (holes) called latent failures. When holes line up, adverse drug events occur. ADR = adverse drug reaction.

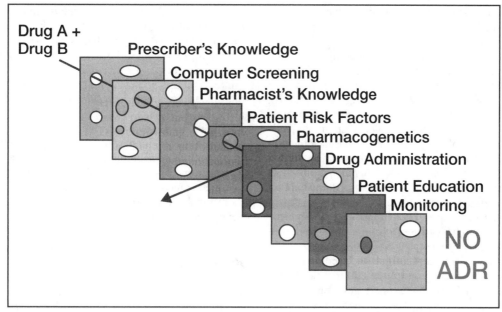

Figure 7–3. Swiss cheese model of adverse outcomes. PharmER Pyramid implemented, and an adverse event is avoided.

she referred to the Institute of Medicine (IOM) report on quality and safety in healthcare.[2] Maine also warned that if pharmacy as a profession does not step forward to lead needed changes to improve the medication use, someone else will. Establishing a clinical pharmacy service in the emergency department requires courage, leadership, and advocacy, and it's time has come.

The PharmER pyramid is composed of five rows, with each row building on the other leading to the apex of the pyramid, which represents the outcome of a safe medication use system.

The initial row is designed to support the pharmacy navigate the establishment of clinical pharmacy services within the ED. Each block in the row builds the framework and leads to the ultimate outcome of establishing a safe medication use system, which is customized for the unique and specific ED. This book is presented in a manner to permit the pharmacists interested in initiating pharmacy services in the ED a step-by-step process to laying the foundation for a sustainable clinical pharmacy service.

Part II of this textbook represents the first row of the pyramid. These chapters will assist clinical pharmacists in establishing the foundation of a clinical pharmacy service. If each element of the pyramid is implemented, it is likely to assure best practices for a safe medication use system within the ED. For example, in chapter 8 we describe methods for developing a collaborative relationship with emergency staff including medicine and nursing, while chapter 9 describes how to implement information technology to facilitate pharmaceutical care. Chapter 10 describes a customized unit of medication use formulary and unit dose distribution for the ED, and in Chapter 11, we describe current controversies with prospective review of medication orders in the ED and our approach.

The second and third rows of the PharmER pyramid (reviewed in Part III) will assure quality of pharmacotherapy within the emergency department. For example, Chapter 12 describes the implementation of antimicrobial stewardship in the ED that facilitated achieving pay-for-performance initiatives, continuity of care while avoiding overuse. In

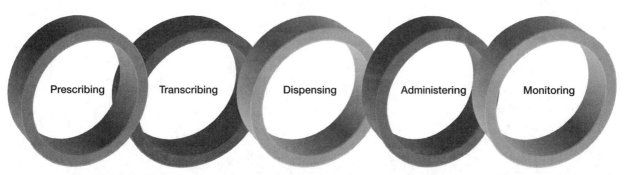

Figure 7–4. Five stages of drug ordering and delivery process expressed as links in a chain.

chapter 13, we describe the clinical significance of drug interactions in the ED. In Chapter 14, we discuss the use of antidotes in brief and the role of pharmacotherapist in implementing optimal antidotes and responding to public health emergencies. Chapter 15 describes what to expect during the emergency care of the critically ill patient and provides critical care tools to expedite care. In chapter 16, we describe the role of the ED clinical pharmacy services in informatics to building a decision support system that facilitates implementation of emergency care pharmacotherapy protocols and instructs on procuring, administering, and dispensing critical care drug therapy. Our approach to hospital-wide reconciliation and the role of targeted medication reconciliation to assure safety and quality within the ED setting are reviewed in Chapter 17. Chapter 18 describes the emergency department consideration of the geriatric, pediatric, and obstetric patient and the EDP role.

Clinical pharmacy services navigate the medication use system and give it direction and mobility. In chapter 19, we describe the PGY1 and PGY2 pharmacy practice residents and their role in the day-to-day operations of each stage of the drug order and delivery process.[3] Their roles and their activities will be described, and the academic-based clinical pharmacy services role in fostering this involvement will be reviewed. In chapter 20, we describe an emergency medicine pharmacy intern practice model to foster postgraduate training in emergency care pharmacotherapy. In chapter 21, we describe the role of board-certified pharmacy technicians who facilitate clinical pharmacy services in the ED.[4] The PharmER Pyramid will perpetually adjusts itself to assure safety and quality of emergency care pharmacotherapy.

In chapter 22, the frontiers chapter in emergency medicine clinical pharmacy services will be proposed, such as the future of ED clinical pharmacy services including establishing emergency department based medication therapy management services, obtaining reimbursement for clinical pharmacy services in the ED, and establishing a pharmacy-based immunization delivery and other wellness activities.

The PharmER pyramid model provides a primer to those seeking a career in areas of emergency medicine and is not meant to be all encompassing to the practice of emergency care. Ultimately, this textbook provides those interested in emergency medicine pharmacy with the tools that will help them break down barriers to quality of care in the emergency department.

References

1. Horn JR, Hansten PD. Sources of Error in Drug Interactions: The Swiss Cheese Model. Pharmacy Times. 2004 March; http://www.pharmacytimes.com/issues/articles/2004–03_1029.asp accessed 10.2007
2. Maine LL. Finding leaders among us. In Boyel CJ, Beadsley RS, Holdford DA, eds. *Leadership and Advocacy for Pharmacy*. American Pharmacists Association 2007;15–26.
3. The 2005 Model of Clinical Practice in Emergency Medicine http://www.abem.org/public/_Rainbow/Documents/2005%20Model%20-%20Final.doc. Accessed in October, 2007.
4. Purcell K. How to develop, implement, coordinate and monitor an introductory or advanced internship program. In Cuellar LM, Ginsburg DB, eds. *Preceptor's Handbook for Pharmacists*. Bethesda, MD: ASHP, 2005.

8

Establishing Relationships in the Emergency Department: A Pharmacy Leadership and Advocacy Role

I am a man of fixed and unbending principles, the first of which is to be flexible at all times.

Everett Dirksen

Objectives
- Stress the importance of TEAM
- Review the management and leadership concept of Sharpen the Saw and its relationship to ED pharmacy services
- Review management tools
- Discuss multidisciplinary approach to system change
- Review how to establish win-win relationships
- Describe how to establish clinical and administrative presence in the ED

THE IMPORTANCE OF "TEAM"

Lucinda Maine writes that the phrase "TEAM stands for Together Everyone Achieves More." This rings true when it comes to establishing pharmacy services in the ED.[1] The clinical pharmacist must be prepared to participate in multidisciplinary team activities to improve ED services that include both medication and non-medication issues. The benefit of this participation is establishing a pharmacy presence, demonstrating that the pharmacist is a team player, and that the pharmacist has value as an administrator for emergency care.

Administratively, the EDP must be skilled in developing independent collaborative relationships between nursing and medical administrators of the ED while not losing sight of the service of the pharmacy department. The team approach will favor quality of care provided to the patients. As the EDP is the patient's most important advocate, the patient is the EDP's most important customer.

SHARPEN THE SAW: LEADERSHIP AND PEAK PERFORMANCE

It is essential for a pharmacist initiating clinical pharmacy services in the ED to avoid being overly aggressive; pharmaceutical care or pharmacotherapeutic principles do not need to be implemented immediately. Instead observe the emergency department, its needs, the operational gaps, and the available infrastructure. Management tools help identify areas in need of quality improvement and will be described.

Sharpen the Saw[4] is a life management skill that requires a person to consider their own physical, mental, spiritual, emotional, and social goals before career obligations, on a weekly basis, to assure that you are achieving a quality of life for yourself. If you "sharpen the saw," it assures peak performance when helping others. As this concept is applied to establishing ED pharmacy services, you must strike a balance between your career goals with the needs of the department. Avoid overcommitting yourself. Creating a balance between career goals and the service you can provide is essential.

MANAGEMENT TOOLS

Early in the establishment of the clinical pharmacy service, we conducted a detailed system analysis of the current drug order and delivery process and the degree of pharmacy oversight and incorporated safeguards. We created a

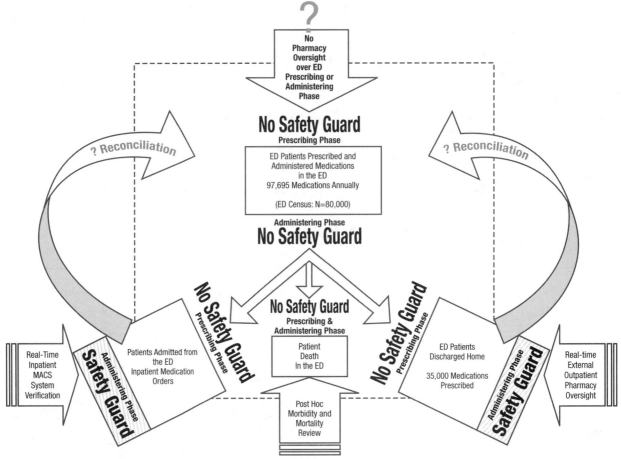

Figure 8–1. Conceptual model of the gaps in pharmacy oversight of Emergency Department medication use.

conceptual model of all areas in which pharmacotherapy is ordered and delivered in the ED (Fig. 8-1) and identified areas where there were no safety guards. This depiction assisted in rationalizing and justifying the need for pharmacy oversight.

We then used a modified form of a Failure Mode Effect Analysis (FMEA) to highlight current gaps in good medication use practices. The FMEA illustrated all good medication use practices missing before implementation of an academic-based clinical pharmacy service was appointed to the ED (Fig. 8-2) and highlighted all elements implemented after the appointment of a clinical pharmacy service (Fig. 8-3).

FAILURE MODE EFFECT ANALYSIS

An FMEA is a method that hospitals use to comply with requirements of The Joint Commission and includes at least one proactive risk assessment of a high-risk process each year. FMEA is a step-by-step approach to identify all possible failures in design, manufacturing or assembly process, or product or service. An FMEA has five steps as seen in Table 8-1.

Although not the classic process used in traditional FMEA,[2–3] we chose to analyze those processes associated with exit and entry into the ED where pharmacotherapy may be involved. We identified all **critical steps and processes**

associated with medication use within the emergency department and identified where gaps existed in assuring optimal pharmaceutical care.

There are multiple entries and exist points (**modes**) to which pharmacotherapy is implemented with little to no official pharmacy oversight and review. The risk of error with medication use is estimated at 3%, and 70% of these are due to negligence (**the effect**). Opportunities to implement safeguards (**mitigation strategies**) exist; however, unlike the critical care arena that may have 12–20 beds, an average emergency department contains 50–100 beds and has a diverse mix of patient problems. This makes any process in this area a challenge to implement and manage. Furthermore, variations in acuity from lower acuity to emergent and critical requires unique strategies that may not have been described.

MULTIDISCIPLINARY APPROACH TO SYSTEM CHANGE

The ED clinical pharmacists alone cannot be expected to safeguard all areas of the emergency department against medication error. Systems approach are needed to be

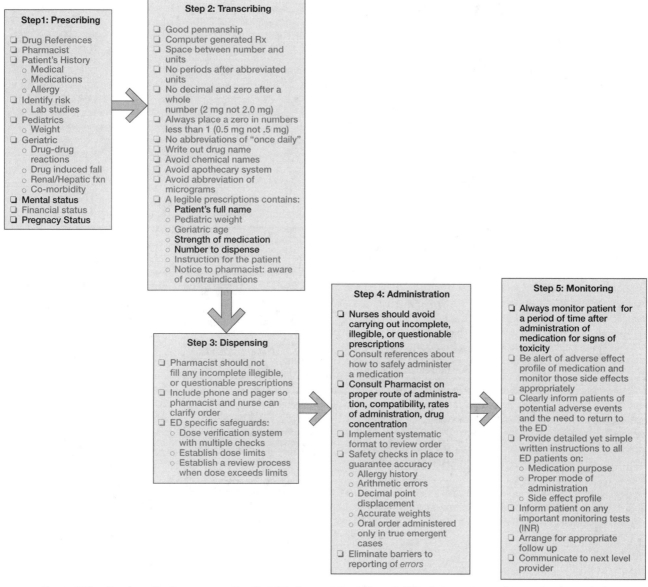

Step1: Prescribing

- ❏ Drug References
- ❏ Pharmacist
- ❏ Patient's History
  - o Medical
  - o Medications
  - o Allergy
- ❏ Identify risk
  - o Lab studies
- ❏ Pediatrics
  - o Weight
- ❏ Geriatric
  - o Drug-drug
    reactions
  - o Drug induced fall
  - o Renal/Hepatic fxn
  - o Co-morbidity
- ❏ **Mental status**
- ❏ Financial status
- ❏ **Pregnacy Status**

Step 2: Transcribing

- ❏ Good penmanship
- ❏ Computer generated Rx
- ❏ Space between number and
  units
- ❏ No periods after abbreviated
  units
- ❏ No decimal and zero after a
  whole
  number (2 mg not 2.0 mg)
- ❏ Always place a zero in numbers
  less than 1 (0.5 mg not .5 mg)
- ❏ No abbreviations of "once daily"
- ❏ Write out drug name
- ❏ Avoid chemical names
- ❏ Avoid apothecary system
- ❏ Avoid abbreviation of
  micrograms
- ❏ A legible prescriptions contains:
  - o **Patient's full name**
  - o Pediatric weight
  - o Geriatric age
  - o **Strength of medication**
  - o **Number to dispense**
  - o Instruction for the patient
  - o Notice to pharmacist: aware
    of contraindications

Step 3: Dispensing

- ❏ Pharmacist should not
  fill any incomplete illegible,
  or questionable prescriptions
- ❏ Include phone and pager so
  pharmacist and nurse can
  clarify order
- ❏ ED specific safeguards:
  - o Dose verification system
    with multiple checks
  - o Establish dose limits
  - o Establish a review process
    when dose exceeds limits

Step 4: Administration

- ❏ **Nurses should avoid
  carrying out incomplete,
  illegible, or questionable
  prescriptions**
- ❏ Consult references about
  how to safely administer
  a medication
- ❏ **Consult Pharmacist on
  proper route of administration, compatibility, rates
  of administration, drug
  concentration**
- ❏ Implement systematic
  format to review order
- ❏ Safety checks in place to
  guarantee accuracy
  - o Allergy history
  - o Arithmetic errors
  - o Decimal point
    displacement
  - o Accurate weights
  - o Oral order administered
    only in true emergent
    cases
- ❏ Eliminate barriers to
  reporting of *errors*

Step 5: Monitoring

- ❏ Always monitor patient for
  a period of time after
  administration of
  medication for signs of
  toxicity
- ❏ Be alert of adverse effect
  profile of medication and
  monitor those side effects
  appropriately
- ❏ Clearly inform patients of
  potential adverse events
  and the need to return to
  the ED
- ❏ Provide detailed yet simple
  written instructions to all
  ED patients on:
  - o Medication purpose
  - o Proper mode of
    administration
  - o Side effect profile
- ❏ Inform patient on any
  important monitoring tests
  (INR)
- ❏ Arrange for appropriate
  follow up
- ❏ Communicate to next level
  provider

Figure 8–2. Good medication use practice (bold) before academic-based clinical pharmacy service was implemented.

implemented with use of existing infrastructures, automation, and skilled personnel to develop a sustainable safe medication use system. Thus, a multidisciplinary effort must be used; the team should include leaders of nursing, medicine, and administration to provide system changes needed to create safeguards against medication errors within the ED.

WIN-WIN RELATIONSHIPS

Stephen Covey[4] in the *Seven Habits of Most Highly Effective People* states that one element to achieving success is to always go into situation with the goal of "win-win." Win-Win is a leadership skill that enables all parties to leave the negotiations feeling as if they won; this creates great partnerships

and credible relationships. Pharmacists who are establishing services must negotiate using the win-win approach.

For example, despite the findings of the FMEA, the clinical pharmacist must be cautious not to overwhelm the ED administration on fixing problems that seem significant from the pharmaceutical care perspective but not a priority of nursing or medicine. It may prove more helpful to establish credibility by supporting nursing or medicine with their process-related problems. Routinely problems of the ED impact processes associated with pharmaceutical care anyway.

ESTABLISHING A CLINICAL AND ADMINISTRATIVE PRESENCE WITH NURSING

Despite the misconceptions that emergency care pharmacy services may irritate the emergency nursing staff or be a

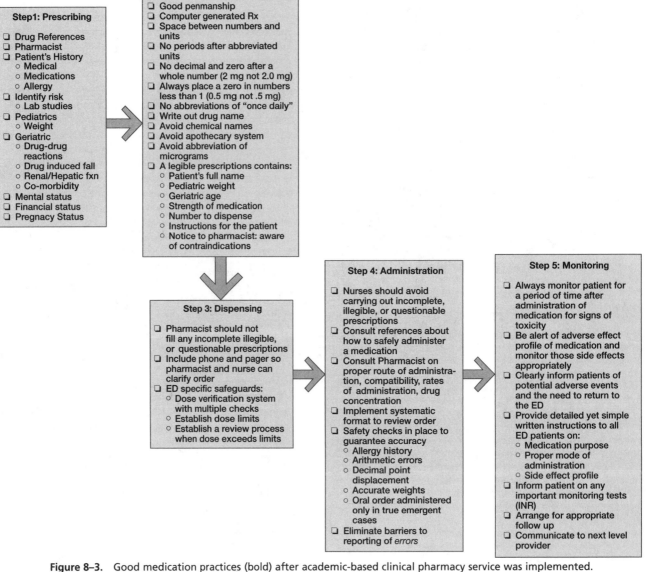

Figure 8–3. Good medication practices (bold) after academic-based clinical pharmacy service was implemented.

TABLE 8-1

Steps in a FMEA

1. Identify the failure **modes** in a process.
2. Establish the risk and consequences of the failure modes called **effects.**
3. Identify potential **mitigation strategies** for the effects.
4. Assess the **success** of mitigating strategies for the effects.
5. Implement modifications to hospital procedures as appropriate.

Adapted from Failure mode and effect analysis: A hands–on guide for healthcare facilities. *Health Devices* 2004;33(7):233–243.

barrier, this is in contrast to published data.[5–8] Elenbaas reported that 13 of 17 nurses who were surveyed responded positively toward the pharmacist as a benefit to patient care, educational activities, and research.[6] Czajka reported that 8 of 9 nurses surveyed about a clinical toxicology consultation program provided by the pharmacist to the ED, that 90% of nurses strongly agreed the pharmacist suggestions improved patient care, information provided was practical, the pharmacist was a benefit to patient care, and this consultation would be requested for a poisoned member of their own family.[7] Most recently, Fairbanks et al. described a web-based survey that was sent to 182 eligible staff members of which 82% returned; 42 were nurses. The investigators used a 5-point Likert scale where 1 represented strongly agree, 2=agree, 3=neutral, 4=disagree, and 5=strongly disagree. Nurses on average strongly agreed that the pharmacist improves quality of care in the ED and that the emergency pharmacist is an integral part of the ED team. They also reported that when the pharmacist is accessible in the ED, he or she is used more as compared to if the nurse has to call pharmacy; the presence of the pharmacist during trauma and codes helps deliver enhanced safe quality care to patients; the emergency pharmacist is a valuable educator; the pharmacist helps select an alternative medication; the emergency pharmacist is useful with consulting on drugs used in pregnancy and regarding toxicology; and the emergency pharmacist helps make decisions on medication based on efficacy. Nurses agreed or were neutral on the following: helpfulness of emergency pharmacist in checking medication orders before they are carried-out, whether the emergency pharmacist should conduct mandatory review of all routine orders for patients less than 1 year of age or weighing less than 10 kg to improve patient safety; whether the emergency pharmacist was helpful in selecting antibiotics; and whether the emergency pharmacist was helpful in making medication decisions based on pricing.[8] This data may be positively biased toward the benefits of the emergency pharmacist as this survey was conducted in a single academic medical center with an emergency pharmacist service. A more national nursing view on benefits of the ED pharmacist is needed. Despite the limitation of the surveys, it does appear that nursing values the ED pharmacist role and presence, and pharmacy appears to provide services helpful to good nursing care within the ED.

Despite the current position of the Emergency Nursing Association on mandatory pharmacist-conducted prospective review of medication orders and MM4.10 standard, in academic medical centers where emergency pharmacists are involved in the ED, nursing values the collaboration.

Clinically, we have observed that nursing will immediately see the benefit of pharmacy involvement because the pharmacist improves speed of acquisition, preparation, and monitoring of medications, acts as a check and balance to avoid risk, provides support when there is a dispute with physicians in management of the patient, and is a resource to important drug information. The pharmacist is an essential team member to nursing in cases of pediatric and adult code support and assures appropriate procurement and titration of complex high-risk medications. In-services and education on operational considerations with medication use, new medications, new indications, and formulary modifications is another area for acceptance and collaboration, and we frequently provide these services on a weekly and monthly basis.

Demonstrating the collaborative relationship of nursing and pharmacy, we developed several activities. Currently, nursing and pharmacy conduct medication management rounds throughout the ED three times weekly. Using a tracer form of elements of performance, the mangers of nursing and pharmacy tour the ED and survey each region for compliance with medication management standards. A tracer form with a listing of elements that must be in compliance is evaluated and documented, and actions for improvements are planned and assigned (Fig. 8-4).

ESTABLISHING A CLINICAL AND ADMINISTRATIVE PRESENCE WITH EPs

Based on survey data, physicians also value the emergency pharmacist role.[5–8] Initially, however, the emergency physi-

cians may be unclear on how to employ or collaborate with the clinical pharmacist, and although the knowledge base of pharmacists differs from that of the emergency physicians, pharmacists' mastery of pharmacotherapy of emergency care and non-emergent yet specialized pharmacotherapy and management of toxicologic emergencies can be incredibly valued and helpful.

It is the ED pharmacist's responsibility to assert during medical emergencies the preferred pharmacotherapeutic options during a medical emergency. He or she must communicate and facilitate that information and action without hesitancy to gain credibility as a clinician among emergency physicians. We illustrate this in the following case study.

■ Case Study

Clinical Presence with Emergency Physicians

Several pulmonary attending, cardiology attending, and an emergency department attending and residents huddled around a cardiology fellow who was experiencing sustained breathing difficulty due to a severe bronchospasm. The 30-year-old cardiology fellow was given continuous bronchodilators such as albuterol, metaproterenol, terbutaline, steroid therapy, such as methylprednisolone, magnesium sulfate, and was on 100% FIO2 without resolution. This happened to be the second day of the ED pharmacist's appointment into the ED; the clinical nurse specialist was providing a tour to the ED pharmacist in the resuscitation room. She pointed out that the patient (our own cardiology fellow) may need to be intubated because he was becoming lethargic and asked for recommendations. The ED pharmacist recommended a loading dose of intravenous aminophylline. Though skeptical because ED use of aminophylline for status asthmaticus has gone out of favor, the ED attending said to do whatever would work. The ED pharmacist initiated an aminophylline loading dose, and within 15–20 minutes, the cardiology fellow appeared to become alert and suggested that he felt that his breathing had become easier. The cardiology fellow was convinced that the aminophylline was temporally related to his improvement. After 12 hours in the intensive care unit resting comfortably without need of mechanical ventilation, the cardiology fellow praised this intervention as the cause for preventing his intubation.

PHARMACIST CAN FACILITATE KNOWLEDGE-TRANSLATION

Another area to establish a win-win relationship with the administration is through knowledge-translation. A pharmacist may play a role in reducing gaps in knowledge-translation. Implementation of new knowledge or guidelines has been reported to be very difficult.[9–11] Translation within a large department takes time because the changes affect the normal routine workflow of the emergency department staff. The gap in knowledge translation may affect care, delay implementation of change, increase risk of non-compliance with standards, and increase risk of error and confusion.

Maimonides Medical Center
Emergency Department
JCAHO Mock Survey

Area: _____   Date: _____

Answer each question Yes, No, or Not Applicable (N/A). Additional comments or actions taken will be documented on the reverse side of this survey.

1. All medications/admixtures are labeled and in date. ☐ Yes ☐ No ☐ N/A

2. Multi-dose vials are stored properly and contain expiration date and initials of nurse that opened the vial ☐ Yes ☐ No ☐ N/A

3. Stock cabinet and/or refrigerator are locked when not in use. ☐ Yes ☐ No ☐ N/A

4. External drugs are stored separately from internal drugs ☐ Yes ☐ No ☐ N/A

5. Stock IV solutions are in date and useable ☐ Yes ☐ No ☐ N/A

6. All medications are secured in medication room or locked cabinet ☐ Yes ☐ No ☐ N/A

7. Medication room door is closed and locked, combination is not readily visible for non-employees to use, and room is free from clutter ☐ Yes ☐ No ☐ N/A

8. Pyxis® machine is clean and uncluttered ☐ Yes ☐ No ☐ N/A

9. Syringes are secured in medication room or cabinet away from patient/family access ☐ Yes ☐ No ☐ N/A

10. Partially used single-dose vials are discarded ☐ Yes ☐ No ☐ N/A

Controlled Substances

11. Narcotic cabinet is locked when not in use or Pyxis® machine is logged off when not in use ☐ Yes ☐ No ☐ N/A

12. Controlled substances are properly labeled and in date. ☐ Yes ☐ No ☐ N/A

13. Schedule II official NYS prescription pads or printer paper are properly secured in narcotic box, Pyxis® machine, or locked printer. ☐ Yes ☐ No ☐ N/A

Food and Refrigerator

14. The medication refrigerator temperature is 4-8 °C (36-46 °F) and daily log is kept with a record of actions taken. ☐ Yes ☐ No ☐ N/A

15. All refrigerators are labeled "Medications only, No Food" and "Not for storage of Explosive Materials" and are clean. ☐ Yes ☐ No ☐ N/A

16. Food or unauthorized drugs are not present with medications in refrigerator or in medication room. ☐ Yes ☐ No ☐ N/A

Emergency and crash cart

17. The emergency medication cart is sealed (lock numbers match), in date, and checked every day for readiness (log documentation. ☐ Yes ☐ No ☐ N/A

18. No unsecured medications are present at patient's bedside ☐ Yes ☐ No ☐ N/A

19. Alteplase (tPA) kits for myocardial infarction are sealed, in date, and secured. ☐ Yes ☐ No ☐ N/A

Actions taken to remedy any items that were checked "No":

_____
_____
_____
_____
_____

Additional comments:

_____
_____
_____
_____
_____
_____

Reviewer: _____   Life Number: _____

Supervisor: _____   Life Number: _____

Figure 8–4. JCAHO mock survey used during nursing-pharmacy medication management rounds.

■ Case Study

Achieving Success with Island Peer Review Organization (IPRO) Guide for CAP

Emergency physicians initially identified a problem with significant delays in antimicrobial acquisition because infectious disease approval was required. The clinical pharmacy service reviewed methods for facilitating and streamlining the use of antimicrobials. The clinical pharmacy service initiated an ED-specific modified antibiotic stewardship that would prevent delays in antimicrobial administration, assure compliance with IPRO and The Joint Commission standards, and assure EPs that antimicrobial therapy was being initiated appropriately. Physician feedback was extremely positive.

Pharmacists became a participant in a multidisciplinary clinical operations team to meet and discuss any medication or pharmacy-related change that required department-wide process modifications. A task list is delegated, and a timeline is established. This enables all parties to brace for changes and assures that changes are seamless, with minimal disruption of ED staff workflow. It also ensures that performance improvement activities are being phased in and achieved. We have observed this collaboration and provide two case studies to demonstrate how we established clinical pharmacy services through facilitating the management of infectious diseases. The first case illustrates how we assisted the ED with antibiotic use and assured their timely acquisition. In the second case study, we illustrate how we implemented prescribing of Tetanus Diphtheria-Acellular Pertussis (Tdap) Adacel as an option for vaccination in the ED based on annual changes of adult vaccination schedules by the CDC due to emerging infectious risks.

■ Case Study

Adacel Vaccine

New CDC recommendations related to the requirement of vaccinating patients for pertussis were presented to the ED pharmacists. The clinical operations team set forth to educate the staff on these changes, develop new order sets on the computerized physician order entry, purchase and store the vaccine, post alerts throughout the ED to assure staff are identifying patients who should receive Tdap in place of just a tetanus booster (DT), instruct on administration, and provide decision support on who should and should not receive it.

PHARMACIST ASSURES COMPLIANCE WITH TJC's NPSG AND MEDICATION MANAGEMENT STANDARDS

The ED pharmacists inevitably take on responsibilities of assuring compliance with multiple Joint Commission standards, National Patient Safety Goals, and CDC recommendations. Through strong partnership, pharmacists facilitate compliance and implementation with these standards.

SUMMARY

In summary, with regulatory standards changing annually and performance improvement activities now an expectation, dialogue for continuous change must be established. Establishing a multidisciplinary team approach helps solve problems of complying with standards and national patient safety goals. Clinical pharmacy services support emergency departments who are already understaffed and overwhelmed to adjust to the continuous evolution to optimal emergency care.

The clinical pharmacist, using these leadership and management tools, is not seen as an intruder on the emergency physicians domain. Support is gained from both nursing and medicine. Economic constraints, however, have precluded the incorporation of ED-based clinical pharmacists, but because of the enormous economic burden associated with adverse drug events, it may be more cost effective to incorporate high-level expertise with an in-house clinical pharmacist. Although potentially cost effective, an in-house clinical pharmacist who is not present in the ED and does not experience the nuances of emergency care may not implement practices that are efficient, feasible, or sustainable. An experienced ED pharmacist is ideal.

References

1. Maine LL. Finding Leaders Among Us. In Boyel CJ, Beadsley RS, Holdford DA, eds. *Leadership and Advocacy for Pharmacy.* American Pharmacist Association, 2007;15–26.
2. No authors listed. Failure mode and effect analysis: A hands-on guide for healthcare facilities. *Health Devices* 2004;33(7): 233–243.
3. Fetcher RJ, Barba JJ. Failure Mode Effect Analysis Applied to the Use of Infusion Pumps. Proceedings of the 26th Annual International Conference of the IEEE EMBS San Francisco, CA, USA. September 1–5, 2004; 3496–3499.
4. Covey S. *The Seven Habits of Highly Effective People.* New York: Simon & Schuster, 1990.
5. Case L, Paparella S. Safety and benefits of a clinical pharmacist in the emergency department. *J Emerg Nursing* 2007; 33:6:564–566.
6. Elenbaas RM, Waeckerle JF, Kendall WK. The clinical pharmacist in emergency medicine. *Am J Hosp Pharm* 1977;34:843–846.
7. Czjaka PA, Skoutakis VA, Wood GC, Autian J. Clinical toxicology consultation by a pharmacist. *Am J Hosp Pharm* 1979; 36(8):1087–89.
8. Fairbanks RJ, Hildebrand JM, Kolstee KE, et al. Medical and nursing staff highly value clinical pharmacist in the emergency department. *Emerg Med J* 2007;24:716–719.
9. Lenfant C. Clinical research to clinical practice: Lost in translation? *N Engl J Med* 2003;349(9): 868–874.
10. Davis D, Evans M, Jadad A, et al. The case for knowledge translation: shortening the journey from evidence to effect. *Br Med J* 2003;327:33–35.
11. Hedges JR. The knowledge translation paradigm: Historical, philosophical, and practice perspectives. *Soc Acad Emerg Med* 2007;14(11):924–927.
12. Peth H Jr. Medication errors in the emergency department: A system approach to minimizing risk. *Emerg Med Clin North Am* 2003;21:141–158.

9

Improving the Drug Order and Delivery Process in the Emergency Department with Information Systems

Objectives

- Discuss the high-risk nature of prescribing and transcribing medication orders in the emergency department (ED)
- Define computerized physicians order entry (CPOE) and clinical decision support systems (CDSS) and their advantages on stages of the medication use process
- Review implementation of CPOE/CDSS and the EDP role and activities
- Discuss integrating pharmaceutical care considerations into the ED-electronic medical records (EMR)

PRESCRIBING AND TRANSCRIBING MEDICATION ORDERS: HIGH RISK IN ED

Seventy-one percent of serious medication errors occur at the prescribing stage of the drug ordering and delivery process,[1] and nearly one in five patients suffers an adverse drug reaction, irrespective of whether a medication error occurred.[2] The two most common factors associated with prescribing errors are lack of knowledge pertaining to the drug prescribed and lack of knowledge regarding the patient for whom the drug is prescribed.[3–4]

A transcribing error can occur when there is a breakdown in communication between the prescriber and the person dispensing or administering the medication. In the ED, this may be caused by a verbal order being misinterpreted or ambiguous or the building of an order in a CPOE system. In an outpatient pharmacy, it may be due to poor penmanship. Transcribing errors constitute a serious breakdown in the system of drug delivery, but they are 100% preventable.[5] Advances in information technology hold great promise in countering the effects of these two important sources for error.

DEFINING CPOE AND CDSS AND THEIR ADVANTAGES TO THE MEDICATION USE PROCESS

Many EDs are transitioning from paper systems to CPOE and CDSS, as federal mandates are now requiring health systems to ensure information systems are available to reduce medication errors.

CPOE is defined as a computer application that allows physicians to electronically enter medication orders.[6] CDSS has been defined as a system designed to aid directly in clinical decision making, in which characteristics of individual patients are used to generate patient-specific assessments or recommendations that are then presented to clinicians for their considerations.[7] A well-designed CPOE system can reduce medication-related errors and potentially and significantly impact the medication delivery system.

Advantages of implementation of CPOE towards a safe medication use system includes reducing adverse events by 55% due to transcribing errors[7] and standardizing care through improved adherence to evidence-based care. In one report, CPOE reduced inappropriate antibiotic use by 11%[8], and in another study, CPOE improved efficiency through increased documentation and communication, which reduced medication turnaround time by 64%.[9] The use of CPOE may also enhance formulary compliance, as in one study in which the preferred H_2 receptors antagonist increased from 15.6% to 81.3%.[10] CPOE can affect the medication workflow, as in one study in which turnaround time was reduced from 64 to 58%, and time spent clarifying orders by a pharmacist was reduced by 33%.[11]

CPOE IS NOT A MAGIC BULLET

Disadvantages of implementation of CPOE, however, have also been described. For example, time spent on verifying and editing orders by pharmacists increased by 13%.[12] Pharmacist workload was also impacted in one study in which pharmacists increased time spent educating prescribers on CPOE by 46%.[12]

CPOE implementation failures have been well documented. Dosing calculators, which simplify dosing, may also introduce new errors with calculations. The net effect of CPOE systems may be that it slows clinicians.

Although CPOE reduces the rate of medication error, an even more significant problem is diagnostic error, which can be exacerbated if physicians are using CPOE and CDSS because this may reduce the time spent with the patient to obtain an adequate history and physical.

Although CPOE/CDSS hold great promise for reducing medication error, streamlining workflow, and ensuring optimal compliance with medication management standards, implementation requires significant multidisciplinary commitment and the EDP may play a significant role.

We describe our Emergency Department Information System (EDIS) multidisciplinary approach to converting from a paper system to an electronic medical record with CPOE and CDSS and the role of the ED clinical pharmacy service in assuring medication management standards would be addressed.

IMPLEMENTATION OF CPOE/CDSS AND CLINICAL PHARMACY SERVICE

KNOW THE CAPACITY OF THE TECHNOLOGY

To assure pharmaceutical care and medication management considerations are integrated within the CPOE/CDSS, the pharmacist must be aware of available technology specific to the ED and which applications are best to integrate pharmaceutical care within the workflow and operation of the current systems. The ED pharmacist must be aware of current limitations of information technology to make appropriate decisions.

Pharmacists who are not computer literate or not interested in integrating automation into their ED practice will not be able to assure medication management to all ED patients. Thus, integrating technologies to facilitate pharmaceutical care is an essential component to developing a

---

TABLE 9-1

Emergency Medicine Documentation Systems

- Allscripts HealthMatics ED
- Cerner Millennium FirstNet
- Eclipsys Sunrise ED Manager
- Mckesson Horizon Emergency Care
- Picis ED Pulsecheck
- Wellsoft EDIS
- MEDHOST EDMS

Adapted from KLAS Enterprises, LLC; accessed from www.KLASresearch.com, March 25, 2008.

---

safe medication use system, and the ED pharmacist must embrace this change.

TYPES OF ED INFORMATION SYSTEMS

There are numerous emergency medicine documentation systems as listed in Table 9-1.

The pharmacist must be familiar with their system and know what to consider to successfully integrate pharmaceutical care infrastructure within the electronic systems.

HOW DO I KNOW WHICH SYSTEM IS BEST FOR THE ED?

An excellent resource to use when the ED is considering a purchase of an electronic information system is the KLAS Enterprise. KLAS was named after the founders Kent Gale, Leonard Black, Adam Gale, and Scott Holbrook, using their first initials of each of the first names, and pronounced "Class." KLAS helps healthcare providers make informed technology decisions by offering accurate, honest, and impartial vendor performance information. KLAS independently monitors vendor performance through the active participation of thousands of healthcare organizations. KLAS uses a stringent *methodology* to ensure all data and ratings are accurate, honest, and impartial. Numerous key questions are asked within the software evaluation and then rated. Indicators are rated by those who have implemented the application and are asked to rate the following questions; was it worth the effort? and did the company do a good job in selling? They are asked to rate the quality of the product, ease of use, system response time, quality of implementation staff, system implementation deadlines, speed of error correction, quality of release of updates, quality of custom work, quality of documentation, ease of implementation and support, technology support integration goals, and how well the 3rd party products work with the vendor product. The ratings are averaged and then depending on the score, a red, yellow, or green indicator is noted in similar manner to consumer reports rating.[13] This data is used to derive an overall performance score and ranking as illustrated in Figure 9-1.

	Rank	Vendor	Performance Score (out of 100)
Overall Performance Scores	1st	Wellsoft	89.8
	2nd	Allscripts	88.7
	3rd	EmpowER	87.5
	4th	Epic	87.4
	5th	T-System	86.3
	6th	MEDHOST	84.0
	7th	Picis	82.5
	Avg	**Emergency Department Average**	**81.1**
	Avg	**KLAS HIT Average**	**80.1**
	8th	Meditech	77.4
	9th	Cerner	73.4
	10th	McKesson	69.7
	11th	Eclipsys	69.2

Figure 9–1.   Primary indicators in full performance report. Courtesy of KLAS Enterprise, LLC. July 2008.

The ED informatics director manages the applications and can help assess whether modifications can be implemented as it pertains to medication management.

FAVORABLE VERSUS UNFAVORABLE ELEMENTS OF TECHNOLOGY

Handler et al. provided recommendations based on an EDIS consensus conference as it pertains to the implementation of CPOE and CDSS.[14–15]

The ED pharmacist must be familiar with these recommendations to understand how decisions are made as to the choice of EDIS. Also these recommendations help the ED pharmacist identify what elements of medication management within the information systems are present and what should be requested before implementation.

INTEGRATING PHARMACEUTICAL CARE CONSIDERATIONS INTO THE ED-EMR

Transitioning from Paper to Electronic Medical Records

We transitioned from a paper-based system to HealthMatics ED (HMED) [Allscripts, Chicago, IL], an information system that offers information management for patient registration, triage, patient tracking, order entry, and clinician documentation and disposition. During this transition to a new EDIS, we incorporated safeguards at the point of prescribing and transcribing to reduce the risk of medication error.

Improving Prescribing by Knowing the Patient

Based on the 2015 ASHP health–system pharmacy initiative that requires pharmacists to use the medication portion of the electronic medical records to manage patient medica-

tions, we requested that the pharmacist be given a location for documentation. Despite the EMR not coming standard with a portion for pharmacy documentation of clinical consultation, we requested and subsequently integrated pharmacy documentation elements to assure information is available for review.

The EDP has a location to enter the patient-specific medication information, including allergies, medication history, renal function, comorbid conditions, potential drug interactions, and any consultation provided to the patient while in the ED. The location within the EMR for pharmacy documentation is seen in Figure 9-2 and a sample of a space for documenting a clinical consult by the pharmacist is also illustrated (Fig. 9-3).

Improving Prescribing by Limiting Drug Use and Improving Access to Prescribing Information

An inadequate knowledge base pertaining to the use of medications has been cited as one of the most common causes of medication prescription errors.[5] The number of medications available on the market has skyrocketed in the past few decades, and it is impossible for physicians, nurses, and pharmacists to master the important details of every drug used in emergency medicine. Furthermore, each year dozens of new drugs are added to physicians' armamentarium, each with its own side effects profile and potential for toxicity. In addition to each drug having its own potential for toxicity, the occurrence of adverse drug interactions when two or more medications are combined can be difficult to predict. This can be especially problematic for geriatric patients who are usually taking two or more concurrent medications before treatment is administered in the ED.[14–16]

To reduce this factor as a cause for prescribing errors, we developed a unit of use formulary for the ED incorporated into the EMR as seen in Figure 9-4.

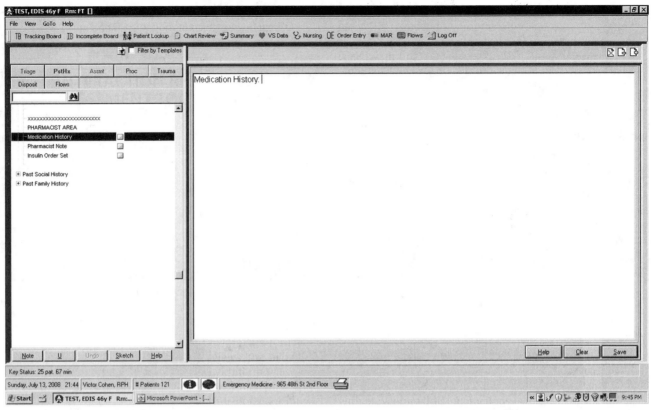

Figure 9–2. EMR portion for documentation of pharmacist-conducted medication history.

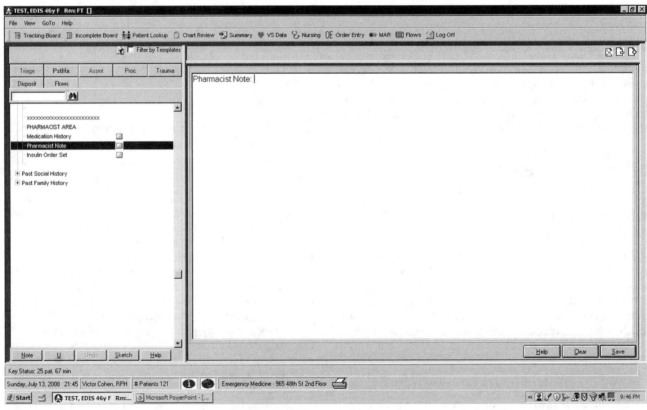

Figure 9–3. Pharmacist consult note.

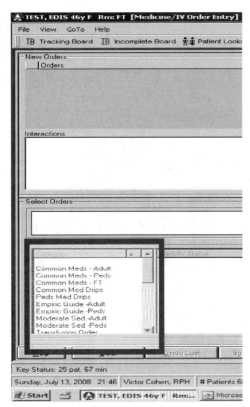

Figure 9–4. Common medication use: unit of use formulary.

During transition from paper to CPOE, the ED clinical pharmacy service was tasked to identify all ED adult and pediatric commonly used medications, intravenous medications, common critical care drips, and discharge prescription lists. These lists were compiled, and their associated doses, available routes, and regimens were listed so elements of the prescription were constructed into preformed orders with monitoring or procurement instructions, as they pertain to the ED. These preformed orders were transformed into electronic orders for the emergency physicians to use when prescribing.

Preformed orders provided clinicians with a one-step selection of the commonly used medication as opposed to a 5–10 step order-building process for each prescription. Preformed orders have been designated "Common Meds," and when selected, the prearranged order occupies the ordering area without any need for the clinician to build the order as illustrated in Figure 9-5.

Furthermore an institutional-specific antimicrobial algorithm has also been incorporated into the CPOE system as a category for selection by the emergency medicine physician. This is an example of CDSS embedded within the CPOE system for improved prescribing. A description of the antimicrobial algorithm and its contents will be reviewed later in this book (see chapter 12).

To improve prescribing knowledge of medications, the institution has also made available a cadre of electronic drug references easily accessible via the hospital intranet to provide real-time research capability.

Despite these resources, emergency physicians may not have the time to research the pharmacotherapy issues; however, these resources become invaluable to ED pharmacists

and facilitate the implementation of evidence-based pharmacotherapy and emergency care in real time.

Implementing Safeguards During the Transcription Stage

The preformed orders also results in a reduced risk of transcription errors and permits the ED to be in compliance with MM3.20 medication management standard that requires that medication orders are written clearly and interpreted or transcribed accurately. The preformed orders prevent inappropriate transcription or misinterpretation of orders and reduce the time required for order entry by the emergency physicians.

Further enhancements were made through the development of preformed order-sets that were incorporated into the CPOE component of the electronic medical record by the information technology specialist. The preformed medication orders were incorporated into order sets to streamline the physicians' workflow and expedite implementation of protocol orders.

The implementation of preformed medication orders expedites identification of transcription error. For example, compare and contrast the difference in appearance of preformed orders in Figure 9-5 to those "built" in Figure 9-6. The errors and omissions are easily detected during pharmacy review of medication orders. Furthermore, there is no instructional support for administration in the "built" orders. This surveillance prompts the need for a brief educational intervention on the use of the technology and what elements should be included in a prescription. Furthermore, this was an opportunity for the ED clinical pharmacist to intercept a faulty medication order. Built orders routinely are inappropriately transcribed, not interpretable by the nurse, or do not conform to current accepted ED formulary and may increase the risk for error (Fig. 9-6).

Implementing Safeguards Facilitates Prospective Review of Medication Orders

Prior to the transitioning from paper to CPOE/CDSS, the ED pharmacist was involved in constant surveillance in real-time of medication orders. Paper-written medication orders were flagged on to medical charts, and the pharmacist would review each flagged order for appropriateness. During transition to the CPOE system, the EDP requested the need to integrate this flagging mechanism into an automated process to alert the EDP that a medication order has been written for a patient. An electronic pill bottle icon was added to the tracking board to alert the pharmacist of emergent and non-emergent medication orders. The EDP surveys the tracking board for medication orders to assure safety and appropriateness. When placing the computer cursor over the pill bottle, the medication orders appear (Fig. 9-7).

The EDP was alerted that inpatient medication orders for boarded patients were prescribed by using a "MACS" icon, which designates the inpatient CPOE system as seen in Figure 9-7.

This EDIS was made available and accessible through the hospital-wide intranet and through virtual project network as seen in Figure 9-8 and thus can be viewed during on-call 24 hours, 7 days a week.

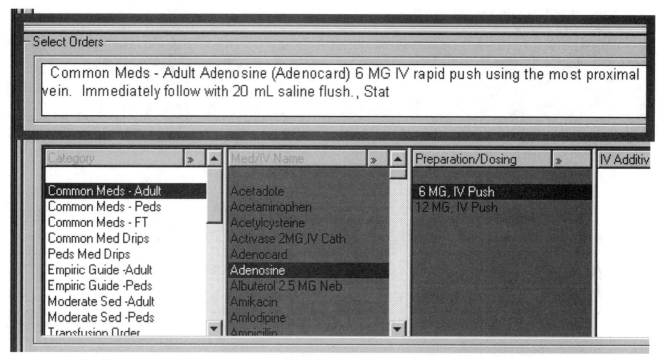

Figure 9–5. Preformed orders.

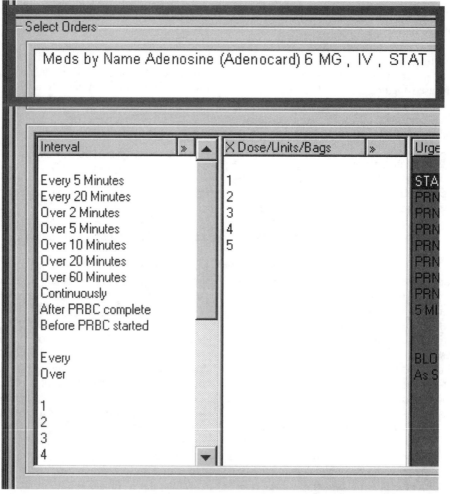

Figure 9–6. Example of a physician order using multiple steps to build the order. Compare with Figure 9-5, a preformed order. Compare and contrast preformed vs. built orders.

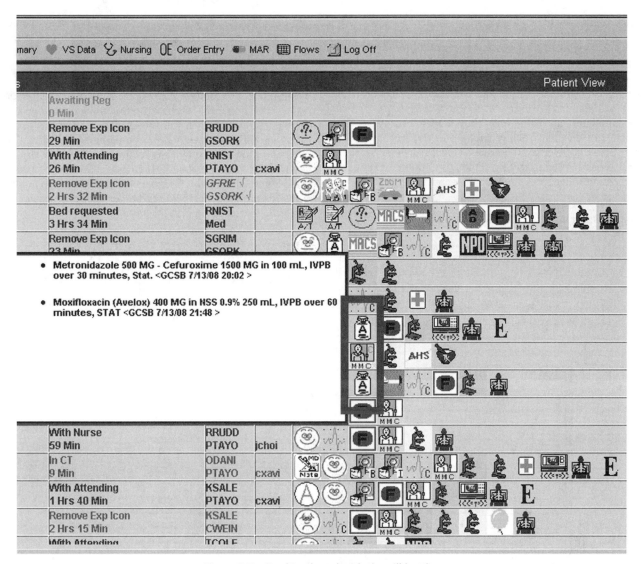

Figure 9-7. Tracking board with the pill bottles.

Figure 9-8. Virtual Project Network (VPN) access into the Institutions Network for on-call surveillance or for use during public health disruptions.

To further facilitate prospective review, we have also created clinical prompts that warn the ED pharmacist that the use of the medication being prescribed has been designated a high-risk medication by the institution. This designation requires enhanced screening of its use; such precautions have been recommended by the Institute of Safe Medication Practices. High alert medications are drugs that bear a heightened risk of causing significant harm when they are used in error. This includes medications such as enoxaparin and various antibiotics that require dose adjustments (Figs. 9-9, 9-10). A double asterisk is used to trigger clinicians to double verify the medication order for appropriateness and safety.

Dispensing and Administering Medications: High-Risk Processes

Dispensing medication is the process of providing the medication to the person who will administer the drug. Among other recommendations, Peth recommends confirming one last time that the patient is not allergic to the medication being dispensed and checking the patient's wristband before dis-

pensing medication.[5] Patients are often moved from one bed to another in the ED, creating the potential that a medication intended for the "patient in Bed A" is given to another unintended patient.

Administration of a drug is the act of physically placing the drug into the body of a patient. Administration errors occur when either the wrong drug is administered, the right drug is administered in the wrong dose or via the wrong route, or with an incompatible co-administered drug. An administration error may also occur when the right drug is given to the "wrong" patient, such as a patient who plans to drive home but is given a narcotic injection.[5] When administration errors occur, they can be very serious, especially when they occur via the IV route.

Implementing Safeguards Improves Dispensing Administration and Monitoring of Drug Therapy

To reduce the risk of error during the administration, dispensing, and even monitoring stages of the medication use

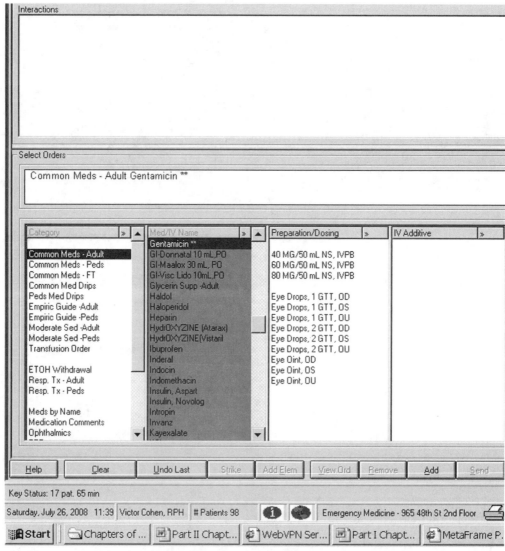

Figure 9-9. High-risk medication identifier seen here with a double asterisk, i.e. gentamicin.

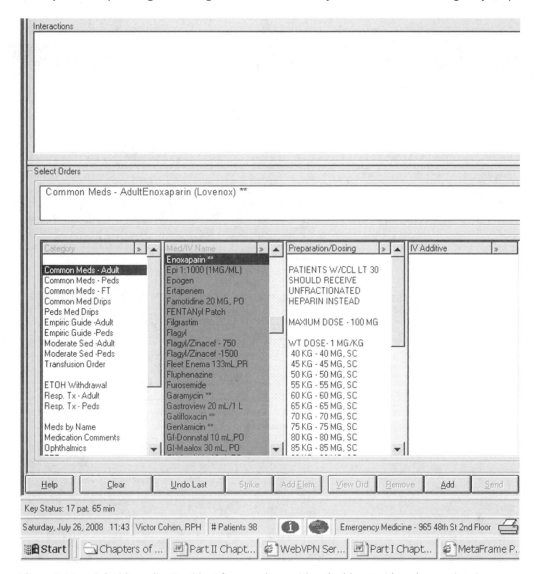

Figure 9-10. High-risk medication identifier seen here with a double asterisk and a warning, i.e. enoxaparin.

process, icons have been included to alert clinicians of "allergies," "pain intensity by using the Wong-Baker pain scale that uses faces to approximate the intensity of pain," and "similar names" to ensure safeguards against error as seen in Figure 9-11.

We have integrated standard dosing concentrations of all intravenous infusion orders with SMART pump technology to assure standardization throughout the hospital. Working with the information technology team, the SMART pump was programmed with dosage concentrations and drip rates, and we created preformed orders that correspond within the ED CPOE system. The list of these commonly used critical care infusions will be described in Chapter 15. An illustration of the pre-formatted critical care infusion order is seen in Figure 9-12.

Note that the order provides instructional support to the nurse for administration and monitoring, which creates a feedback loop as needed to reduce the risk of medication errors.

SUMMARY

In summary, various safeguards have been put into place at the prescribing, transcribing, dispensing, administration and monitoring stages of drug ordering and delivery to preempt any medication-related errors.

As part of the EDIS committee, the ED pharmacist plays a role in the implementation and maintenance of the CPOE system as updates in the drug database, protocols, and preformed orders are frequently required. The ED pharmacist provides to the responsible information technology leader new drug approvals, recent shortages or recalls, identifies the need for additions, deletions, or modifications of medication, and alerts that may need to be applied to specific orders as they are made available.

Automation can facilitate the provision of pharmaceutical care and application of pharmacotherapy principles in

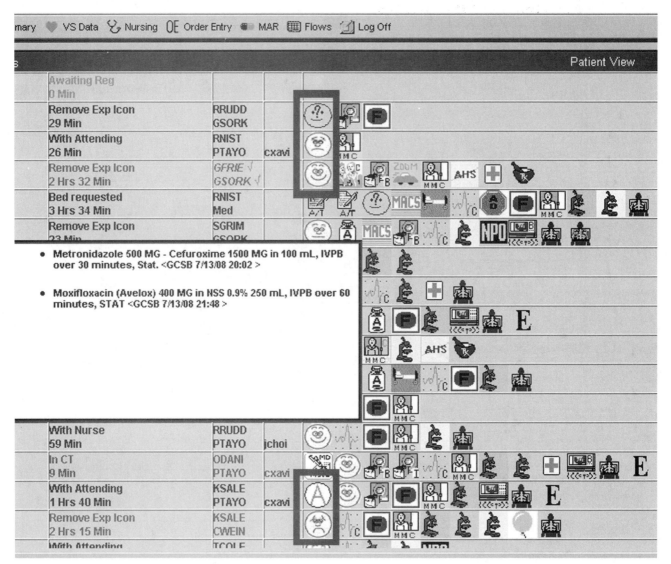

Figure 9-11. Icons to alert clinicians of allergies, pain score, and duplicate name.

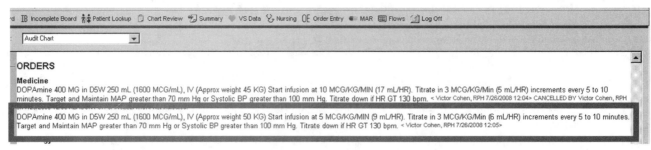

Figure 9-12. Preformed critical care infusion order that corresponds to SMART pump technology to assure standardization.

the ED. Ideally, to ensure a safe medication use system, the ED would be outfitted with a closed-loop electronic prescribing and administration system. A closed–loop system includes automated dispensing, barcode scanning to confirm patient identity, and electronic medication administration records, which has been associated with reducing errors in other inpatient units.[8] Thus more work is still to be done to achieve this standard; however, significant reduction in risk of medication error has been accomplished, and the ED pharmacist has been a catalyst toward this improvement and successful implementation.

References

1. Senst BL, Achusim LE, Genest RP, et al. Practical approach to determining costs and frequency of adverse drug events in health care network. *Am J Health-Syst Pharm* 2001;58: 1126–32.
2. Gandhi TK, Burstin HR, Cook EF, et al. Drug complications in outpatients. *J Gen Intern Med* 2000;15:149–54.
3. Leape LL, Bates DW, Cullen DJ, et al. Systems analysis of adverse drug events. *JAMA* 1995;274:35–43.
4. Lesar TS, Briceland L, Stein DS. Factors related to errors in medication prescribing. *JAMA* 1997;277:312–7.
5. Peth HA Jr. Medication errors in the emergency department: A system approach to minimizing risk. *Emerg Med Clin North Am* 2003;21:141–158.
6. Lai S J, Yokoyama G, Louie C, Lightwood J. Impact of computerized prescriber order entry (CPOE) on clinical pharmacy practice: A hypothesis-generating study. *Hosp Pharm* 2007; 42(10):931–938.
7. Bates DW, Leape LL, Cullen DJ, et al. Effect of computerized physician order entry and a team intervention on prevention of serious medication errors. *JAMA* 1998;280(15):1311–1316.
8. Holroyd BR, Bllard MJ, Graham TAD, Rowe BH. Decision support technology in knowledge translation. *Acad Emerg Med* 2007;14(11):942–948.
9. Samore MH, Bateman K, Alder SC, et al. Clinical decision support and appropriateness of antimicrobial prescribing: A randomized trial. *JAMA* 2005; 294(18):2305–2314.
10. Mekhjian HS, Kumar RR, Kuehn L, et al. Immediate benefits of physician order entry at an academic medical center. *JAMA* 2002;9(5):529–539.
11. Manzo J, Sinnett BS, Ssowski F, et al. Case study: Challenges successes, and lessons learned from implementing cope at two distinct health-systems; implications of cope on pharmacy and the medication se process. *Hosp Pharm* 2005; 40;420–429.
12. Murray MD, Loos B, Tu W, et al. Effects of computer-based prescribing on pharmacists work patterns. *J Am Med Inform Assoc* 1998;5(6):546–553.
13. KLAS Enterprises. Full Performance Report. www.KLASresearch.com. Accessed March 25, 2008.
14. Handler JA, et al. Computerized physician order entry and online decision support. *Acad Emerg Med* 2004;11(11):1135–1141.
15. Handler JA, et al. Emergency medicine information technology consensus conference: Executive summary. *Acad Emerg Med* 2004; 11(11):1112–1113.
16. Beers MH, Storrie M, Lee G. Potential adverse drug interactions in the emergency room: an issue in the quality of care. *Ann Intern Med* 1990;112:61–4.
17. Chan M, Nicklason F, Vial JH. Adverse drug events as a cause of hospital admissions in the elderly. *Intern Med J* 2001;31: 199–205.
18. Schneitman-McIntire O, Farnen TA, Gordon N, et al. Medication misadventures resulting in emergency department visits at an HMO medical center. *Am J Health-Syst Pharm* 1996;53:1416–22.
19. Franklin BD, O'Grady K, Donyai P, et al. The impact of a closed-loop electronic prescribing and administration system on prescribing errors, administration errors, and staff time: A before and after study. *Qual Safe Health Care* 2007;16:279–284.
20. Motov S. Emergency medicine documenting systems. In: *Emergency Medicine 1001.* New York: Xlibris, 2007.
21. Committee on Identifying and Preventing Medication Errors. Preventing Medication Errors: Quality Chasm Series. Washington, DC: National Academy Press, 2006.

10

Emergency Department Unit of Use Formulary and Drug Distribution System

*For the most part, patients are not known and their illnesses
are seen through only small windows of focus and time.*

—*Dr. Patrick Croskerry*

Objectives
- Describe the high-risk nature of the dispensing and administration stages of the medication use process in the ED.
- Discuss how to remove barriers toward restricting formulary and reducing emergency department (ED) drug stock
- Review dispensing in the ED and compare with the "old system"
- Describe how to design an ED unit of use formulary
- Rationalize the need for a unit dose distribution system in the ED

PREVENTING ERRORS DURING DISPENSING AND ADMINISTRATION

The dispensing and administration stages are the absolute last chances to correct or prevent an impending medication error. The wrong drug may be administered when a transcription error occurs, when two drugs with similar sounding names are confused with each other, or when two drugs are packaged alike and the wrong drug is pulled off the shelf.[1] Emergency departments (EDs) without a pharmacy rely on nursing to pull and administer medications, losing an important safeguard of the pharmacist check.

To prevent diversion, dispensing and subsequent administration errors and at the same time assure medications are available during medical emergencies, The Joint Commission

(TJC) standards MM2.10, MM2.20, and MM2.40[2] require that a hospital have defined criteria to create a formulary, that medications are properly and safely stored throughout the hospital, and that a system that identifies the drugs available in response to a medical emergency is in place.

EDs need to strike a balance between achieving the medication management standards of providing easy acquisition of emergent and urgent medications while still assuring safe dispensing, administration, and minimizing drug diversion.

BARRIERS TOWARD RESTRICTING FORMULARY AND REDUCING ED DRUG STOCK

Emergency departments employ many physicians and specialty consultants that may have differing preferences when it comes to pharmacotherapy. Translating a formulary into practice in the ED with high clinician turnover is a challenge. Clinicians will prescribe based on what they are routinely comfortable with. Furthermore, the broad mix of patients and those that may become inpatients may need exotic specialty medications that are difficult to predict. A vast floor stock is a recipe for medication error during dispensing and administration. The ED clinical pharmacist must take the lead toward designing a customized unit of use formulary. Drugs not needed on an emergent or urgent basis should be stocked out of the ED to prevent dispensing and administration errors.[1]

DISPENSING IN THE ED: THE "OLD SYSTEM"

Dispensing in the old system required the ED nurse to execute a handwritten order from the EDP. A floor stock of medications was available in a small self-locking medication room where the nurse would procure the medication. This procedure was used for both boarded and emergency care patients. In the event that the prescription required a medication not on the floor stock list, the nurse would have to transcribe the written physician order onto an interdepartmental prescription order form and send it to central pharmacy by the Translogic pneumatic tube. The centralized pharmacy staff pharmacist would then dispense the medication with no review for appropriateness. Delays in therapy occurred due to inappropriate transcriptions, pharmacy-related delays, and the tube system periodically malfunctioned. Another problem with controlling drug distribution was that any medication on the hospital formulary may have been requested. There were minimal controls, despite a limited floor stock. In fact, the limited floor stock enticed the clinicians to prescribe by preference instead of cost-consciously, which followed the hospital formulary guidelines.

UNIT OF USE FORMULARY: CUSTOMIZATION OF ED DRUG USE

In accord with MM2.10 that states that hospitals should have a defined criterion to create a formulary and with the goal of preventing dispensing and administration errors, we set out to customize the floor stock by creating a unit of use formulary for the ED. Lists of medications were constructed for those required to be stored in the ED for emergency and urgent conditions.

First, we assembled historical data described by Elenbaas et al. for what drug contents should be stored in the ED.[3–5] Nursing and medicine administrators were surveyed as to medications that should be stored in the ED medication room. Lists were generated and compiled by the clinical pharmacy service, and inventory lists with par levels were generated. The EDP then developed ratings for level of acuity of the clinical situation and the required timely administration of the medication as it pertains to a positive outcome benefit (Table 10-1).

Medications such as chemotherapy were given a level 5 rating and restricted from use completely within the ED setting. Nitroglycerin and aspirin were given level 1 ratings because they are required immediately to relieve ischemic pain during an acute coronary syndrome. Level 1 medications were stored in the ED, and levels 2–5 were excluded unless other circumstances required storage within the ED. For all level 1 medications, par lists were created for the central pharmacy to assure that the quantities were available to the ED at all times, inventory was tracked and replenished daily, and that medications being requested were appropriate for use within the scope of ED care.

This exercise allowed us to reduce the ED formulary to what is essential for initial emergency and primary care

TABLE 10-1

Level of Acuity for Medication Use

Acuity Level	Described
1	Clinical situation requires immediate administration to relieve acute pain and suffering.
2	Clinical situation requires timely administration within 1 hour for improved outcomes.
3	Clinical situation requires treatment within 1–4 hours for improved outcomes.
4	Clinical situation requires treatment within 4–6 hours for improved outcomes.
5	There is no time dependency for the use of these medications or these medications are beyond the scope of emergency care and they require approval before use within the ED setting.

management. The ED formulary was reduced to include 50–100 medications as seen in the medication floor stock tables in Appendix B.

The ED clinical pharmacy service is responsible for maintaining the ED unit of use formulary, monitoring and record diversion, pilferage, and inappropriate use.

We collaboratively designed the formulary to avoid any false impression that emergency physicians were being manipulated to prescribe the formulary items. This collaborative approach was enforced by the department's leading physician and nurse and maintained and monitored by the ED clinical pharmacy service.

Conners et al.[6] support this contention and strategy of drug availability and how it may indirectly affect prescribing behaviors. The investigators conducted a retrospective observational study to identify the effects of ED automated medication management systems (AMMS) on physicians' prescribing to determine if the availability and location of the drug affects prescribing frequency. The study found that drugs previously available only from central hospital pharmacy made available in the AMMS in the ED showed large increases in their frequency of prescription. Rates of usage were calculated using orders per month and compared pre and post ED AMMS. Four drug preparations met the study entry criteria including Moxifloxacin 400 mg injection and tablets azithromycin 500-mg injection, and pantoprazole 40-mg injection. Rates of use pre-ED AMMS were 0.5, 0.5, 0.83, and 0.5, and increased post-ED AMMS to 2.0, 3.6, 5.4, and 12.5, respectively. The investigators concluded that adding drugs to an AMMS may influence physician prescribing behaviors.[6]

Restricting availability of commonly used medications in the ED is associated with increased prescribing of unavailable nonformulary items. Expanding, but customizing, the ED floor stock availability is likely to improve formulary compliance.[6]

CPOE ENHANCES COMPLIANCE WITH PRESCRIBING OF FORMULARY ITEMS

Another strategy used to improve compliance with the unit of use formulary was to incorporate these drugs into the common medications tab of the CPOE system as described in Chapter 9. The technology provided a further enhancement in the translation of the agreed formulary into practice.

The clinical pharmacy service maintains the unit of use list and updates it during times of shortage and new drug approvals. Frequent turnover of emergency medical staff makes it difficult to maintain control of the formulary. Emergency physicians frequently request the storage of a medication that they may prefer. The clinical pharmacy service acts as a formulary reviewer to provide feedback of whether the request is justified or if the current unit of use formulary already has an alternate medication that serves the same purpose as the requested medication.

STORAGE OF MEDICATIONS IN THE ED

According to MM2.20, TJC mandates that medications are properly stored throughout the hospital. All controlled substances were originally stored in double-locked cabinets and now are in automated dispensing machines (Pyxis) as seen in Figures 10-1 and 10-2.

Non-narcotic medication floor stock are stored in locked cabinets or Herman-Miller carts inside of push-combination locked medication rooms to accommodate quick access to these urgent, emergent and primary care medications (Figs. 10-3, 10-4, 10-5).

Medications used during resuscitative care are stored in various code carts located in the resuscitation rooms immediately available for use.

AUTOMATED STORAGE AND DISPENSING TECHNOLOGIES

Technology in the workplace is broadly defined as how an organization transforms its inputs into outputs thereby accomplishing its goals.[7] For pharmacy, this process is producing dramatic revolutions in daily processes and procedures.

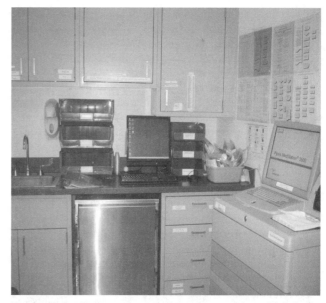

Figure 10–2. Pyxis automated dispensing machine within barcoded security locked entry. Access is given to pharmacy and nursing only.

Various technologies are being introduced to process and distribute medications from point A to point B. The ED is a prime location for implementation of these technologies. Storage of medication in the ED that is devoid of a satellite pharmacy or a clinical pharmacist may require innovative approaches; many have gone to the use of automated dispensing machines.

ED clinical pharmacy services should be familiar with automated dispensing technologies so they can make the best choices as to purchases for each individual ED. Although a complete description of benefits of all technologies is beyond the scope of this chapter, we summarize our and others experience with Pyxis MedStation and Medstation Rx. As seen in Table 10-2, smaller automated systems are available.

Automated storage and dispensing machines provide secure storage of medications. Profiling by patient and physician allows nursing to access the required medica-

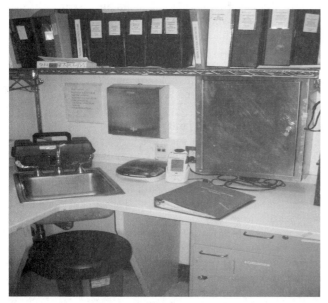

Figure 10–1. Double-locked cabinet within a self-locking medication room. The red binder is the Controlled Drug Substance Abuse record.

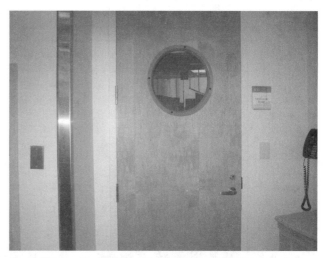

Figure 10–3. Medication room in the new ED. ID bar coded entry, with access given to pharmacy and nursing only.

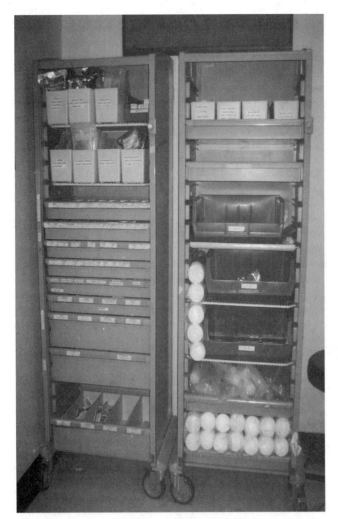

Figure 10–4. Herman-Miller carts within self-locking medication room in the existing ED. Floor stock medications are alphabetically arranged and categorized by dosage form.

tions, and during off-hours when pharmacy may not be available, it provides the ED with the medications immediately. Automated dispensing machines may also enhance drug capture for reimbursement purposes and provide actual use data. Furthermore, it interfaces with the CPOE

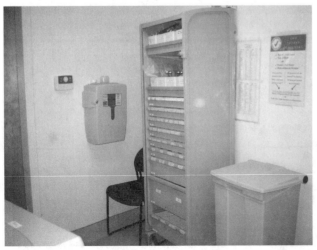

Figure 10–5. Herman-Miller carts within self-locking medication room in the new ED.

TABLE 10-2

Smaller Automated Systems

Argus
Automated 250FD
Automated Pharmacy Station
Baxter ATC-212
Baxter ATC 240
Baxter Sure-Med
Management Systems
Pyxis Medstation and Medstation Rx
ScriptPro, LLC
ScriptPro 200 Vial Filling System
Selectrac-Rx

*Adapted from reference Szeinbach et al.

system so it can be a part of the closed loop system that assures verification of medication orders before accessing by the nurse.

Several disadvantages of the automated dispensing machine exist. For example, the potential loss of pharmacy oversight may occur because an ED nurse can over-ride the system to obtain any medication needed. Pharmacy review is then bypassed. Risk of error exists as medication errors have been reported because of look-a-like and sound-a-like medications, and the nurse selecting the wrong drug vial. Furthermore, there are a significant number of discrepancies that may arise associated with the drug count in each cubby (bin), the access (forefinger print), and this may require a significant amount of time for the pharmacist to reconcile these discrepancies.

Although there is perceived inventory control with automated dispensing machines, nurses can access more than one medication from a bin, despite selecting only one item. This creates problems with par level counts of inventory that need to be reconciled, and this could also be labor intensive. The labor required to maintain the inventory of the automated dispensing machines is significant. Automated dispensing machines require the staff to be constantly educated as needed to assist nursing in its proper use. Also, the ED physician names must be updated frequently due to turnover. The maintenance of an automated dispensing machine can be a full-time job.

UNIT DOSE DISTRIBUTION SYSTEM FOR BOARDED PATIENTS

Although the floor stock system was a tool used to control inventory, ensure compliance with hospital formulary, and check that medications available for emergent conditions were easily accessible, this only supports the emergency medicine patients. Most EDs board patients. We have on average 30–60 boarded patients at any one time, with predominantly an elderly population taking 10–12 medications each. This was a problem that needed a resolution. There are no published reports of a best practice drug delivery process for boarded patients within the ED.

The ED clinical pharmacy services needed to devise a system that provided a safe, efficient, timely, and effective drug distribution system that quickly mobilized distributed and tracked boarded patient medications 24 hours a day, 7 days a week.

To solve this problem, the ED clinical pharmacist led a multidisciplinary team to design a unit dose distribution system for boarded patients as illustrated in the Figure 10-6.

We have designated our boarded patient region in the ED as "KRB1," which happens to be a virtual floor within the inpatient CPOE system and not a real space. In fact, holding patients may be scattered over the existing and new ED.

Drug Ordering

The designated admitting team will see their patient within the ED and enter orders, which then will print in the pharmacy department.

Prospective Verification of Boarded Medication Orders

The staff pharmacist will verify the medication order for therapeutic appropriateness within the CPOE system. Drug labels with required information such as brand and generic name of drug, dose, route, frequency, allergy information, initials of verifying pharmacist or requesting nurse (or if stat medications, the physician's initials), location of the patient, quantity of drug to be dispensed and date of verification of order are printed via the Zebra Z4M+ printers in both the pharmacy and the ED medication room. The pharmacy technician retrieves the drug labels and dispenses a 24-hour drug supply to the ED. The ED nurse retrieves the labels printed in the medication room and places it on a medication administration record and documents when given. This form is subsequently

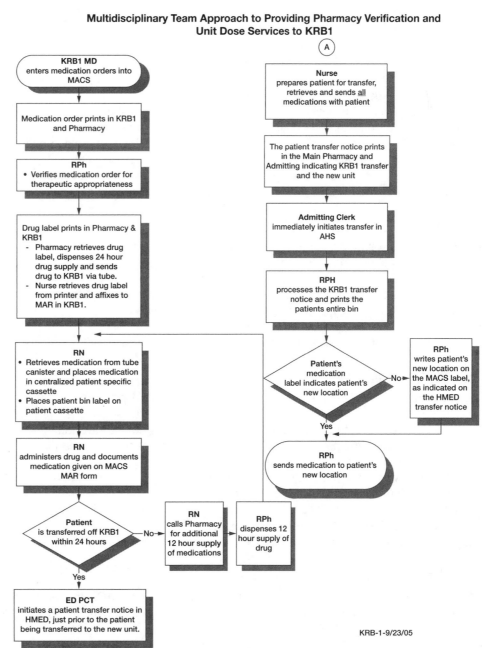

Figure 10–6. ED unit dose distribution system.

Policy for Prospective Review of Medication Orders in the Emergency Department for <u>Boarded Patients</u>

KRB1/2 Background, Policy, and Procedure Statement

Background: Historically the ED nursing staff has requested from pharmacy 1st dose of medications for boarded (KRB1) patients. Delay and ever expanding number of boarded patient have made this process overwhelming, and at risk for medication error.

Policy: To assure safety of medication use and reduce delay in receiving prescribed medications, the pharmacy will provide a 24 hour/7 days a week unit dose dispensing service for KRB1/2 patients boarded in the ED.

Pharmacy Procedures

Medication Order Processing/Computer/Entry

1. Pharmacists as routinely have done by current policy will verify KRB1/2 medication order.
2. Thirty **minutes will be provided** for order verification.

Filling Unit Dose Medication Bags

1. Pharmacy will provide a continuous 24 hour supply of medications for each KRB1/2 patient.
2. At 7:00 am a designated pharmacy technician will print the KRB1 cart fill labels (as routinely done) for KRB1 and KRB2, fill the medication orders to supply sufficient medications until 9:00 am the next day (A 24 hour supply), the pharmacist will check the correctness of the cart-fill.
3. 9:00 am the pharmacy technician will deliver all medications, and place patient specific cassette of medications in one of three alphabetically designated blue bins in the ED.
4. Beyond 9:00 am, the pharmacy will fill continuously a 24 hour medication supply up until 9:00 am the following morning, and sent via the tube system.

Unit Rounds and Deliveries

5. Medications will be delivered via the Translogic tube system continuously.
6. Pharmacy will provide these services 24 hours a day and 7 days a week.
7. During unit dose rounds the pharmacy technician will
   a. Deliver stat medications, new medications, and controlled drugs
   b. Placing the medications directly into the patients bin
   c. Remove the discharged patient medications
8. Pharmacy upon receiving returns will put back into stock all intact unit doses medications.

Nursing Procedures

1. Nursing will administer medication upon delivery to KRB1 patients at 9:00 AM.
2. During the day KRB1 designated nurses will check the Translogic tube system for their patient's medications.
3. Once delivered via the tube, nursing will remove the batch of medication from the canister, and place the medications into the patient specific bag if one exists, or place the bag into the alphabetically designated blue bin of the patients.
4. Upon transfer of the patient, the nurse will attach to the file of the patient all medications and the receiving nurse will sign off on receipt of these items.
5. Upon discharge of the patient from KRB1-the nurse will place all medications from that patient into the bin designated **"Returns"** located in the medication room.
6. Stat dose medications will be transferred from the canister to the designated "stat" bin.

MIS Procedures

1. MIS will transform the current designation of KRB1 unit in MACS to a Nursing-unit. This will permit the technician to run the cart fill once and print the entire units labels, as opposed to printing each patients bin of medications individually.

Figure 10–7. Policy and procedures for ED boarded patient unit dose distribution.

scanned into the automated emergency record and is viewable as a hyperlink.

Boarded Patient Cart Fill, Exchange and Order Verification

As part of the unit dose distribution system, the ED clinical pharmacy service will conduct daily morning 7:30 AM cart fill rounds for all patients in the ED to be delivered by 8:30 AM so the nurses can administer all nine o'clock orders. The ED clinical pharmacy service provides a 24-hour supply of these medications. Concurrently, the ED clinical pharmacy service is verifying all new boarded patient orders until nine o'clock.

Drug Delivery

The ED clinical pharmacy services delivers a 24-hour supply of patient-specific medications for all boarded patients in the ED and places these patient-specific baggies into an alphabetically arranged blue bin labeled "Patient medications" A-G, H-P, R-Z.

After nine o'clock, all new medication orders for boarded patients are verified and processed by the central staff pharmacist and pharmacy technicians and the ED clinical pharmacists serve to assist the verification for complicated orders if more patient-specific information is needed. During the day until 11 PM a 24-hour supply is being delivered by the pharmacy technician to the ED medication room at the designated round times. We call this technician, the pharmacy expeditor. From midnight until the next morning at eight, a 24-hour supply of medications is delivered via the pneumatic tube. Regardless of the time of the day, when a new medication order is placed, the pharmacy will always dispense a supply to last until 8 AM the next morning.

Nursing Administration

The nurse retrieves medications from the blue bins located in the medication room and administers the medication and documents on the medication administration record. The nurse places the remaining drug supply into the designated blue bin for future use. In the event, the patient stays in the ED for longer than 24 hours, an additional supply of 12 hours of medications will be sent to the ED if the patient has a longer than usual stay in the ED. The average length of time boarded in our ED is 7 hours, but can be for as long as 24 hours.

Continuity of Care (Managing Patient Transfers and Discharges)

The ED patient care technician initiates a patient transfer notice before the patient is physically transferred to a new unit. It is the nurse's responsibility to retrieve those medications in the patient medication blue bins and include it as part of the chart for transfer. A patient transfer notice prints in the central pharmacy and admitting department indicating a KRB1 transfer to a new unit. The pharmacist now processes the KRB1 transfer and prints an entire bin of medication labels for that patient. The patient's medication labels indicate a new location; the pharmacist sends the medications to the receiving nursing unit within the hospital.

Besides transfers to other locations within the hospital, transfer may occur within the physical structure of the ED; the nurse will make sure to transfer those medications with the patient and place the medications in the designated patient-specific medication blue bins. The pharmacy expeditor will conduct the usual rounds and make sure that medications have been transferred.

When a patient is treated and released (discharged) form the ED, the nurse will remove the patient's medications from the medication bin and place the medication into the "discharge medication bin" located in the medication room. The nurse will write the letters "DSG" on the label, designating that the patient was discharged. Again, during delivery rounds, the pharmacy expeditor removes all discharged medications and returns them to pharmacy.

Stat Medications and Now Doses

All stat medications are delivered via the tube by pharmacy upon request by the nurse and placed in a designated bin. Usually the EDP expedites the "stat" and "now" doses that may be urgent or emergent.

Policy and Procedure

To assure implementation of this process is sustained and there is commitment from the ED and pharmacy staff, a policy and procedure was written and includes those responsible for ensuring compliance with this process (Fig. 10-7).

SUMMARY

Customizing and standardizing the emergency department formulary and delivery process are essential components to assuring a safe medication use system. Many processes may be needed, and no one strategy works for all EDs. Pharmacists are encouraged to evaluate their own ED setting to analyze what would work best for their organization, based on their ED characteristics. We have provided one strategy.

References

1. Peth HA Jr. Medication errors in the emergency department: A system approach to minimizing risk. *Emerg Med Clin North Am* 2003;21:141–158.
2. Hoying MR. *The Compliance Guide to JCAHO's Medication Management Standards. 2ⁿᵈ Edition.* Massachusetts: HCPro; 2005,
3. Ellenbass RM. The pharmacist in emergency medicine. In Majerus TC, Dasta JF, eds. *Practice of Critical Care Pharmacy.* New York: Aspen, 1985; 219–239.
4. Mar DD, Hanan ZI, Lafontaine R. Improved emergency room medication distribution. *Am J Hosp Pharm* 1978;35(1):70–3.
5. Schiavone JD. Developing a unit of use drug distribution system for the hospital emergency room. *Hosp Pharm* 1981; 16(4): 208–9, 214–15, 219.
6. Conners GP, Hay DP. Emergency department drug orders: Does drug storage location make a difference? *Ann Emerg Med* 2007; 50(4):414–8.
7. West DS, Szeinbach SL, Prescription Technologies: Keeping Pace. *J Am Pharm Assoc* 2002;42(1):21–25.

11

Reviewing Medications for Appropriateness in the Emergency Department

*"It would slow things down and force hospitals to use resources
for something that wasn't necessary."*
"That means something else wouldn't get the resources it needed"

—on JCAHO Standard MM.4.10

Objectives

- Describe the impact of a pharmacist on preventing adverse drug events that rationalizes prospective review
- Evaluate whether prospective review is the correct strategy in the ED by reviewing the barriers associated with this standard
- Describe alternative methods of quantifying the impact of prospective review of medication orders
- Compare alternative PharmER Model to the traditional prospective review of medication orders as a means to improve quality healthcare in the ED
- Review medication order in the ED at Maimonides
- Propose pharmaco-surveillance or pharmacist prospective review

PHARMACIST IMPACT ON PREVENTING ADVERSE DRUG EVENTS

Many studies have shown that pharmacists working in conjunction with other healthcare providers reduces the number of preventable adverse drug events (ADEs).[1-4] Pharmacist participation in hospital rounds in an intensive care unit reduced preventable ADEs by 66–78%.[5-6] Based on this medication safety data (formerly TX.3.5.2, most recently MM.4.10[7]), The Joint Commission (TJC) on Accreditation of Healthcare Organizations standards related to medication use states that all prescription orders should be reviewed for appropriateness by a pharmacist.[8] TJC has attempted to apply a patient safety standard found effective in other set-

tings to the ED. However, this standard was not met kindly by emergency medicine societies and has significant roadblocks to its implementation.

PROSPECTIVE REVIEW: CORRECT STRATEGY IN THE ED?

BARRIERS TO PROSPECTIVE REVIEW: DELAYS IN THERAPY AND PHARMACISTS IN SHORT SUPPLY

The American College of Emergency Physicians (ACEP), American Academy of Emergency Medicine (AAEM), and the Emergency Nursing Association (ENA) were part of an interdisciplinary task force convened by the Joint Commission on this issue. The interdisciplinary task force argued that as originally stated the MM4.10 standard that requires a pharmacist review of all medication orders before their administration in the emergency department would create a barrier to treating patients quickly and efficiently in already stressed emergency department, and this standard ignores the fact that pharmacists are already in short supply.[9]

As a result in January 2007, TJC issued proposed revisions to MM4.10 that clarified the expectation for prospective medication order review by a pharmacist in the emergency department and introduced a requirement for pharmacist retrospective review of medication orders. An interim standard was implemented; this standard stipulates elements of performance for retrospective review within 48 hours and the development of a list of non-urgent medications that could be used without prior pharmacist review. The interim standard mirrored the Center for Medicare and Medicaid Services requirements for prospective order review, and those of the state board of pharmacy.[10–11] However, as quoted by Dr. Weiss from the Joint Commission who stated "that retrospective review did not lessen the burden and would take a huge amount of pharmacist's time, some have estimated that it would take six hours of a pharmacist's day and with the current shortage, this is not currently possible."[9] TJC subsequently suspended the interim standard indefinitely, and the original version of MM4.10 was reinstated.

BARRIER #2: LACK OF EVIDENCE OF PROSPECTIVE REVIEW TO REDUCE ERROR

A letter sent to Dennis O'Leary, current president of the TJC, on behalf of ACEP, ENA, AAEM, stated there was deep concern with the recent reversal of the interim medication standards. They noted that they have not been able to identify, nor has TJC been able to identify, any research that indicates prospective pharmacist review would reduce medication errors in the ED, and that medication administration does not require prospective pharmacist review because the ordering physician is in attendance and has ordered the medication based on his/her assessment of the patient. They also reference the USP database that notes very low rates of medication errors in the ED based on a 5-year review.[12] They contend that ED medications are typically not danger-prone drugs, and that when danger-prone drugs are used, protocols developed by interdisciplinary teams are implemented. They also state that pharmacists typically are and should continue to be available for consultation should it be sought by the emergency physician and/or nurse.

Exceptions to MM4.10

As a result, TJC issued an urgent bulletin notifying hospitals that, until an interdisciplinary task force proposes revisions that will then be field reviewed, liberal interpretations of MM4.10 will apply during survey of the two exceptions provided for compliance to MM4.10.

For example, one exception occurs when a licensed independent practitioner in the emergency department controls the ordering, preparation, and administration of the medication and further loosens the regulations by allowing a registered nurse or other licensed staff with medication administration responsibilities, such as respiratory therapist to process and administer the medicine as long as a physician remains available to provide immediate treatment if the patient has a problem. Furthermore, the MM4.10 standard has been suspended for urgent situations when a delay would harm the patient. This allows the doctor caring for the patient to define "urgent." Dr. Weiss has stated that current modifications to the MM4.10 standard does not deal with all the issues and that the Joint Commission is in the process of putting together a task force to see how pharmacists can be used in the emergency department in a way that improves quality and safety without burdening the system or the physician.

BARRIER #3: DOCTOR-NURSE TEAM ALONE CAN MAKE DECISIONS ON MEDICATIONS

Representatives of ENA and ACEP cited grave concerns that TJC rules would make care slower and potentially more dangerous. Furthermore, they stated that the Joint Commission's insistence on prospective pharmacy review of ED prescriptions was probably unnecessary, especially when a doctor-nurse team was capable of making good decisions about when to give medications. They suggest emergency rooms are so busy that adding anything into the equation can put the system into gridlock. This task force is currently in the process of finding an alternative solution to medication safety and quality.[10]

AMERICAN SOCIETY OF HEALTH-SYSTEM PHARMACISTS STATEMENT ON MM4.10 AND ALTERNATIVE APPROACHES

The American Society of Health-System Pharmacists (ASHP) has agreed with current exceptions of MM4.10; however, they do believe that prospective pharmacist review of ED medication orders is ultimately the best method to ensure that ED patients receive the same level of care as other patients.[11] However, ASHP supports alternative strategies that achieve safe and effective medication use as an acceptable approach as well.[10] Examples of these alternatives include electronic decision support, pharmacy and medical staff committee-developed protocols and treatment algorithms, adjustments to floor stock inventory, mandatory double checks, and standardization of concentrations. More advanced automation, such as barcoding, and adding a pharmacist to the interdisciplinary ED care team have been well received as effective strategies in a growing number of hospitals.[11]

ASHP has recommended that retrospective medication order review be a standard component of the quality improvement plan required by MM8.10 and supports the design of an individualized data collection and quality plan. However, time restrictions have been eliminated, and hospitals may use representative sampling rather than 100% review for large quantities of data. ASHP's guidelines for conducting medication use evaluations should be used when conducting medication use quality improvement.[12]

Few studies have been conducted that report pharmacist outcome benefit as it pertains to reducing preventable ADEs and patient outcomes within the emergency department; however, recent reports provide data on pharmacist interventions in the emergency department and related cost avoidance.

In one study, 2510 interventions were documented in 1042 patients triaged to the resuscitation area of the ED with cost avoidance during the study of $1,029,776 for a 3-month period. The most common activities of the pharmacists included providing drug information, dose recommendations, dosing adjustments, formulary interchange, and suggestions for initial therapies.[13]

We qualitatively described life-saving impact of the pharmacist interventions during active surveillance within the ED during emergency care.[14] However, current data that support prospective review as a medication error prevention strategy in the ED measured in a standard method across multiple hospitals is needed to identify the impact of this strategy in improving patient safety and quality.

It is also worth noting that because diagnostic error is an even greater problem than medication error within the ED setting, conducting prospective review of all medication orders may expose the "elephant in the room." Emergency physicians, because of the complexity of undifferentiated clinical presentations, may make mistakes, as described by the SATO effect (speed over accuracy tradeoff). Because of the acuity of the patient situation, the emergency physician (EP) may correct their mistakes, at the expense of more invasive procedures, overuse of resources, or specialty consultation, which may include a clinical pharmacist during a drug-induced event. Acceptance that EPs make mistakes and that they are not all equally trained or skilled in providing emergency care may remove barriers to safeguards, such as pharmacy-conducted prospective review of medication orders. From a public health perspective, this goal could improve transparency, accountability, and assure safety and quality.

Furthermore, as discussed in the systematic review of pharmacy services, because of the broad mix of patients, varying acuity, and different needs, medication error alone is not an appropriate measure for assessing the impact of the EDP on patient care. An alternative approach would be more appropriate. This alternative approach may include a bundle of safety and quality measures associated with medication management and quality emergency care. We contend that there are more feasible approaches to patient safety than strict all-or-nothing prospective review of orders in the ED to impact patient care, and there should be a threshold level of orders that should be prospectively reviewed.

ALTERNATIVE TO PROSPECTIVE REVIEW: PHARMER MODEL APPROACH

As described in previous chapters, we have implemented the PharmER Model, with multiple safeguards to medication use, to illustrate our approach to medication safety for our ED patients. With these safeguards in place, i.e., limited floor stock, eliminated chemotherapy use, implementation of CPOE/CDSS, implementation of drug interaction check software, preformed order sets, an intranet resource available to clinicians, and safety alerts, we created safeguards that streamline medication order review.

Based on motion studies that we conducted in our ED, on average, excluding acute stabilization where the EDP is present as part of the emergency care team managing pharmacotherapy, the time to initial EP-initiated therapeutic medication order from the time of initial arrival in triage is approximately 81 minutes, with an interquartile range from 53–129 minutes. This amount of time permits the EDP to generate data associated with the patient and the event to conduct a prospective review, thus streamlining this process.

The clinical role of the pharmacist has been described earlier; however, logistically and operationally in conjunction with the safeguards described, the clinical pharmacist fills the gaps where needed and when needed. The EDP responds to medical emergencies, such that medication orders during resuscitation are managed by the pharmacist within the team approach. These orders are proactively selected and verified by the pharmacist and entered into the CPOE system. The experienced clinical pharmacist can make a difference in these critical times and can expedite and facilitate care, in contrast to what has been purported that there may be a delay. Pharmacists trained in responding to medical emergencies are a perfect resource at the bedside to provide reassurance, conduct real-time documentation of order entry, and ensure medication information is optimal for decision making during patient management. As described by Schwerman and Schwartau in the 1970s, the involvement of a pharmacist during cardiac arrest allows for the physician to focus on the diagnosis and immediate treatments needed while the pharmacist focuses on the preparation and appropriateness of dosing of therapy, thus making this a collaborative team-oriented activity that results in a high rate of success.[1]

PROSPECTIVE REVIEW OF MEDICATION ORDER IN THE ED AT MAIMONIDES

Although we had already been providing a form of active surveillance of medication review within the ED, we believed we had to formalize a policy and procedure and ensure a workflow in response to MM4.10. Thus, we conducted several multidisciplinary meetings to identify the current workflow for the medication use process and for prospective review of medication orders by the ED pharmacist team.

Several aspects unique to the emergency department were taken into account that needed to be formally organized and supported: 1) the ED holds boarded patients (patients who remain in the ED from 7–12 hours on average) and who have been admitted to a team in the inpatient setting but remain in the ED; medication orders are entered in the inpatient CPOE system; and 2) the ED inputs medication orders for emergency care situations on a separate electronic medical record system.

It was agreed that the central pharmacy would be responsible for inpatient medication order verification for boarded patients, as part of the unit dose distribution service described previously. Verification of emergency medication orders was the responsibility of the clinical pharmacy team present in the ED. Because the pharmacists respond to emergent care situations, verification is facilitated because they observe first hand what the problem is with the patient. Furthermore, we recommend already prepared on-hand medications for administration by the emergency care team at the bedside or in anticipation of need; thus, verification is in real-time when emergently needed and requires no additional process other than pharmacist participation in the emergent care. Also, the pharmacist may assist and expedite processes such as order entry and code reporting of medications administered during an event. Despite this, many patients seen in the ED have primary care issues that require initial management within the ED and then subsequent follow up in the community. For these patients, prospective medication order review is most beneficial as traditionally conducted.

PHARMACY VERIFICATION IN THE ED

When we transferred from paper to an electronic medical record, it facilitated the review of emergency medication orders, which may be reviewed, clarified, and modified by the pharmacist for safety and quality.

The initial pill bottle that the ED pharmacist surveys while in the ED workstation or at any computer terminal within the ED is shown in Figure 11-1. The ED pharmacist then conducts a prospective review of this order using the seven-step emergency care pharmacotherapy verification form, as illustrated in Figure 11-2.

If a discrepancy or a problem medication order (PMO) is identified, the EP is contacted; and the pharmacists warns the EP about the potential risks and the original order is cancelled as seen in Figure 11-3.

A rationale for the cancellation is requested (Fig. 11-4). The medication order is modified by the ED pharmacist (Fig. 11-5). Once the action is completed, a yellow pill bottle appears on the tracking board with the letter "v" for verified (Fig. 11-6). The cancellation time stamp and entry of the more appropriate order populates several fields in the chart (Fig. 11-7).

A policy and procedure for verification of emergency care medication order was agreed upon (Fig. 11-8).

Since the inception of the requirements for prospective review of pharmacy orders in the ED, we have complied with this standard and now verify all boarded patients' medication orders in the emergency department. However, less emphasis is placed on prospective review of medication orders for emergency patients because the exceptions to MM4.10 have essentially removed the momentum for change. Using elements of the PharmER Model may provide an alternative approach to the traditional all-or-none prospective pharmacy review of medication orders. Pharmaco-surveillance or vigilance should be done by an EDP at all times and while in the ED (Fig. 11-9). This alternative may be more cost effective and permit the pharmacist to engage in other parts of the PharmER Model, as compared to prospective review as a sole responsibility for the pharmacist in the ED.

SUMMARY

Prospective review of medication orders in the ED as traditionally conducted is an important safeguard against medication errors from the prescribing and transcribing stage. Current barriers to acceptance of prospective review have

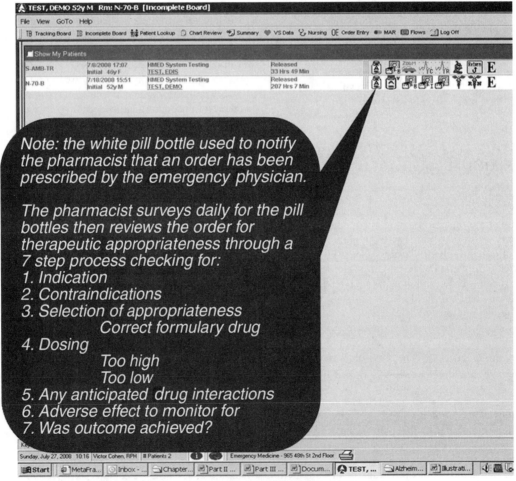

Figure 11–1. The white pill bottle appears and notifies that a medication order is prescribed.

Patient Name   *JJ*   *MR#*   *123456*   *EP*   *Dr. D*   *CC: Chest pain*   *DX: Pending*   *CRCL:Pending*   *Ht 5'6"*   *ABW*   *85 kg*

Medication History Upon Arrival	Taken Within 12 hours of Visit to ED	Patient-Problem Indication	Treatment to be Rendered in ED	Medication Transcribed Correctly	Dose Is optimized	Any Conflict with Active Co-morbid States	DI	Management
Metoprolol	Yes (No)	*Chest Pain*	*Aspirin 81 mg Chewable Po Stat x 1*	(Yes) No	Yes (No) *Change to 162–324 mg*	Yes (No)	Yes (No)	*Cancel initial ASA order Re-enter ASA with correct dose*
Aspirin	Yes (No)			Yes No	Yes No	Yes No	Yes No	
	Yes No			Yes No	Yes No	Yes No	Yes No	
	Yes No			Yes No	Yes No	Yes No	Yes No	
	Yes No			Yes No	Yes No	Yes No	Yes No	
	Yes No			Yes No	Yes No	Yes No	Yes No	
	Yes No			Yes No	Yes No	Yes No	Yes No	

> *Academic Prescription:*   *What is the importance of aspirin dosing during acute chest pain in the ED?*

Figure 11–2.   Seven-step emergency care pharmacotherapy screening form.

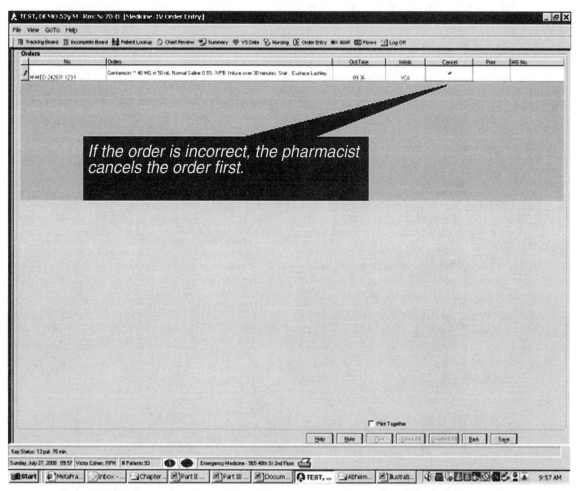

Figure 11–3.   Order entry cancellation through the pharmacy verification pathway.

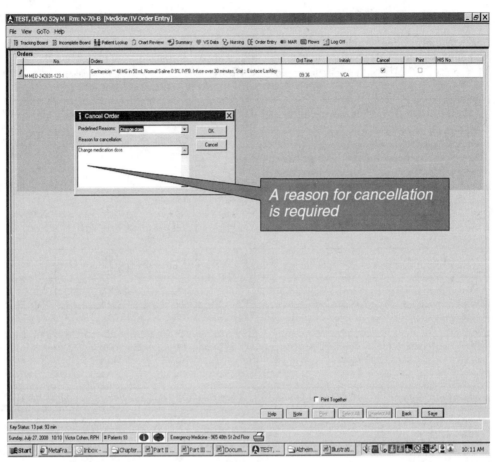

Figure 11–4.   A dialogue box is used to describe why the order is being cancelled.

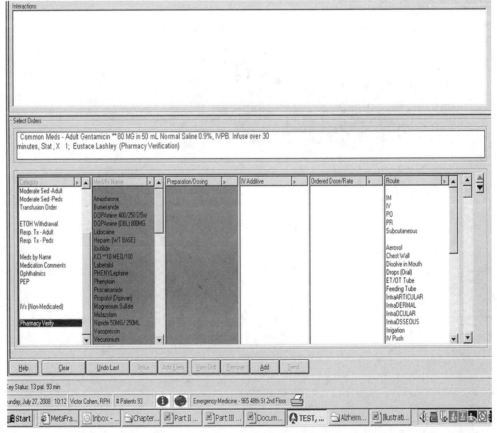

Figure 11–5.   ED pharmacist re-enters the medication order into the EDIS order entry pathway.

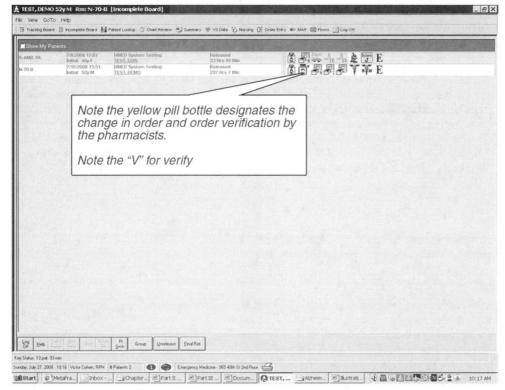

Note the yellow pill bottle designates the change in order and order verification by the pharmacists.

Note the "V" for verify

Figure 11–6. Yellow pill bottle designates a re-entry and verification of the medication order.

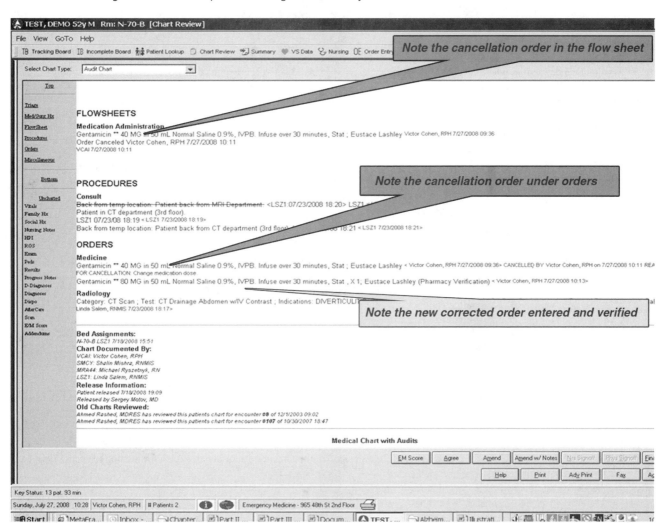

Figure 11–7. Modification documentation on the EMR.

Policy for Prospective Review of Medication Orders in the Emergency Department for Emergency Patients

Background: To comply with the JCAHO's medication management standard MM4.10, requiring all medication orders be reviewed for appropriateness.[1] "A pharmacist must review all medication orders before dispensing a medication, removing it from floor stock, or removing it from an automated storage and distribution device". It further states that, "All concerns, issues, and questions must be clarified with the prescriber before dispensing the medication."

Policy: To achieve the standard MM4.10 a Pharmacist will be stationed in the ED satellite to review all medication orders entered into the electronic medical record (EMR) before dispensing or removed from floor stock or automated dispensing machine. The pharmacist will clarify any issues before dispensing.

Procedures:

Physicians:

1. Emergency physician will enter orders into the EMR as routinely done.
2. Emergency physician will clarify any order in question.

Pharmacist:

1. Pharmacist will verify all medication order entry into the EMR within 15 minutes.
2. Pharmacist will expedite emergent orders and verify them as priority
3. Pharmacist will clarify any issues before dispensing or before nurse is able to remove from automated dispensing machine.
4. Pharmacist will prepare the medication for administration.
5. Pharmacist or designee will deliver medication to the bedside.

Nursing:

1. Nursing will execute order once verified.
2. Nursing will administer medication.
3. Nursing will document medication given.
4. Nursing may override verification if not completed within 15 minutes.
5. Emergent care situations where medication orders that may be received verbally; the nurse may override the pharmacy verification if elect to do so.
6. Any over-rides will be recorded and audited for evaluation.

ER Pharmacy Team:

1. Will meet monthly to review over-rides
2. Identify delays in the process.
3. Reports on compliance with policy
4. Interventions identified
5. Modification to the EMR pharmacy verification system

Satellite Pharmacy Operations:

1. A satellite pharmacy will be available only to the pharmacists to verify medication orders and procure first doses needed.
2. Space will be allotted for this operation.
3. The satellite will be opened only when a pharmacist is present.
4. A locked door will secure the satellite contents and medication inventory.
5. Two dual monitor dell computers will be dedicated for the pharmacist to verify medication orders, equipped with all drug databases search engines, and clinical intervention software
6. A laminar flow hood will be present for procurement of first dose IV medication orders.
7. A refrigerator will be provided for refrigerated medications.
8. Gravity –shelving system will be prepared to store medication inventory.
9. Counter space will be available to package and label medications.

Satellite Hours of Operation:

1. During the initial phase the satellite will be covered from 7am–11PM.
2. During night shift the satellite door remains closed, but the external medication room remains open for nursing to access floor stock or automated dispensing machine medication.
3. Weekends the satellite will be in operation from 7am–7pm.

Figure 11–8. Policy for prospective review of medication orders in the emergency department for emergency patients. *(continued)*

Policy for Prospective Review of Medication Orders in the Emergency Department for Emergency Patients *(continued)*

Pharmacist Coverage:

1. The satellite will be covered by a PGY2 Pharmacist from 7:30 am–3:30 pm Monday through Friday.
2. The satellite will be covered from 3 pm–11pm Monday through Friday by one of four PGY1 or PGY2 pharmacy residents.
3. Pharmacy coverage will be provided from 7am–7pm weekends, and main pharmacy will take over from that time on.
4. Holidays and vacation time will be covered by the main pharmacy.
5. Schedule and hours of operation will be posted outside of the satellite, and any variation will be provided a week in advance.

MIS-HMED:

1. MIS will provide the automated verification pathway.
2. MIS will attend monthly meeting to identify any issues concerning the EMR pharmacy verification pathway.
3. MIS will provide reports of order-entry to verification time and verification time to administration time.
4. MIS will address in a timely fashion any disruption in the verification process.

RESPONSIBILITY:
Pharmacy

1. The Clinical Pharmacy Manager is responsible to supervise and audit process.
2. The Clinical Pharmacy Manager is responsible for scheduling meetings and report findings as pertaining to the process and achievement of goals

Figure 11–8. *(continued)*

Description of Code for Mandatory Prospective Review of Medication Orders

Red	Full 7-step prospective review is required for error prevention, improve quality, cost avoidance, cost savings, prevent over and under use, or continuity of care issues and assurance of outcome achieved
Yellow	Modified pharmacy review for specific issue must be checked and recorded that it has been reviewed, i.e. enoxaprin and renal function. View policy for specific drugs and required parameters to review.
Green	No review is mandated due to urgency of situation, lack of significance of risk, or low cost, however review may occur under the discretion of the pharmacist

Figure 11–9. Pharmaco-vigilance codes for an alternative approach to prospective review of medication orders.

convinced TJC to allow for exceptions to remove the momentum towards an important safeguard. Future research is needed to dispel the contention that prospective review in the ED is too time consuming, potentially dangerous and is not associated with medication error reduction. Alternative strategies as we have suggested may provide a window towards a compromise.

References

1. Kaushul R, Bates DW. The clinical pharmacist's role in preventing adverse drug events. In: *Making Healthcare Safer: A Critical Analysis of Patient Safety Practices.* Rockville, MD: Agency for Healthcare Research and Quality, 2001.
2. Foli HL, Poole RL, Benitz WE, et al. Medication error prevention by clinical pharmacists in two children's hospitals. *Pediatrics* 1987;79;718–722.
3. Scarsi KK, Fotis MA, Noskin GA. Pharmacist participation in medical rounds reduces medication errors. *Am J Health-Syst Pharm* 2002;59:2089–92.
4. Leape LL, Cullen DJ, Clapp MD, et al. Pharmacist participation on physician rounds and adverse drug events in the intensive care unit. *JAMA* 1999;282: 266–270 [erratum, *JAMA* 1999;283:1293].
5. Leape LL, Berwick DM. Five years after to err is human: what have we learned? *JAMA* 2005;293:2384–2390.
6. Lee AJ, Boro MS, Knapp KK, et al. Clinical and economic outcomes of pharmacist recommendations in a Veterans Affairs medical center. *Am J Health-Syst Pharm* 2002;59: 2070–7.
7. Rich DS. New JCAHO medication management standards for 2004. *Am J Health-Syst Pharm* 2004;61:1349–1358.
8. SoRelle R. EM groups persuade Joint Commission to temper pharmacy review policy. *Emerg Med News* 2007;29(9): 42–45.
9. Santell JP, Hicks RW, Cousins D. http://www.usp.org/hqi/patientSafety/resources/posters/posterEmergencyDept5yr.html. Accessed January 2008.
10. American Society of Health-System Pharmacists. http://www.ashp.org/s_ashp/docs/files/JC_ED_DraftComments 061307.pdf. Accessed January, 2008.

11. Thommaset KB, Faris R. Survey of pharmacy services provision in the emergency department. *Am J Health-Syst Pharm* 2003;60(15):1561–1564

12. American Society of Health-System Pharmacists. http://www.ashp.org/s_ashp/bin.asp?CID=6&DID=5423&DOC=FILE.PDF. Accessed January 2008.

13. Lada P, Delgado G Jr. Documentation of pharmacists' intervention in an emergency department and associated cost avoidance. *Am J Health-Syst Pharm* 2007;64:63–68.

14. Cohen V. Chapter 40 The Emergency Department Pharmacist. In: O'Donnell J, 2nd ed. *Drug Injury Liability, and Analysis.* Tucson, Arizona; Lawyers & Judges Publishing Company, Inc., *2005:733–742*

15. Cohen V Jellinek SP, Likourezos A, et al. Variation in the medication information for elderly patients during initial interventions by emergency department physicians. *Am J Health-Syst Pharm* 2008;65:60–64.

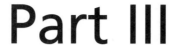

Part III

Assuring Quality of Emergency Care Pharmacotherapy: Focus on Quality Measures, High-Risk, High-Cost Medication, and Response to Medical Emergencies

In Part III, we describe quality of care medication management activities and tools that translate into safe and cost-effective practices when using pharmacotherapy in the ED.

In Chapter 12, we describe the implementation of antimicrobial stewardship in the ED that facilitated achieving pay-for-performance initiatives and continuity of care. In Chapter 13, we review the clinical significance of drug interactions in the ED, and in Chapter 14, we discuss the use of antidotes in brief and the role of the pharmacotherapist in ensuring optimal implementation of antidotes and responding to public health emergencies. In Chapter 15, we describe what to expect during the emergency care of the critically ill patient and provide critical care tools to expedite care. We describe the role of ED clinical pharmacy services in informatics (Chapter 16) and how to build a decision support system that facilitates implementation of emergency care pharmacotherapy protocols and instructs on procurement, administering, and dispensing of critical care drug therapy. Chapter 17 focuses on our approach to hospital-wide reconciliation and the role of targeted medication reconciliation to assure safety and quality within the ED setting, and in Chapter 18, we discuss geriatric and pediatric patients and the ED pharmacist role in caring for these special patient groups.

In 1998, President Clinton commissioned a study on quality care that resulted in the document "Quality First: Better Health Care for All Americans."[1] This report noted that the likelihood that any one American will get the best possible care varies considerably, and that national aims should be set to focus quality improvements efforts.[2] Quality of healthcare is predicated on safe care.[2] The national patient safety foundation notes that "Patient safety is an important subset of quality."[3]

Assessing and measuring quality includes three characteristics related to patient safety: 1) structure, 2) process, and 3) outcomes. *Structure* is the capacity to provide high quality care including incorporating resources in the healthcare system that protect patient safety, such as licensure. *Process,* also referred to as *performance,* relates to clinical and technical aspects of care processes including those that contribute to or compromise patient safety, such as errors in drug administration.[2] *Outcomes* is defined as changes in patient's status attributable to care processes.[2,4] Safe patient care as an outcome can be influenced by structure and process characteristics.

This relationship between healthcare quality and patient safety has been described in three different quality problems: 1) overuse: too much care, i.e., overuse of antibiotics that may put patient safety at risk; 2) underuse: too little use of effective and appropriate care that, when applied, decreases unnecessary complications, such as noncompliance with ordering pneumococcal vaccination in asthma or COPD patients; and 3) mis-use: inferior care that results when health care providers perform inadequately, resulting in unnecessary injuries, delayed care, or mortality, such as seen with delay in antimicrobial use and goal-directed therapy in sepsis patients. Misuse results in preventable harm from medical treatment and compromises patient safety.[5]

HOW CAN WE ENHANCE QUALITY AND PATIENT SAFETY?

Internal and external forces to healthcare systems are used to promote healthcare quality and patient safety. External competition, pertaining to achievement of quality of care, improves quality of healthcare and patient safety. Improving processes internally ensures safe care and thus improves quality.

External pressures have been created through the efforts of the Centers for Medicare & Medicaid Services (CMS), the Department of Health and Human Services, and other members of the Hospital Quality Alliance that have set numerous hospital quality measures for comparison between hospitals [6] (Table III-1).

Several of these quality measures include emergency care and pharmacotherapy, for example, AMI-1, AMI-3, AMI-4, AMI-6, AMI-7, AMI-8, AMI-8a, HF-3, HF-4, PN-1, PN-2, PN-3a, PN-3b, PN4, PN-5, PN5a-c, PN6, PN-7, SCIP-1. In Part III, we describe the clinical pharmacy services role in the development of processes that we term "rubrics" implemented within the ED setting to remove barriers toward achieving optimal performance of quality measures and that permit for performance to be evaluated.

TABLE III-1

Quality Indicators

Code	Hospital Quality Measure
AMI-1	Aspirin at arrival
AMI-2	Aspirin prescribed at discharge
AMI-3	ACEI- or ARB for LVSD
AMI-4	Adult smoking cessation advice and counseling
AMI-5	Beta Blocker at discharge
AMI-6	Beta blocker at arrival
AMI-7	Median time to thrombolysis
AMI-7a	Thrombolytics within 30 minutes
AMI-8a	PCI within 90 min of arrival
AMI-8	Time from arrival to PCI in patients with ST inc. or LBBB on ECG
HF-1	Discharge Instructions
HF-3	ACEI- or ARB for LVSD
HF-4	Adult smoking cessation advice and counseling
PN-1	Oxygenation assessment
PN-2	Pneumococcal vaccination
PN-3a	Blood culture within 24 hours
PN-3b	Blood cultures before first antibiotics
PN-4	Adult smoking cessation advice and counseling
PN-5	Time from arrival to admin. of antibiotic for patients with pneumonia
PN-5a	Initial antibiotics within 8 hours of arrival
PN-5c	Initial antibiotics received within 6 hours
PN-5b	Initial antibiotics received within 4 hours
PN-6	Initial antibiotic selection in CAP patients
PN-7	Influenza vaccination Oct.-Mar. At discharge
SCIP-1	Prophylactic antibiotics received within 1 hour prior to surgical incision
Mort 30-AMI	AMI-30 day mortality
Mort 30-HF	HF 30 day mortality

References

1. Advisory Commission on Health Consumer Protection and Quality in the Health Care Industry. *Quality First: Better Health Care for All Americans.* Washington DC: US Government Printing Office; March 1998.
2. Zipper L, Cushman S. The relationship between quality and patient safety. In: *Lessons in Patient Safety.* National Patient Safety Foundation, 2001.
3. Cooper JB, Gaba DM, Liang B, Woods D, Blum LN. National Patient Safety Foundation agenda for research and development in patient safety. *MedGenMed* 2000;2(4). Available at www.medscape.com/MedGenMed/PatientSafety.
4. Donabedian A. Evaluating the quality of medical care. *Milbank Q* 1966;44:166–203.
5. Donaldson M. *Measuring the Quality of Health Care.* Institute of Medicine. Washington DC: National Academy Press, 1999.
6. U.S. Department of Health & Human Services [Homepage on the internet] Hospital Compare Available from: http://hospital qualityalliance.org/hospitalqualityalliance/aboutus/aboutus.html. Accessed December 2008.

12

Antimicrobial Stewardship in the Emergency Department

Objectives
- Review ED pharmacist (EDP) role in expediting administration of antibiotics
- Explain importance of early antibiotic therapy
- Discuss how to ensure optimal selection and prevent overuse or underuse of antimicrobials
- Review outcomes of implementation efforts

ED PHARMACIST ROLE IN EXPEDITING ADMINISTRATION OF ANTIBIOTIC

The EDP can improve quality and reduce preventable deaths by achieving recommended timely antibiotic therapy and pay-for-performance incentives.[1]

There are no published reports that describe the role of an EDP in managing antibiotics and how the EDP can improve timely administration of antibiotics within the emergency department. Using the description of an antimicrobial stewardship,[2-5] we implemented a variety of activities consistent with this role to prevent overuse and underuse of antimicrobial agents and to assist in achieving pay-for-performance incentives within the ED.

Antimicrobial stewardship is defined as an activity that includes appropriate selection, dosing, route, and duration of antimicrobial therapy. The multifaceted nature of an antimicrobial stewardship has led to a collaborative review and support of implementation by many infectious diseases organizations.[6] Antimicrobial stewardship programs can be financially self-supporting and improve patient care because these programs have demonstrated annual cost savings of $200,000 to $900,000 in both larger academic and smaller community hospitals. Clinical pharmacists with infectious disease training are part of the core members of this multidisciplinary stewardship team; however, customization to specific units or departments, such as the ED, are not normally represented, and therefore, having a liaison to communicate ED needs and assure implementation provides another enhanced element to this multidisciplinary approach.

Because of the speed in evaluation and management and the lack of available and reliable information, i.e., no blood cultures, inaccurate medication or allergy histories, translation of infectious disease principles in the ED is daunting and nearly impossible without appropriate clinical operations and automation that support such activity. The emergency department clinical pharmacy service in collaboration with emergency medicine, infectious disease, and information systems were the catalyst to creating sustainable changes in operations to assure optimization of infectious disease quality standards.

In 1998 corresponding with the EDP academic appointment with the Arnold Marie Schwartz College of Pharmacy and Health Science to initiate clinical pharmacy services in the ED at Maimonides Medical Center; it was evident there was a need to improve the safe and effective use of antimicrobials in the ED. Although there was an inpatient-restricted antimicrobial program and antibiotic surveillance committee within the hospital, there was no such program in the ED. Consultation by the infectious disease team was informal and by phone only, which delayed care. Antibiotics were selected based on emergency physician (EP) preference, despite the institutional antibiogram, host factors, or drug factors that may have suggested otherwise, and if selection was restricted, an extensive delay in treatment was observed. Furthermore, the antimicrobial budget would spontaneously spike, creating concern from the Pharmacy Administration. The knowledge of the preferred cost effective antimicrobials was not shared with the EP due to a lack of collaboration.

Over the next several years, the ED clinical pharmacy service set in motion a goal to assure provision of quality antimicrobial pharmaceutical care while assuring expedient antimicrobial delivery. First, the EDP provided a 24-hour on-call consult service to gain understanding of antimicrobial prescribing needs. The EDP was tasked with the following duties and responsibilities as seen in Table 12-1.

- Develop a process to expedite acquisition of broad spectrum antimicrobial
- Obtain approval privileges for the ED for restricted antimicrobials
- Recommend preferred antimicrobial based on host and drug factors and institutional antibiogram and previous cultures
- Procure antimicrobial
- Adjust dose based on organ function and severity of illness
- Streamline therapy over the subsequent 24–48 hours
- Assure appropriate continuation
- Act as a liaison to infectious diseases for restricted antimicrobials that require direct ID consult
- Conduct quality improvement projects to assure compliance with performance indicators and time to administration of antibiotics
- Advocate for immunization and vaccinations

Second, the antibiotic surveillance committee, with the input from emergency medicine leadership, infectious disease, and pharmacy leadership, designed an antimicrobial guideline for acute severe infectious diseases commonly seen within the ED. An initial guideline in the form of a yellow card (Figs. 12-1, 12-2) was used as a tag for follow up.

The yellow card evolved into a pocket guide (Fig. 12-3) and then into a clinical decisions support system, embedded into the order-entry pathway for adult infections (Figs. 12-4 and 12-5).

PROCEDURES FOR ED-BASED ANTIBIOTIC STEWARDSHIP PROGRAM

The clinical pathway was initially formatted into a yellow prescription card that included the antimicrobial of choice, an alternative choice for frequently seen infectious diseases based on host factors, i.e., allergy risk, and their corresponding indications. We included infections such as pneumonia

Empiric Antibiotic Request Form
NOTE: This card is only to be used to request restricted antibiotics as outlined in MMC's Adult Guidelines for Initial Empiric Treatment of Common Infections. Restricted Antibiotics to be used for indications other than those outlined require ID approval. This request is valid only while the patient is in the ED. Once the patient is admitted, ID approval is required to continue a restricted antibiotic.

DRUG	INDICATION/REASON FOR USE
☐ Moxifloxacin 400 mg PO	Mild – moderate community acquired pneumonia (Patient with co-morbidities or Cephalosporin/PCN allergy)*
☐ Moxifloxacin 400 mg IV	Severe CAP (Patient with co-morbidities or Cephalosporin/PCN allergy)*
☐ Piperacillin / Tazobactam 4.5 g IV + Amikacin ODA[1] +/- Vancomycin 1g IV	Nosocomial Pneumonia/Sepsis (Vancomycin if MRSA suspected)
☐ Cefepime 1-2 g IV+/- Metronidazole + Amikacin +/- Vancomycin 1g IV	Nosocomial Pneumonia/Sepsis (Vancomycin if MRSA suspected)
☐ Vancomycin 1g IV+ Aztreonam 1-2 g IV + Amikacin +/- Metronidazole	Nosocomial Pneumonia/Sepsis w/ severe PCN/Cephalosporin allergy
☐ Ceftriaxone 2 g IV + Vancomycin 1 g IV +/- Ampicillin 2 g IV	Suspected Meningitis
☐ Cefotaxime 2 g IV + Ampicillin 1-2 g IV	Biliary Tract Infections with intolerance to Aminoglycosides
☐ Ampicillin 1-2 g IV + Ceftriaxone 1-2 g IV + Metronidazole 500mg IV	Bowel Infection with intolerance to Aminoglycosides
☐ Vancomycin 1g IV + Cefepime 1-2 g IV +/- Metronidazole +/-AG	Surgical Wound Infections
☐ Vancomycin 1g IV + Piperacillin/Tazobactam 4.5 g IV +/- Aminoglycoside	Surgical Wound Infections
☐ Vancomycin 1g IV + Aztreonam 1g IV +/- Metronidazole +/- AG**	Surigcal Wound Infections w/severe PCN/Cephalosporin allergy
☐ Cefepime 2 g IV+/- Vancomycin 1 g IV +/- Aminoglycoside	Neutropenic Sepsis
☐ Piperacillin / Tazobactam 4.5 g IV + Aminoglycoside +/- Vancomycin 1 g	Neutropenic Sepsis
☐ **STD KIT** (Azithromycin 1g PO + Cefixime 400 mg PO)	Coverage for *Chlamydia trachomatis* + *Neisseria gonorrhoeae*
☐ Ceftriaxone 250 mg IM + Doxycycline PO 100 mg BID x 14 days	PID Outpatient

* Mild – moderate community acquired pneumonia (CAP) – Hemodynamically stable/able to tolerate PO.

** AG – Aminoglycoside
[1] Once Daily Aminoglycoside

Place Decal Here	MD Stamp & Signature/Date/Time of order

Figure 12–1. Empiric antibiotic request form before CDSS and CPOE.

FOR OFFICE USE ONLY

1. **Door to antibiotic time:**   ☐ < 4 hours   ☐ > 4 hours

2. **Was the initial antibiotic consistent with Medical Center guidelines?** ☐ Yes   ☐ No

3. **Were blood cultures collected prior to antibiotic administration?**   ☐ Yes   ☐ No

4. **Was patient screened and/or given Pneumococcal Vaccine?**   ☐ Yes   ☐ No

5. **Outcome of Therapy:**   ☐ Treatment Success   ☐ Treatment Failure

6. **Length of Stay:**   ☐ 1-4 days   ☐ 4-8 days   ☐ > 8 days

7. **Any reported Adverse Drug Reaction (describe/discuss):** _____

    _____

    _____

ADDITIONAL COMMENTS: _____

    _____

    _____

Figure 12–2. Backpage of empiric antibiotic request form for utilization review and quality assurance.

(Community acquired pneumonia (CAP), Hospital acquired pneumonia (HAP), Ventilator associated pneumonia (VAP), and Healthcare associated pneumonia (HCAP)), skin and skin structure infections, urinary tract infections, meningitis, intraabdominal infections, surgical wounds, and neutropenic sepsis. The yellow prescription card was entitled Empiric Antibiotic Request Form, and it was used by the EP to acquire the recommended antimicrobial. The yellow prescription card also included a location to justify the need for the antimicrobial by the EP, i.e., "positive infiltrate on chest x-ray," was written to request a fluoroquinolone for community-acquired pneumonia. Upon receipt of the yellow card, pharmacy dispensed the initial antimicrobial requested. The yellow cards were stored in the pharmacy for the EDP to pick up the next morning. On daily morning rounds, the EDP would follow up to streamline use and assure continuity of care over the next 24–48 hours. When necessary and at the request of the EP, the EDP initiated the empiric antimicrobial request form and this would expedite the management. Additionally upon review if the antimicrobial was prescribed without initiating a request, the EDP would intervene.

With the use of the ED antibiotic request form, otherwise restricted antibiotics would be approved for 24 hours without ID approval.

Subsequently, the inpatient or admitting physician had to request approval from infectious disease (ID) to continue or discontinue therapy, or switch to alternative therapy that also was restricted.

CONTINUITY OF CARE

Led by the ID pharmacy specialist and the antibiotic surveillance committee, an inpatient computerized physician order entry (CPOE) CAP pathway was developed to further assure the continuity of care. This interactive decision support CPOE CAP pathway required the physician to consider and select therapy based on renal adjustments, allergies, or comorbid conditions. In addition, the clinician was required to initiate an automatic switch from IV to PO therapy (minimum time permitted was within 48–72 hours).

INCORPORATING INFECTIOUS DISEASE GUIDE INTO ED-SPECIFIC CPOE/CDSS

Conversion from a paper to an automated electronic medical record within the ED permitted the ED clinical pharmacy service, in collaboration with information systems, to

INFECTION	COMMENTS	FIRST CHOICE	ALTERNATIVE CHOICE	SIGNIFICANT ALLERGIES	ORAL CONVERSION
COMMUNITY-ACQUIRED PNEUMONIA	Sputum Gram stain encouraged to guide therapy	Moxifloxacin IV × 2 days Followed by oral formulation (If quinolone used within past 3 months, use	Ceftriaxone ◆ & Azithromycin ◆ (Preferred regimen for ICU admission)		Moxifloxacin or Cefpodoxime + Azithromycin ◆
HOSPITAL-ACQUIRED, VENTILATOR-ASSOCIATED, AND HEALTHCARE-ASSOCIATED PNEUMONIA	Sputum Gram stain & Culture encouraged to guide therapy. Legionella Sputum Culture and Urinary Antigen Assay	Cefepime ◆ + Aminoglycoside *ODA + Azithromycin ◆ +/- Metronidazole +/- Vancomycin	Piperacillin/Tazobactam ◆ + Aminoglycoside *ODA + Azithromycin ◆ +/- Vancomycin	If significant Cephalosporin allergy: Aztreonam ◆ + Aminoglycoside + Moxifloxacin ◆ +/- Vancomycin	Step down determined by the isolated pathogen, culture results, and clinical status. Call ID for recommendations
SOFT TISSUE INFECTION (e.g. CELLULITIS)	Surgical evaluation encouraged for aggressive skin and soft tissue infection. Gram stain & culture recommended	Cefazolin (+ Clindamycin for aggressive Infection)	Nafcillin (+ Clindamycin for aggressive Infection)	Cephalosporin allergy: Clindamycin	Cefadroxil or Dicloxacillin +/- Clindamycin
MIXED SOFT TISSUE INFECTION (e.g. diabetic foot, ischemic, or decubitus ulcer)	Surgical evaluation encouraged for aggressive skin and soft tissue infection. Gram stain & Culture recommended.	Cefuroxime + Metronidazole Or Cefuroxime + Clindamycin	Cefazolin + Metronidazole Or Cefazolin + Clindamycin	For severe Cephalosporin allergy: Clindamycin + Aztreonam	Cefadroxil + Clindamycin Or Amoxicillin/ Clavulanate
PYELONEPHRITIS	Urine culture and Urine analysis	Ampicillin + Gentamicin	Cefuroxime + Gentamicin	β-Lactam allergy: Gentamicin If Gram-positive organisms suspected, call ID for recommendations.	Trimethoprim/SMX Or Cefpodoxime according to urine C&S
BACTERIAL MENINGITIS	Lumbar Puncture essential	Ceftriaxone ◆ + Vancomycin +/- Ampicillin (> 50 y/o or the presence of risk factors for Listeria monocytogenes) + Steroids		Anaphylaxis to Cephalosporins: Call ID for recommendations	
BILIARY TRACT		Cefuroxime +/- Gentamicin*ODA		For severe Cephalosporin allergy: Moxifloxacin ◆ +/- Gentamicin *ODA	
BOWEL RELATED INFECTIONS	Gram stain & culture	Cefuroxime+ Metronidazole +/- Gentamicin *ODA		For severe Cephalosporin allergy: Moxifloxacin ◆ +/- Gentamicin *ODA	Determined by isolated pathogen, Culture results, & clinical status. Call ID for recommendations.
SURGICAL WOUND INFECTIONS	Gram stain & culture	Vancomycin + Cefepime ◆ +/-Metronidazole +/- Aminoglycoside	Vancomycin + Piperacillin/Tazobactam ◆ +/- Aminoglycoside	Cephalosporin allergy: Call ID for recommendations	Determined by isolated pathogen, Culture results, & clinical status.
NEUTROPENIC SEPSIS	Cultures recommended	Cefepime ◆ (2gm IVPB q8h) +/- Aminoglycoside +/- Vancomycin	Piperacillin/Tazobactam (4.5gm IVPB q6h) + Aminoglycoside +/- Vancomycin	Cephalosporin allergy: Call ID for recommendations	

* Amikacin ODA (15mg/kg/day), Gentamicin ODA (4-7-mg/kg/day); take level 6–14 hours after the dose is initiated
◆ Requires ID Physician approval
Guidelines are provided to assist in selection of appropriate initial empiric therapy. They are not intended to be all-inclusive and may be modified according to individual patient requirements. For further advice and recommendations contact a physician from the division of infectious diseases.

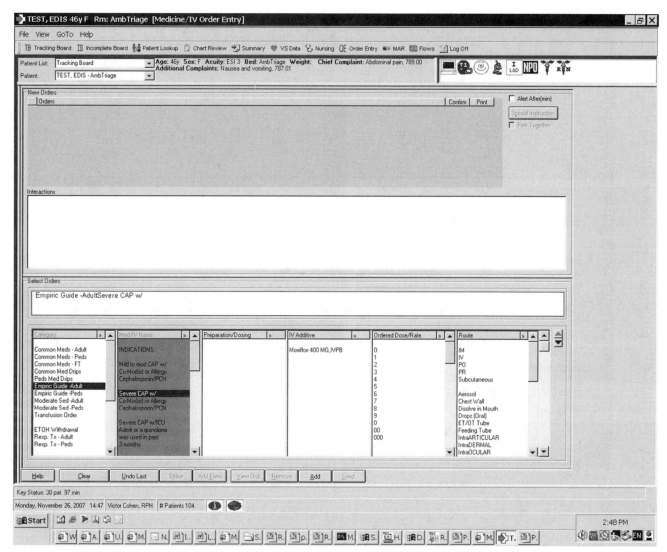

Figure 12–4. Clinical decision support system for antimicrobials embedded in order entry system.

automate this antimicrobial guideline into the ED-specific electronic medical record as part of our decision support. Incorporation of the antimicrobial guide embedded into the ordering process enhanced compliance with recommended antimicrobials, increased ease of use for EPs, and increased the speed of acquisition and preparation of the antimicrobial agents for nursing.

The EDP conducts a risk assessment to narrow the likely source of infection and the likely etiological agent to go from an empiric approach to a presumptive approach for prescribing antimicrobials during infectious emergencies. At the request of the EP, the EDP enters infectious disease orders into the ED-specific CPOE system.

During prospective review the EDP screens for allergies, adjusts doses as needed, and modifies initial prescribing by the EP when a discrepancy arises.

RATIONALIZING THE IMPORTANCE OF EARLY ANTIBIOTIC THERAPY

Empiric antibiotic therapy aimed at the likely source of infection are the cornerstone in therapy for patients who have

acute life-threatening infections presenting to the ED.[7] Early antibiotic therapy for these severe infections makes sense because destroying the offending agent may reduce the progression to multisystem organ failure (MSOF), as it deters the physiological response to infection that causes MSOF and subsequent death. A delay in antibiotic therapy coupled with a significant bacterial load can result in a dramatic cytokine release, when antibiotic therapy is begun, which actually increases the likelihood of progression to MSOF. A delay worsens the clinical condition.[7]

Despite this consideration of the importance of early antibiotic therapy, studies are conflicting. Several studies have reported improved outcomes associated with early administration whereas others have not, and there is a lack of quality randomized controlled trials in humans on the timing of antibiotics, which has made evidence-based decision making on early antibiotic therapy a challenge.[8]

PAY FOR PERFORMANCE INCENTIVES

Despite conflicting data, quality improvement organizations, such as the Joint Commission (TJC), Centers for

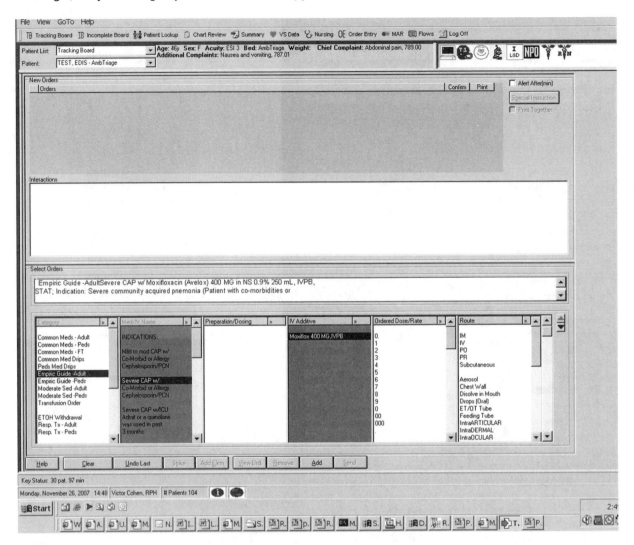

Figure 12–5. Clinical decision support system for antimicrobials embedded in order entry system.

Medicare and Medicaid have used early administration of antibiotics as a measure of quality care. For example, antibiotics must be administered within 4 hours (6 hours with subsequent writings) from the time of arrival to the ED to define a key measure for quality of pneumonia care.[9] TJC and CMS have named this measure **PN-5b** as part of the bundle of quality indicators for pneumonia. PN-5b has gained significantly more attention because of the CMS inclusion of this element as part of a pay-for-performance incentive to U.S. hospitals.[10] The PN-5b program enables hospitals to receive financial incentive for ensuring that a high percentage of patients admitted with pneumonia receive antibiotics within 4 hours of hospital arrival.

The surviving sepsis campaign, which recommends goal-directed therapy for hemodynamic support with early antibiotics to be administered within 1 hour of diagnosis of sepsis or septic shock to reduce rates of mortality is another quality measure associated with early antibiotic administration.[11] This quality improvement initiative was based on a landmark study by Rivers et al. that implemented a protocol for hemodynamic support. Rivers et al. reported results on 263 enrolled patients, 130 were randomly assigned to early

goal-directed therapy and 133 to standard therapy; there were no significant differences between the groups with respect to base-line characteristics. In-hospital mortality was 30.5 percent in the group assigned to early goal-directed therapy, as compared with 46.5 percent in the group assigned to standard therapy (P=0.009).[12]

Meningitis carries a high risk for significant morbidity and mortality. Prompt recognition and antibiotic therapy for patients with bacterial meningitis are the standard of care because meningitis is such a rapidly progressing illness.[13] Delay in meningitis antibiotic treatment may stem from the presentations; in one group, the patient may have clear signs and symptoms and is considered high risk whereas in the second group, the patient may present as low risk with nonspecific symptoms. In the high-risk patient, early antibiotics is associated with reduced mortality; however, in the low-risk group, early antibiotics is questionable.[12] In summary, due to the rapid progression of various infectious diseases, early administration of antibiotic therapy in the ED is warranted; however, risk of overuse may occur. Because of this complexity of care, a multidisciplinary collaborative approach is warranted.

POOR PERFORMING QUALITY INDICATORS IN THE ED: NEED FOR A MULTIDISCIPLINARY APPROACH

These quality initiatives pose significant challenges to EPs.[13] EPs must balance the goal of providing timely antibiotics with preventing overuse. Historically, hospitals have poor performance on the pneumonia quality measure for a variety of reasons, including ED overcrowding, long wait times for physician evaluations, radiograph performance and interpretation, and delays in antibiotic administration; thus, hospitals have struggled to improve compliance with these guideline.[14–16] A recent national study on quality of emergency department care in treatment of pneumonia reported that there were 14.2 million visits for pneumonia. Patients with pneumonia received appropriate antibiotics and pulse-oximetry measurement 69% and 46% of the time, respectively. There were an estimated 1.7 million annual opportunities to improve care for the patient with pneumonia, and an estimated 7,000 excess deaths per year. Thus, nationally, emergency department quality of care in the management of pneumonia is below national goals and accounts for significant preventable deaths; a multidisciplinary approach is indicated.[1]

BARRIERS TOWARD OPTIMAL INFECTIOUS DISEASE MANAGEMENT IN THE ED

There are multiple barriers to achieving these early antibiotic initiatives. They include presentation-level factors, patient-level factors, and system-level factors. For example, patients presenting to the ED may not have a definitive diagnosis; diagnostic testing creates time lags (hours); if culture results are required, identification of a definitive source can take days. All of these barriers are exacerbated by overcrowding in the ED, and those patients with co-morbidities that predispose them to atypical presentations.

Also unintended adverse consequences of these initiatives include operational solutions that hospitals may implement that may not be in the best interest of patient safety, such as encouraging overuse of antibiotics and prioritization of selected patients solely to meet performance goals.[8,17]

TOOLS TO ENSURE OPTIMAL SELECTION AND PREVENT OVERUSE AND UNDERUSE OF ANTIMICROBIALS

CONSTRUCT OF EMERGENCY DEPARTMENT BASED INFECTIOUS DISEASES GUIDELINE

Hans et al. reviewed several rapidly fatal infections that EPs may encounter including bacterial meningitis, toxic shock syndrome, methicillin-resistant necrotizing pneumonia, severe acute respiratory syndrome, and avian influenza. Many of these infectious diseases may manifest similarly to stable infections and then proceed rapidly to a more sinister infection. The challenge to EPs is to identify and initiate pharmacotherapy as rapidly as possible.[18] We incorporated the needed antimicrobial agents into the empiric antibiotic guide for these infections. We also facilitated a rapid response for these infectious diseases by making the indicated antimicrobial agents available as floor stock or including these antimicrobial agents as part of the CDSS empiric guide. This inclusion into the order entry pathway enabled rapid turnover because once the prescription is selected and entered into the CPOE system, a label is transmitted to the pharmacy with a "red boarder" which alerts the central pharmacist to release a stat dose.

The empiric guide depicted is specifically for adults who are hospitalized for infections. Treatment recommendations are based on likely organism current guidelines modified by age, allergy history, co-morbid conditions, antibiogram, the pharmacy department's preference for IV admixtures, and marketing agreements. Caution should be used to adopt this guideline to other EDs; however, this guide may serve as a template to construct an ED-specific guide for each unique ED.

An in-depth review of pharmacotherapy of infectious diseases is beyond the scope of this chapter.

Our goal is to describe the rationale for emergency care antimicrobial pharmacotherapy that we have selected, which should be stored in the ED for various rapidly fatal infectious diseases. For the more indolent infectious commonly seen in the ED setting that require early antibiotic management, but do not require storage within the ED, rationale for the preferred antimicrobial is provided. Furthermore, we describe the various clinical scoring systems that the emergency care pharmacotherapist uses to confirm the presence and severity of infection; these systems allow the pharmacotherapist to make better decisions and recommendations about the initial empiric choice selected by the emergency physician.

REVIEW OF RAPIDLY FATAL INFECTIONS THAT REQUIRE MANAGEMENT IN THE ED

With an increasing incidence of sepsis, increasing use of the emergency department by populations at risk, and an increase in time spent in the emergency department awaiting hospital admission, emergency medicine practitioners have an opportunity to make a significant difference in the fight against sepsis. By administering appropriate antibiotics in a timely manner, removing possible sources of infection, practicing early goal-directed hemodynamic optimization, using lung-protective ventilation strategies, and judiciously using corticosteroids and intensive insulin therapy, the goal of reducing mortality from sepsis can be achieved.

Sepsis

Selection of antimicrobial therapy for patients presenting with severe sepsis and septic shock depends on a number of factors including the source or focus of infection, whether the infection is community- or hospital-acquired, knowledge of local antimicrobial resistance patterns, presence of indwelling catheters, and immunologic status of the patient.

Initial empirical anti-infective therapy should include one or more drugs that have activity against the likely pathogens (bacterial or fungal) and that penetrate into the presumed source of sepsis.

A combination of a beta lactam, such as piperacillin/tazobactam plus an aminoglycoside, such as amikacin or gentamicin, is usually initiated for sepsis. This approach broadens the coverage of the beta lactam in the case of multidrug resistant gram negative organisms.

Brooklyn has become known for the origin of multidrug resistant Klebsiella *pneumonia*, which is resistant to all beta lactam antibiotics and only susceptible to aminoglycosides and polymixin B. In addition, if the cause of infection is health care associated, vancomycin may be initiated. Monotherapy with broad spectrum beta lactams has also been effective. Despite theoretic advantages of combination therapy, such as enhanced broad spectrum coverage, potential for synergism, and prevention of emergence of resistance, a recent Cochrane review conducted by Paul et al. concluded that combination therapy offers no advantage and may increase the risk of toxicity. The investigators reviewed the literature for all studies of patients with sepsis comparing the treatment of a beta lactam, which included a penicillin or cephalosporin as monotherapy, to that of a beta lactam combined with an aminoglycoside. The aminoglycoside may have included gentamicin, tobramycin, or amikacin. The investigators compiled 64 trials including 7586 patients hospitalized for a variety of infections (i.e., urinary tract, intra-abdominal, pneumonia, source of unknown origin, skin and skin structure). When comparing beta lactams of

similar spectrum (20 studies), no difference was observed between groups with regard to all-cause fatality RR 1.01 (95% CI 0.75–1.35) and clinical failure RR 1.11 (95% CI 0.95–1.29).[19] When comparing monotherapy with beta lactams of broader spectrum compared with those with a narrower spectrum and aminoglycoside, there was an advantage to monotherapy. Investigators noted that there was no evidence of an increase in emergence of resistance, and no overall significant difference in toxicity amongst groups. However, there was an increase in adverse events associated with nephrotoxicity as one would expect in the combination therapy.[19] Based on this data, the emergency care pharmacotherapist may be able to simplify empiric therapy, increase speed of delivery, and perhaps reduce costs associated with the management of sepsis.

Acute Meningitis

Case fatality rates of bacterial meningitis remain at 20–25%. Sequelae may result in hearing loss, brain damage, learning disabilities, and mental retardation. Thus, empiric antibiotics is indicated despite the risk of resistance.

As seen in the empiric guide, ceftriaxone plus vancomycin, and if Listeria monocytogenes is suspected, ampicillin (patients > 50 years) is recommended. A recent Cochrane review conducted in 2007 supports steroid therapy (dexamethasone) to reduce mortality and accompanying sequalae.[20] Vancomycin is included because of drug-resistant streptococcus pneumonia. Furthermore, when suspecting a gram-negative organisms, cefepime or ceftazidime may be

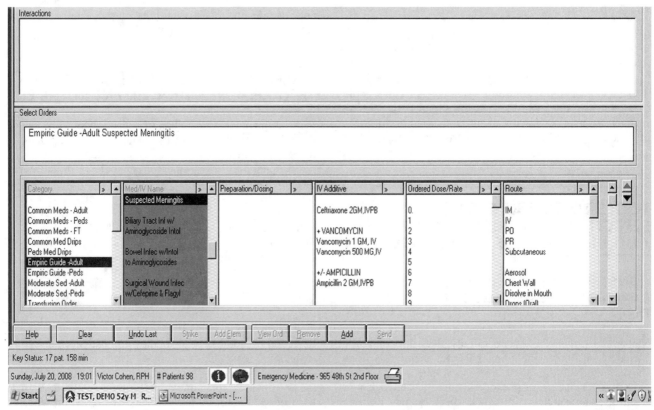

Figure 12–6. Embedded empiric antimicrobial pathway for acute meningitis.

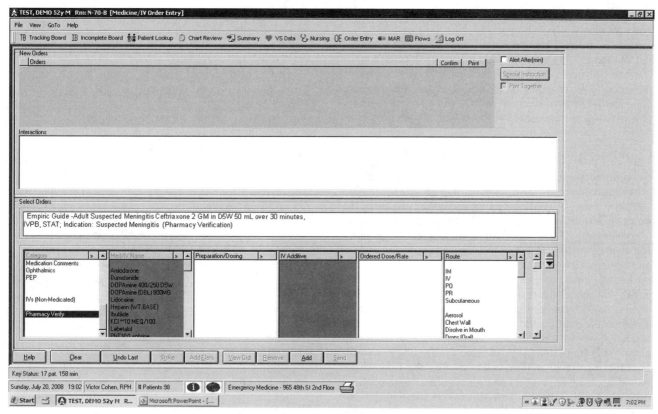

Figure 12-7   Embedded empiric antimicrobial pathway for acute meningitis verified by pharmacy.

warranted. Meropenem is indicated for multidrug resistant organisms, unless severely allergic to penicillin, then aztreonam is recommended. The EDP is integral at risk assessing the patient for true cephalosporin allergy as this class of agents is superior in meningitis because of their superior penetration. The empiric guide assured bactericidal antibiotics that penetrate the blood brain barrier utilized at the appropriate doses. Meningitis may also be due to a viral pathogen. There is no antiviral therapy currently available so all efforts are toward supportive care and notification of public health authorities. Fungi and parasites are associated with a more diffuse inflammatory process of the meninges and brain parenchyma. Antifungal therapy is usually initiated by a consulting intensive care team.

Case Study

Pharmacy Intervention on Life-Threatening Acute Meningitis

A patient with a brain abscess on CT scan was initially managed with ceftriaxone 2 g IV only. Pharmacy surveillance of this case by the ED Pharmacist suggested that this patient is at risk of drug resistant Streptococcus Pneumonia, and anaerobic organisms. The EDP recommended ceftriaxone to be dosed at 2 grams every 12 hours and metronidazole and vancomycin to assure broad-spectrum coverage. The recommendations were well accepted. Initial empiric therapy was enhanced.

We have identified discrepancies because only ceftriaxone may be selected without consideration of other organisms and without consideration of administration of steroids prior to antibiotics. A case study of a pharmacy intervention during acute meningitis is seen below. To expedite initial management, we embedded the recommended antimicrobials into an order set within the empiric guide. Stat labels are transmitted via Zebra printers in the pharmacy, then the antibiotic is procured by a technician and sent to the ED in a rapid response.

Toxic Shock Syndrome

Toxic shock syndrome (TSS) presents as a sudden onset of fever, chills, vomiting, diarrhea, and rash rapidly progressing to hypotension and multisystem failure and even death. TSS is linked to tampon use, intravaginal contraceptive devices, nasal packing, postoperative wounds, minor trauma, surgical procedures, and viral infections.[21] The mortality rate is 30–70% despite aggressive treatment and is most commonly associated with staphylococcus aureus and group A streptococcus. Supportive therapy is the mainstay of treatment with large volumes of fluids needed to manage the hypotension. A surgical intervention including debridement or fasciotomy is usually required. Despite data that suggest no alteration in the course of treatment with antibiotics for acute staphylococcus aureus and that TSS may resolve on its own, the recurrence rates are reduced with antibiotic therapy.[18]

Clindamycin hypothetically suppresses toxin production whereas beta lactams are associated with increased toxin production because of cell wall lysis.[22] Other in vitro data suggest clindamycin and linezolid reduces toxin production more than vancomycin and beta lactams.[23] Thus current antibiotic therapy should include clindamycin and vancomycin or linezolid for staphylococcus aureus and clindamycin and a beta lactam for group A streptococcus.[24] If cultures and sensitivities support methicillin-sensitive staphylococcus aureus (never available immediately), then nafcillin or oxacillin is preferred.[20] We currently include clindamycin, vancomycin, and nafcillin as floor stock in the ED, which is easily retrievable to expedite treatment of suspected TSS.

Community-Acquired MRSA

Necrotizing pneumonia may be attributed exclusively to community-acquired MRSA strains that initiated as a skin infection. Hans et al. describes that mortality rate is in the range of 35–75%. CA-MRSA is the predominant producer of penton-valentine leukocidin (PVL), which is a pore-forming cytotoxin associated with leukocyte destruction and tissue necrosis that causes soft tissue infections and necrotizing pneumonia[25–27] Necrotizing pneumonia is not easily distinguishable from other CAP, with the exception of its rapid progression and severity of symptoms.[27] Younger patients, presenting with a history of viral illness, sudden onset of cough and hemoptysis, leukopenia, and chest x-ray consistent with pneumonia should be considered for aggressive antibiotic therapy covering CA-MRSA including vancomycin or linezolid, with clindamycin as drug of choice. There are currently no studies that demonstrate superiority of one over another. ID would be consulted to further guide the use of these agents.

Indolent Infections That Require Initial Treatment in the ED

Common infections that are treated initially in the ED and can have indolent progression include urinary tract infections, pneumonia, and skin and soft tissue infections. Preparation to guide selection of therapy is essential to prevent over- or underuse.

UTI

Because many patients with urinary tract infections may be treated as outpatients, one of the first tasks to consider is whether the patient should be admitted. Norris and Young described patients with the following symptoms as possible candidates for admission: unable to maintain oral hydration or medication by mouth, diagnosis is uncertain, suspected sepsis or other severe illness, urinary tract obstruction, progression of uncomplicated UTI, pregnancy, significant dehydration or acute renal insufficiency, age >60 years, immunocompromised, and baseline debilitation. Often a patient with less severe clinical presentations of UTI and none of the conditions indicating admission will be treated and released with a prescription of ciprofloxacin 500 mg orally twice daily for 7 days.[8] Not all fluoroquinolones are appropriate; moxifloxacin has limited bioavailability in the urinary tract because only 20% of the drug is excreted unchanged into the urine.

If a patient is hospitalized with acute uncomplicated pyelonephritis, ciprofloxacin may be administered intravenously every 12 hours; however, based on our antibiogram, ciprofloxacin coverage of various gram-negative organisms is extremely limited, and alternative choices include Ampicillin with gentamicin or ceftriaxone as monotherapy. When prior episodes suggest a resistant organism, a broader spectrum will be suggested.

As for dosing, high daily dose gentamicin (5 mg/kg) administered initially and repeated based on a level at 6 to 14 hours may be initiated. However, lack of appropriate execution of blood sampling and interpretation of the nomogram limits its use unless someone is involved to appropriately sample and interpret. The inpatient antibiotic stewardship will streamline therapy using the pocket guide provided by the antibiotic surveillance committee; this guide includes an oral conversion for in-house clinicians.

For acute complicated pyelonephritis, pseudomonas must be considered as a possible organism; we start therapy with ampicillin and gentamicin as an initial approach; an alternative choice for patients who are allergic to penicillin and have credible histories that the allergy was not anaphylaxis, selection includes cefuroxime and gentamicin. Based on –observations, patients with historical penicillin-allergy rarely have cross-allergenicity with a cephalosporin. This combination is provided as floor stock for ease of use and does not require ID consult for use.

If broader coverage is needed, we may start piperacillin–tazobactam because many of these patients may have sepsis as well. The cost of piperacillin–tazobactam, however, may preclude its use, and we may substitute with cefepime. The EDP reviews past episodes to assess risk for a drug-resistant organism and may tailor therapy based on these past cultures. Because immediate urine cultures are usually not available by the time empiric coverage is initiated and their value is questionable, they are not relied upon for initial empiric therapy.

Asymptomatic bacteruria is a common finding among patients presenting to the ED. It may complicate evaluation of geriatric patients because classic symptoms are not always present; the patient is demented and or intubated so treatment decisions are a challenge. Younger women do not require antibiotic therapy because their symptoms do not progress to a UTI. A pregnant patient should be treated because they are at risk of pyelonephritis, premature labor, and pregnancy-induced hypertension. Nitrofurantoin is the drug of choice if the patient has normal renal function; alternatively, cephalexin may be given four times a day for 3 days.[28] We frequently intervene on the use of nitrofurantoin in patients with abnormal renal function.

Pneumonia

Best practice standards for receiving antibiotics for pneumonia in the emergency department are changing according to PN-5c to over a 6-hour window.[29] The 2007 CAP guidelines have changed focus from an absolute time frame to recommending that patients receive an antibiotic dose during their time in the ED before being admitted and that hospitals now should monitor for inappropriate antimicrobial treatment of patients who do not have CAP.[30]

As recommended by national guidelines and as described earlier, we have developed a local pneumonia protocol at our hospital initiated within the ED. Decisions of whether the patient has pneumonia or not must be made clinically and radiographically as the first step in confirmation of the presence of disease. A patient with respiratory symptoms and positive infiltrate on chest x-ray is the obvious presentation; however, respiratory symptoms may also be associated with many other ailments that may masquerade as pneumonia, such as sepsis, bronchitis, asthma, COPD, MI, CHF, PE, CNS diseases, and cancer—all of which confound the diagnosis.[31] Elderly patients also present atypically without classic pulmonary symptoms, i.e., they may have confusion plus other comorbid states concomitantly. These complicated cases are a significant challenge to the ED clinician, and often multiple diagnoses are entertained and treated. For example, pneumonia and CHF are dually diagnosed and treated. The management often results in overuse of antibiotics; however, sometimes this tradeoff is necessary to avoid missing pneumonia.

The second step is to categorize patients based on the type of pneumonia. Patients suspected of pneumonia are stratified to community-acquired pneumonia (CAP) or healthcare-associated pneumonia (HCAP) as defined by 2007 CAP guidelines.[30] Included within healthcare-associated pneumonia stratification are nosocomial pneumonia transfers, recent hospital discharge, chronic care facility, assisted living facility, bed ridden, and or immunocompromised patients [30] It is also important to note that that 2007 CAP guidelines are not all inclusive and numerous patients with comorbidities have been excluded and may require further research and consideration for best treatment, such as those who are transplant recipients, those with lymphatic malignancies, neutropenic patients, patients on chemotherapy and high dose steroids for at least a month, and HIV-infected patients with CD4 <350 cells/mm^3.[30]

The EDP, consulting with infectious diseases, can expedite optimal therapies for these unique CAP patients and HCAP patients because more extensive histories must be obtained to distinguish accurately between CAP and HCAP; this has significance as HCAP patients may receive the wrong antibiotic and have higher rates of mortality as a result.[32] Furthermore, the patient with several acute diseases is at greater risk of mortality from pneumonia; therefore, greater vigilance is needed to treat these patients.

The third step of the protocol includes profiling for disease severity. Profiling includes an assessment of the initial clinical presentation using the mnemonic CURB-65 to assign whether the patient is mild, moderate, or severe. CURB-65 includes an assessment of mental status (confusion such as recent disorientation to person, place, or time); uremia (BUN of >20 mg/dL); respiratory rate (>30 breaths/min or greater); blood pressure (systolic of <90 mmHg or diastolic 60 mmHg or less); and age of 65 years and older. Initial vitals signs recorded by the paramedic should be used to profile the patient. CURB-65 scores of 0 or 1 are considered mild, and the patient should be sent home; a patient for whom CURB-65 = 2 is considered moderate and should be admitted to an inpatient medical ward unless the patient has severe sepsis or respiratory insufficiency; in which case, the patient should be admitted to the ICU; and a patient with CURB-65 >3 is also admitted to the ICU.[33]

Despite the use of profiling as a tool to predict the clinical management, Plouffe and Martin describe that patients with pneumonia who visit the ED typically present with fever, acute cough, with or without sputum production, dyspnea, tachypnea, or chest pain; however, many patients do not present with these classic symptoms, i.e., elderly may present with decreased mentation, patients may present hemodynamically unstable as sepsis and respiratory failure; thus, there is wide variation in presentation, which confounds precise and rapid diagnosis. Initial studies to obtain in the ED include pulse oximetry in all patients with a possible diagnosis of pneumonia. Patients with mild disease to be treated at home do not require additional workup. In the moderate to severely ill patient, laboratory studies should include blood urea nitrogen, CBC and differential, platelet count, and basic admission tests. In COPD patients, ABGs should be done as pulse oximetry is not adequate to define arterial CO_2 content. Urine antigen testing for legionella and pneumococci should be done for the more acute patients, this is not done routinely.

Debate surrounds the need for blood cultures as data suggest they have little impact on changing therapy, with the exception of ICU patients or patients admitted to the ward with multiple comorbid states as cultures do guide therapy in the patient with bacteremia. Current guidelines support obtaining blood cultures before antibiotics are initiated, and even if pretreated, to help identify resistant organisms. Lastly, as MRSA becomes more prevalent on skin infection, it is likely to become a more common cause of CAP, thus sputum gram stain may be an appropriate exam to use to detect it.[29]

ED pharmacists use drug, bug, and patient factors to assist in selecting the empiric antibiotics. For example, if the presenting patient is healthy with no antibiotics use within the past 3 months, a macrolide or doxycycline is considered the preferred choice unless the local geographic area has a resistant streptococcus pneumonia rate >25%, then, respiratory fluoroquinolones or beta lactams with a macrolide are suggested. A patient with underlying diseases and prior antibiotic use within the last 3 months should be given the same regimen as the healthy patient with resistant streptococcus pneumonia.[29] The antibiotic surveillance committee decided to preferentially use intravenous moxifloxacin for mild to moderate CAP, and within 48 hours, to streamline to oral therapy. The advantage of fluoroquinolone is the lack of risk of cross allergenicity with beta lactams. For patients with severe infections, we prefer the use of intravenous ceftriaxone with azithromycin; some suggest in addition a respiratory fluoroquinolone especially if the patient is admitted to the intensive care unit and has COPD to cover for pseudomonas aeruginosa. The severity may be assessed using the mnemonic CURB-65 as described a scoring system developed by the British Thoracic Society.[33]

RESULTS OF ID AND ED CLINICAL PHARMACY SERVICES ON CAP

After 3 months of the initial employment of the empiric antimicrobial request card, 231 restricted antimicrobial cards were sent to the pharmacy by the ED clinicians, with a 95% rate of compliance to the clinical infectious disease pathway recommended by the Antibiotic Surveillance Committee. After 2 years of implementation of the integrated ED–ID approval system and the CPOE CAP pathway, the quality of patient care has improved as demonstrated by a reduction in the average length of stay from

4.3 days pre ED-ID approval system to 3.34 days post ED-ID approval system.

Similar impact on pneumonia outcome has been reported with other institutions implementing pneumonia clinical pathways in the emergency department. In one report, the mean time to antibiotic administration decreased from 315 minutes pre-pathway to 175 minutes in the first post-pathway period (ANOVA p<0.0001). Furthermore, the length of stay was statistically significantly reduced from 9.7 days pre-pathway to 8.9 days for the first post-pathway period, and 6.4 days at 3 years (ANOVA p<0.0001).[34] Unique to our process improvement was the role that the ED clinical pharmacy service played.

The results of pneumonia care measures as they pertain to prevention are as follows; the percent of pneumonia patients assessed and given pneumococcal vaccination if appropriate was 94% (210 patients reviewed), which compares favorably to the United States average of 75% and local area hospital average of 78%. Furthermore 94% (35 patients reviewed) were given initial antibiotics within 6 hours after arrival if appropriate as compared with national averages of 93% and local area hospital average of 92%.[35]

SUMMARY

In summary, one route to facilitating acceptance of ED clinical pharmacy services can be through supporting the emergency department by assuring and expediting optimal infectious diseases pharmacotherapy. Important to the ED is early antibiotic administration for severe infections, such as septic shock, meningitis, and severe pneumonia. The EDP can assist in tailoring the therapy within the time interval required. The EDP can create a consult service within the ED, ensure continuity of care, and assist the antibiotic surveillance committee in development of guidelines. This process can be automated for ease of use into the ED-specific CPOE system. These processes implemented at our institution have helped achieve better than average quality of care measure.

References

1. Cuong J, Garbor K, Pronovost PJ. National study on the quality of emergency department care in the treatment of acute myocardial infarction and pneumonia. *JAEM* 2007;(10)856–863.
2. Freidman K, Kolluri B, Neudecker L. Antimicrobial stewardship stabilizes resistance patterns in a behavioral health setting. *Conn Med* 2007;71(8):457–460.
3. Fishman N. Antimicrobial stewardship. *Am J Med* 2006; 119(6): S53–S61; discussion S62–S70.
4. MacDougall C, Polk RE. Antimicrobial stewardship program in health care systems. *Clin Microbiol Rev* 2005;18(4): 638–656.
5. Owens RC Jr. Fraser GL, Stigsdill P. Society of Infectious Diseases Pharmacists. Antimicrobial stewardship programs as a means to optimize antimicrobial use. Insights from the Society of Infectious Diseases Pharmacists. *Pharmacotherapy* 2004; 24(7): 896–908.
6. Hand K. Antibiotic pharmacist in the ascendancy. *J Antimicrob Chemother* 2007;(60):73–76.

7. Deresinski S. Principles of antibiotic therapy in severe infections: optimizing the therapeutic approach by use of laboratory and clinical data. *Clin Infect Dis* 2007;45(Suppl 3):S177–83.
8. Pines JM, Hollander JE, DatnerEM, Metlay JP. Pay for performance for antibiotic timing in pneumonia caveat emptor. *Joint Comm J Qual Patient Safety.* 2006;32:531–535.
9. Specifications manual for national hospital quality measures, version 1.05. Centers for Medicare and Medicaid Services (CMS) Joint Commission on Accreditation of Healthcare Organizations(JCAHO). 2005. Available at: http:/www.quality net.org/dcs/ Accessed June 27, 2006.
10. Kahn CN, Ault T, Isenstein K et al. Snapshot of hospital quality reporting and pay-for-performance under Medicare. *Health Affairs* 2005;25:148–162.
11. Dellinger RP, Levy MM, Carlet JM, et al. Surviving Sepsis Campaign: international guidelines for management of severe sepsis and septic shock: 2008. *Crit Care Med* 2008;36(1): 296–327. Erratum in: *Crit Care Med* 2008; 36(4):1394–6.
12. Rivers E, Nguyen B, Havstad S, et al. Early goal-directed therapy in the treatment of severe sepsis and septic shock. *N Engl J Med* 2001;345:1368–1377.
13. Van de Beek D, de Gans J, Tunkel AR. Community-acquired bacterial meningitis in adults. *N Engl J Med* 2006;354: 44–53.
14. Pines JM, Hollander JE, Localio AR, Metlay JP. The association between ED crowding and hospital performance on antibiotic timing for pneumonia and percutaneous intervention for myocardial infarction. *Acad Emerg Med* 2006;13:873–878.
15. Thompson D. The pneumonia controversy: hospitals grapple with 4 hour benchmark. *Ann Emerg Med* 2006;47: 259–261.
16. Pines JM, Morton M, Datner EM, Hollander JE. Systematic delays in antibiotic administration for adult patients admitted with pneumonia. *Acad Emerg Med* 2006;13:939–945.
17. Pines JM. Profiles in patient safety: Antibiotic timing and pay for performance. *Acad Emerg Med* 2006;13:787–790.
18. Hans D, Kelly E, Wihelmson K, Katz ED. Rapidly fatal infections. *Emerg Med Clin North Am* 2008;26(2):259–279.
19. Paul M, Silbiger I, Grozinsky S, Soares-Wieser K, Leibovici L. Beta lactam antibiotic monotherapy versus beta-lactam –aminoglycoside antibiotic combination therapy for sepsis (Review). http://mrw.interscience.wiley.com/cochrane/clsysrev/ articles/CD003344/pdf_fs.html. Accessed November 2008.
20. Van de Beek D, de Gans J, McIntyre P, Prasad K. Corticosteroids for acute bacterial meningitis. *Cochrane Database Syst Rev* 2007;(1): CD004405.
21. Laupland KB, Davies HD, Low DE, et al. Invasive group A streptococcal disease in children and association with varicella zoster virus infection. Ontario Group A streptococcal study group. *Pediatrics* 2000;105:E60.
22. Schlievert PM, Kelly JA. Clindamycin-induced suppression of toxic shock syndrome: associated exotoxin production. *J Infect Dis* 1984;149:471.
23. Stevens DL, Wallace RJ, Hamilton SM, et al. Successful treatment of staphylococcal toxic shock syndrome with linezolid: a case report and in vitro evaluation of the production of toxic shock syndrome toxin type 1 in the presence of antibiotics. *Clin Infect Dis* 2006;42:729.
24. Zimbelman J, Palmer A, Todd J. Improved outcome of clindamycin compared with beta lactam antibiotic treatment for invasive Streptococcus pyogenes infection. *Pediatr Infect Dis J* 1999;18:1096.
25. Moran GJ, Krishnadasan A, Gorwitz RJ, et al. Methicillin–resistant S aureus infections among patients in the emergency department. *N Engl J Med* 2006;355:666.

26. Lina G, Piedmont Y, Godail-Gamot F, et al. Involvement of Panton-Valentine leukocidin producing Staphylococcus aureus in primary skin infections and pneumonia. *Clin Infect Dis* 1999; 29(5):1128–32.

27. Boyle-Varra S, Daum RS. Community-acquired methicillin-resistant Staphylococcus aureus: the role of Panton–Valentine leukocidin. *Lab Invest* 2007;87:3.

28. Norris DL II, Young JD. Urinary tract infections: Diagnosis and management in the emergency department. *Emerg Med Clin North Am* 2008;26(2):413–430.

29. Plouffe JF, Martin DR. Pneumonia in the emergency department. Emerg Med Clin North Am 2008;26(2): 389–411.

30. Mandell LA, Wunderink RG, Anzueto A, et al. Infectious Disease Society of America/American Thoracic Society consensus guidelines on the management of community-acquired pneumonia in adults. *Clin Infect Dis* 2005;40: 1288–97.

31. Rosh AJ, Newman DH. Diagnosing pneumonia by medical history and physical examination. *Ann Emerg Med* 2005; 46: 465–67.

32. Micek ST, Kollef KE, Reichley RM, et al. Healthcare associated pneumonia and community–acquired pneumonia: A single center experience. *Antimicrob Agents Chemother* 2007;51:3568–73.

33. WS, van der Eerden MM, Laing R et al. Defining community-acquired pneumonia severity on presentation to hospital: An international derivation and validation study. *Thorax* 2003; 58: 377–82.

34. Benenson R, Magalski A, Cavanaugh S, Williams E. Effects of a pneumonia clinical pathway on time to antibiotic treatment, length of stay and mortality. *Acad Emerg Med* 1999; 6(12):1243–1248.

35. Healthcare Cost and Utilization Project. The Agency for Healthcare Research and Quality. Available at: http://hcup. ahrq.gov/HCUPnet.asp. Accessed Jun 27, 2006.

13

Significance of Drug Interactions in the Emergency Department

Objectives

- Describe the challenges to prevent drug interactions in the emergency department (ED)
- Compare the ideal versus the Maimonides current process for drug interactions
- Discuss the need for a multi-modal approach to drug interaction surveillance
- Review both the safeguards and gaps in safety
- Explain the role of the ED pharmacist (EDP) to survey for drug interactions
- Expedite screening and interventions for potential drug interactions
- Elucidate knowledge translation of drug interactions and safe medication use practices
- Review drug interaction screening tools

The goal of this chapter is to demonstrate the need for a formal standardized multi-modal approach to screening and providing brief interventions as a means to quality assurance and prevention of drug interactions for patients treated in the ED.

DRUG INTERACTIONS IN THE ED

Drug interactions can cause potentially life-threatening or fatal events and permanent disability, and yet drug interactions are often the result of preventable medical errors.[1-4] The challenge in the practice of emergency medicine is to recognize pre-existing clinically relevant medication interactions and avoid introducing any new harmful drug interactions, while providing expedient medical care. This challenge requires knowledge of all drug therapies for which emergency physicians (EPs) are familiar and those that occur beyond their usual scope. This represents a significant challenge.

With more than 3200 prescription drugs, 600 herbal products, more than 300,000 over the counter (OTC) drugs, and new drugs released on a weekly basis in the United States, there may be over a trillion possible drug–drug, drug–herbal combinations and potential interactions.[5] Keeping current on the many pharmaceutical therapies, their pharmacology, and potential drug interactions represents one of the biggest challenges for emergency medicine practitioners and can seem overwhelming. Despite the overwhelming magnitude of potential drug combinations, only a few drug interactions are of life-threatening serious clinical consequence. Lack of continuing education on the risks of drug interactions further perpetuates the problem of physicians' understanding and prevention of drug interactions.

IDEAL VERSUS CURRENT SCREENING FOR DRUG INTERACTIONS IN THE ED

Because of the potential to cause adverse effects, healthcare providers should routinely evaluate patient's medication lists to identify and resolve drug interactions during each patient care encounter.[6] The clinical reality, however, is that few if any EPs have the time and training to systematically screen patients for drug interactions.[6] We suggest a multimodal approach to ensuring safety.

NEED FOR A MULTIMODAL APPROACH TO DRUG INTERACTION SURVEILLANCE

A multimodal approach to surveillance for at-risk drug interactions is needed. Medical errors are still occurring at an alarming rate and may be responsible for 44,000 to 98,000 patient deaths annually in the United States.[8] Drug interactions represent preventable sources of this morbidity in patient care. Because of polypharmacy and the magnitude of medications available, drug interactions along with drug-induced diseases should be considered a public health issue that requires cross-care setting surveillance to screen for, detect, treat, and prevent. Any weakness in the link may result in passage of drug interactions, morbidity, and mortality.

SAFEGUARDS AND GAPS IN SAFETY

EPs are aware of the need of preventive strategies to reduce the risk of clinically significant drug interactions. Limited formulary and unit-specific medication use reduces risk, as described in previous chapters, and the use of CPOE has been shown to outperform emergency medicine residency faculty and expert EPs in detecting drug interactions.[7] Technology provides a solution to detecting drug interactions in the ED. However new drug approvals and lag time for updates of the drug interaction database limit the usefulness in detecting drug interactions with treatment rendered in the ED.

Despite automation, drug interactions still occur as illustrated in the following case study. The case study illustrates that a full-proof strategy to detecting and preventing drug interactions eludes simplicity of automation.

In addition, the sheer lack of time to screen, ensure, and research the risk is overwhelming and attempting to manage the patient is difficult enough. Factors that contributed to this case of a life-threatening adverse drug event include: 1) less than optimal understanding of the patient's medication history, 2) an overcrowded ED that prevented the staff to fully attend to the patient's needs, and 3) the lack of recognition of the risk associated with treatment being rendered. Liability and financial risk associated with these types of drug interactions cost in the range of 20 to 127 million dollars.[9]

■ Case Study

Coronary Vasospasm Secondary to Sumatriptan Interaction

We experienced a case of subcutaneous sumatriptan-induced coronary vasospasm. Sumatriptan was administered for resolution of migraine pain to a patient with a vague history that may have contraindicated the triptans. The history included prior use of cocaine within the last month and recent use of escitalopram, both serotonin-releasing agents that increase the risk of a serotonin syndrome. Furthermore, no history was obtained to determine if the patient had taken an ergot or triptan within the last 24 hours. Although other treatments were not initiated and because the patient had a prescription in her hand for sumatriptan, the ED attending assumed that the primary care physician prescribed a triptan so he prescribed and administered a subcutaneous dose of sumatriptan. This patient required an emergency coronary angiography to rule out any subsequent damage. It was confirmed that the patient had clean arteries, but the patient did suffer a significant event that could have been life threatening.

With problems of overcrowding and the current frenetic nature of EDs, it is difficult for the EPs to study and assess the risk-benefit of drug therapy and to avoid all lethal combinations of medications in the ED. Furthermore, no full-proof successful strategies have been reported in the literature to ensure transparency and screening for all potential drug interactions within an ED setting. With 90,000 to 100,000 ED patient visits, an efficient strategy must be used to screen against drug interactions to fill gaps that may serendipitously arise. Thus, a multimodal system comprised of both automation and human interface is needed.

SURVEYING FOR DRUG INTERACTIONS: ROLE AND RATIONALE FOR ED PHARMACIST

The ED pharmacist assumes the role of screening for drug interactions to detect whether a drug is the cause of an ED visit, to assist with identifying the etiology of presentation, and to help with management. The EDP will also try to prevent drug interactions that may occur when prescribing a drug given via the parenteral route to an unstable patient because this may lead to a potentially catastrophic event. For example, recent use of sildenafil (Viagra®) within the last 24 hours with administration of IV nitroglycerin in a patient with chest pain or acute pulmonary edema is ominous.

As part of a comprehensive surveillance plan the EDP works with the Drug Abuse Warning Network (DAWN),[9] registry sponsored by Substance Abuse and Mental Health Services Administration (SAMSHA) of the United States Department of Health and Human Services, to provide community awareness and education on drug use and inappropriate prescribing as a means of prevention.

Maimonides ED provides charts to the DAWN registry to assess cases for drug-related visits; this includes drug interactions.

Based on a sampling of charts from 2006 to 2008, 2.2% of all the visits to the emergency department per year were classified as Drug Abuse Warning Network (DAWN) cases as seen in Figure 13-1.

The etiology of these cases are reviewed, and education activities are provided to the medical and emergency staff. A DAWN case is defined as any of the following types of visits in which a DAWN substance is involved; suicide attempts seeking detoxification, under 21 years old alcohol abuse, adverse reactions to medication (both OTC and prescription), overmedication, malicious poisoning, accidental ingestion, or abuse of illegal drugs. These data have quality improvement implications by providing community awareness and education on drug use and inappropriate prescribing as a means of prevention.

Similar to other public health efforts, such as smoking cessation and substance abuse screening, there is a role for medication error prevention through drug interaction screening. Drug-induced causes of disease may go misdiagnosed or be inappropriately treated. Currently, no acceptable means of ensuring drug screening and intervention exists because this goes beyond the scope of emergency care and enters into public health or primary care. As a result, the EDP fills this gap.

The role of the EDP is to survey and anticipate for drug–drug, drug–disease interactions that are introduced by

RAW COUNTS OF DATA REVIEWED AND COLLECTED FOR DAWN 2006/2007

Month	Charts Reviewed	DAWN Cases Identified
January	7291	165
February	6382	168
March	7166	149
April	7141	161
May	4929	133
June	4671	153
July	4777	122
August	4380	83
September	4632	113
October	4908	137
November	2840	70
December	0	0
Total	59117	1454

RAW COUNTS OF DATA REVIEWED AND COLLECTED FOR DAWN 2007

Month	Charts Reviewed	DAWN Cases Identified
January	5817	149
February	5078	136
March	5585	155
April	5163	167
May	6045	114
June	5425	106
July	5383	105
August	3684	66
September	3806	62
October	3567	51
November	3825	58
December	4065	109
Total	57443	1278

RAW COUNTS OF DATA REVIEWED AND COLLECTED FOR DAWN 2008

Month	Charts Reviewed	DAWN Cases Identified
January	7857	167
February	7720	181
March	8125	219
April	7683	224
May	8333	215
June	6856	217
July	5972	190
August	5904	187
September	6283	164
October	6096	168
November	6235	186
December	335	14
Total	77399	2132

Figure 13–1. Drug Abuse Warning Network (DAWN) cases presenting to the ED in 2006 to 2008.

new treatments given in the ED by an EP. The EP or specialist may be unfamiliar with the patient, prescribe a medication that may interact with one medication the patient has recently taken upon arrival, or interact with the patient's underlying co-morbidities. This screening also can unmask a drug- induced visit, as experienced in the case of a patient who had serotonin syndrome but it was diagnosed as sepsis.

It is unlikely that this event would have been caught with automation alone. The initial impression of the case was sepsis, and antimicrobial agents were prescribed. Instead, the EDP recommended the use of dantrolene intravenously, and as a result, the patient's clonus and rigidity improved. Antibiotics were discontinued, and the patient was provided supportive care to improve symptoms of serotonin syndrome. The patient subsequently recovered.

Pharmacists attempting to implement the structure to provide this service often ask how can I efficiently help reduce the risk of a significant drug interaction in the ED with all the other responsibilities that they may have clinically?

■ Case Study

Serotonin Syndrome Unmasked

Broad spectrum antibiotics were prescribed for this 75-year-old male who presented with an altered mental status, tremors, and clonus.

The EDP conducted a medication history and recognized that the patient was taking a selective MAO-inhibitor (selegiline), amantadine, and a selective serotonin reuptake inhibitor, all of which may exacerbate a serotonin syndrome.

The EDP recognized this cluster of symtoms as part of the serotonin or neuroleptic malignant syndrome and warned the physician.

Subsequently, antidotal therapy such as dantrolene was initiated and appeared to reduce the tremors and movements, and the EP was convinced.

The patient was admitted to the MICU with a diagnosis of serotonin syndrome instead of the initial diagnosis of sepsis and recovered without being given unnecessary antibiotics.

DEVELOPING AN EFFICIENT SCREENING AND INTERVENTION PROGRAM TO PREVENT DRUG INTERACTIONS

Several factors were identified that increase the risk for drug interactions and were used to identify who may be benefit for screening and brief intervention by a pharmacotherapist (Fig. 13-2).

These factors include older age, taking three or more medications, taking medications with a narrow therapeutic index, or that require therapeutic drug monitoring.[6] Several medications appear to have greatest risk for drug interactions and include warfarin (anticoagulants), digoxin, aspirin, NSAIDS, antibiotics, opioid analgesics, benzodiazepines, antacids, and

---

Name   **Vital signs: HR_____BP_____RR_____SPO2_____FBS_____**

Does patient meet criteria: Yes   No

- Patient >60 years of age
- Patient taking three or more medications
- Patient taking NSAIDS, opioids, ABX, anticoagulants

Screen for potential drug interactions

Circle all of the following medications the patient may be taking:

CYP 450 inhibitors	Serotonin Syndrome medications	Hyperkalemia Drugs	Drugs that Prolong the QT interval
1. Allopurinol	**a. MAOI**	1. Amiloride	**a. Antiarrhythmics**
2. Amiodarone	1. Phenelzine	2. ACE Inhibitors	1. Amiodarone
3. Cimetidine	(Nardil)	3. Beta Blockers	2. Disopyramide
4. Ciprofloxacin	2. Tranylcypromine	4. Cyclosporine	3. Procainamide
5. Clarithromycin	3. Selegiline	5. Digoxin	4. Quinidine
6. Diltiazem	4. Moclobemide	6. Heparin	**b. Quinolones**
7. Erythromycin	5. Isocarboxazid	7. NSAIDS	5. Gatifloxacin
8. Fluconazole	6. Pargyline	8. Penicillin G	6. Levofloxacin
9. Fluoxetine	7. Brofaromine	Potassium	7. Moxifloxacin
10. Indinavir	**b. TCAs**	Infusion	8. Sparfloxacin
11. Isoniazid	8. Amitriptyline	9. Spironolactone	**c. TCA**
12. Itraconazole	9. Clomipramine	10. Succinylcholine	9. Amitriptyline
13. Ketoconazole	10. Imipramine	11. Triamterene	10. Desipramine
14. Metronidazole	11. Nortriptyline	12. Trimethoprim	11. Imipramine
15. Omeprazole	**c. Atypical**		**d. Antidepressants**
16. Paroxetine	**antidepressants**		12. Fluvoxamine
17. Propoxyphene	12. Mirtazapine		13. Nefazodone
18. Quinidine	13. Trazodone		**e. Antipsychotics**
19. Sulfonamides	14. Venlafaxine		14. Droperidol
20. Verapamil	**d. Selective serotonin**		15. Haloperidol
	uptake inhibitor		16. Pimozide
	15. Citalopram		17. Thioridazine
Warfarin	16. Fluoxetine		18. Ziprasidone
	17. Fluvoxamine		**f. P-450 inhibitors**
	18. Paroxetine		19. Macrolides
	19. Sertraline		20. Azole antifungals
	e. Atypical		**g. Protease**
	antipsychotics		**inhibitors**
	1. Risperidone		21. Delavirdine
	2. Olanzapine		22. Indinavir
	3. Lithium		23. Saquinavir
	g. Illicit Drugs		24. Nelfinavir
	1. Cocaine		25. Ritonavir
	2. MDMA		**h. Calcium channel**
			blockers
			26. Diltiazem
			27. Verapamil

Figure 13–2. Drug interaction screening and brief intervention form completed during prospective review.

diuretics. Patients with these factors require a proactive screen and evaluation for drug interactions.[11–12] To be efficient, we use these criteria to identify who is in need of screening. Furthermore, any specialist-consultant prescribed medications in the ED require a review for drug interaction by the EDP.

THE EVALUATION

The evaluation includes conducting a medication history, a risk assessment for drug interactions, and a counseling recommendations to the caregiver or the patient. Although medication histories are obtained by a nurse at triage (Fig. 13-3), they are imprecise, incomplete, and only obtain a list without the dose, route, frequency and last day and time taken.

In a study we conducted at our facility, we demonstrated that medication histories upon EP diagnostic and therapeutic intervention are only complete 13% of the time, and that what is listed in the physician and pharmacy medication profile and what the patient tells you they are taking varies significantly.[13]

An additional medication history is taken by the ED attending (not routinely documented), and it is targeted based on the presentation. Thus, cognitive recognition of risk may not occur if it is unrelated to the presentation. If the medication history does not apply to the presenting symptoms, it is no longer considered clinically relevant. An acutely ill patient may not remember all of his medications upon initial presentation so a more complete medication history including dose, route, frequency, consumption of OTC and herbal products is conducted, perhaps at multiple times to obtain the most precise data from multiple sources. This data is then used to quickly screen for risk and weigh the benefit of therapies during emergency care. The pharmacotherapist will intervene when necessary when the risk-benefit ratio is not favorable for emergency care and provide an alternative approach. This approach is provided when medications are prescribed by the EP or specialist and for outpatient prescriptions for those patients treated and released.

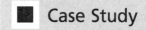

Case Study

Metformin and Elevated Serum Creatinine

A diabetic patient visited the ED because of failure to fill his antidiabetic medications. The ED physicians elected to start metformin. The ED pharmacist identified that the patient's serum creatinine was 1.6 mg/dL and that metformin was contraindicated. The physician was notified, and alternative therapy was recommended and prescribed.

EDUCATION AND KNOWLEDGE TRANSLATION OF SAFE MEDICATION USE PRACTICES

The EDP should also educate new EPs to avoid initiating any nonessential prescriptions, especially in high risk patients, such as the elderly who may be taking multiple medications. EPs are guilty of prescribing for minor symptom relief for conditions without adequate indication because of the perception that this is the patient's expectation; when in fact, providing education, reassurance, and nonpharmacologic interventions has been shown to be more satisfying to the patient.[14] As part of the brief intervention, the pharmacotherapist may provide counseling and reassurances that would help avoid administration of unnecessary therapies.

Except in certain situations where high doses may be required, low doses of medication should be used for high risk patients. Despite differences in old and young individuals, in pharmacokinetic studies for many medications, manufacturer-recommended doses are the same. Many studies have shown clinical effectiveness of low-dose therapy, and this may prevent drug complications in selected patients. Only one high, or

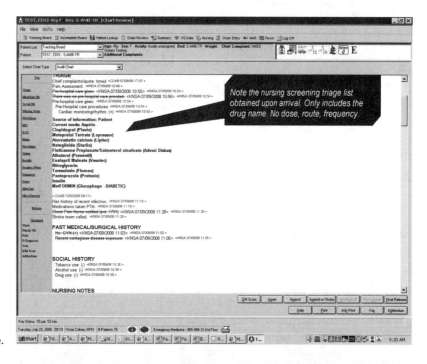

Figure 13–3. Medication list obtained at triage.

even perceived, normal therapeutic dose may induce an adverse drug event and disrupt normal operations in the ED.

DRUG INTERACTION RESOURCES AND RISK ASSESSMENT TOOL

Resources for conducting a risk assessment for drug interactions to the EDP include: a drug interaction handbook (Facts and Comparsions®), PDA software or an intranet site with a drug interaction calculator, such as MicroMedex® or Lexi-comp®. No reference exists that is precise at identifying emergency care drug interactions. References may help identify the risk of the drug interaction and the subsequent management. To expedite risk assessment, an efficient clinical operation must be designed and in place to optimize screening and interventions for drug interactions.

We have employed an efficient screening and evaluation tool for the purpose of screening for life threatening drug interactions. We introduced this form earlier in Chapter 11 as part of a process for prospective review of medication orders as seen in Figure 13-4. This form includes a brief screening form that reviews the patient's medications, highlights those taken within the last 12 hours, the current patient problem, and treatment that is to be rendered in the ED. An assessment for potential interactions that are likely based on treatment rendered in the ED or transition points are recorded and flagged for pharmacovigilance. In addition, assessment of appropriate transcription, dose optimization, and any co-morbid condition that precludes the use of any of the medications used

is highlighted. Management considerations are documented as needed to warn the clinician.

Screening criteria with a list of medications that are associated with life-threatening drug interactions, which may require emergency care, are provided on the back page of this form, and include medications that are potent cytochrome P450 inhibitors, warfarin, agents associated with serotonin syndrome, medications associated with hyperkalemia, drugs that prolong the QT interval (Fig. 13-2). The EDP uses this tool to further expedite the screening process. These tools permit the pharmacotherapist to immediately triage and prioritize those patients who may be at risk of clinically relevant drug interactions. The EDP will conduct this activity as part of a global pharmaceutical care approach to emergency care and the subsequent transitions. The experienced pharmacotherapist is likely to cognitively perform these functions without the documentation; however, it is essential to provide a sampling of risk, near misses, and actual interactions prevented and report these findings as part of quality improvement initiatives.

BARRIER TO ACCEPTANCE: WHAT WE DON'T KNOW, WE CAN'T FIX

Unfortunately, even with enhanced surveillance, risks for drug interactions still exist. The most significant problem with preventing drug interactions is that we do not know the extent or scope of the problem. The true overall incidence of clinically relevant drug interactions that present to the ED or result from medications administered in the ED is unknown. Epidemiology is lacking because most drug interactions go undetected or unreported by patients and clinicians for a va-

Patient Name JJ   MR# 123456   EP   Dr. D   CC: Chest pain   DX: Pending   CRCL:Pending   Ht 5'6"   ABW   85 kg

Medication History Upon Arrival	Taken Within 12 hours of Visit to ED	Patient–Problem Indication	Treatment to Be Rendered in ED	Medication Transcribed Correctly	Dose Is Optimized	Any Conflict with Active Co-morbid States	DI	Management
Metoprolol	Yes (No)	*Chest Pain*	*Aspirin 81 mg Chewable Po Stat x 1*	(Yes) No	Yes (No) *Change to 162-324 mg*	Yes (No)	Yes (No)	*Cancel initial ASA order Re-enter ASA with correct dose*
Aspirin	Yes (No)			Yes No	Yes No	Yes No	Yes No	
	Yes No			Yes No	Yes No	Yes No	Yes No	
	Yes No			Yes No	Yes No	Yes No	Yes No	
	Yes No			Yes No	Yes No	Yes No	Yes No	
	Yes No			Yes No	Yes No	Yes No	Yes No	
	Yes No			Yes No	Yes No	Yes No	Yes No	

Academic Prescription:	*What is the importance of aspirin dosing during acute chest pain in the ED?*

Figure 13–4. Pharmacotherapy prospective review: Screening and brief intervention form.

riety of reasons.[15–17] The clinical manifestations of drug interactions can be misdiagnosed easily andattributed erroneously to the worsening of a patient's underlying condition or new illness.[18] Frequently, there is a time lag before the development of serious consequences of drug interactions. In other cases, causality may be doubted despite multiple case reports because formal studies are unable to prove a drug interaction definitively.

Currently, 100 million patients visit the ED each year in the US. Half of these patients have one or more drug interactions from pre-existing medications. Studies of clinically relevant interactions that result from ED-initiated medications vary in reported incidence from 31–50%.[6,7,12,18] To improve the safeguards, a targeted prospective review of a medication order can avoid a potential lethal interaction, identify a drug-induced consequence that caused the visit, and permit management accordingly. These unknowns alone rationalize the need for pharmacist activity in the ED to assure transparency and to grade the institution on their quality assurance based on the frequency of drug interactions averted, detected, managed, and prevented. A no-tolerance threshold to drug interactions should be the standard.

PROSPECTIVE REVIEW OF MEDICATIONS: ENHANCED PHARMACOVIGILANCE

With current TJC mandates that require a prospective review of medication orders still looming, i.e., MM.4.10, pharmacists will be required to evaluate risk for drug interactions in ED patients. We have described the risk of drug interactions in emergency medicine and discussed ways to make a screening process efficient and practical. Pharmacists should be seen as expeditors of emergency care because they permit speedy verification of medication orders.

SUMMARY

In summary a practical, targeted, approach to drug interaction surveillance and monitoring will prevent delays in treatment and permit for necessary safeguards. Risk of drug interactions have too many unknowns and are too vast a problem to be left to technology alone or a highly skilled practitioner who has enough on his plate. Due diligence is needed to prevent any harm, and the EDP can and must provide these services because it is part of the Hippocratic oath to "first, do no harm."

References

1. Kelly W. Potential risks and prevention: Part 1. Fatal adverse drug events. *Am J Health-Syst Pharm* 2001;58: 1317–1324.
2. Kelly W. Potential risks and prevention: Part 2. Fatal adverse drug events. *Am J Health-Syst Pharm* 2001;58: 1325–9.
3. Leape LL Brennan TA, Laird N, et al. The nature of adverse events in hospitalized patients results of the Harvard medical practice study II. *N Engl J Med* 1991;324:377–84.
4. Juulink DN, Mamdani M, Kopp A, Laupacis A, Redelmeier DA. Drug-drug interactions among elderly patients hospitalized for drug toxicity. *JAMA* 2003;289:1652–8.
5. Prybys KM. Deadly drug interactions in emergency medicine. *Emerg Med Clin North Am* 2004;22:845–863.
6. Gaddis GM, Holt R, Woods M. Drug interactions in at-risk emergency department patients. *Acad Emerg Med* 2002; (11): 1162–1167.
7. Langdorf ML, Fox JC, Marwah RS, Montague BJ, Hart MM. Physician versus computer knowledge of potential drug interactions in the emergency department. *Acad Emerg Med* 2000; 7(11):1321–1329.
8. Kohn LT, Corrigan JM, Donaldson MS (eds). *To Err Is Human. Building a Safer Health-System.* Report of the Institute of Medicine. Washington, DC: National Academy Press, 1999.
9. United States Department of Health and Human Services, Substance Abuse and Mental Health Services Administration. Drug Abuse Warning Network Hospital specific report available from restricted site: https://restricted.dawninfo.net/ login.asp
10. Burt CW, McCraig LF. Trends in hospital emergency department utilization: United States 1992–1999. National Center for Health Statistics. *Vital Health Stat* 2001; 13:150.
11. Holl CM, Dnakoff J, Colacone A, Afialo M. Polypharmacy, adverse drug-related events, and potential adverse drug interactions in elderly patients presenting to an emergency department. *Ann Emerg Med* 2001;38: 666–671.
12. Beers MH, Storrie M, Lee G. Potential adverse drug interactions in the emergency room. *Ann Intern Med* 1990;112: 61–64.
13. Cohen V Jellinek SP, Lkourezos A, Nemeth I, Paul T, Murphy D. Variation in the medication information for elderly patients during initial interventions by emergency department physicians. *Am J Health-Syst Pharm* 2008;65: 60–64.
14. Von Feber L, Koster I, Pruss U. Patient variables with expectations for prescription and general practitioners' prescribing behavior: an observation study. *Pharmacoepidemiol Drug Safe* 2002;11:291–9.
15. Figueiras A, Tato F, Fontainas J, Takkouche B, Gestal-Otero JJ. Physician attitudes towards voluntary reporting of adverse drug events. *J Eval Clin Pract* 2001;7:347–354.
16. Chyka PA, McCommon SW. Reporting adverse drug reactions by poison control centers in the US. *Drug Safe* 2001; 23:87–93.
17. ISMP surveys show weaknesses persist in hospital systems for error detection, reporting, and analysis. *ISMP Med Safety Alert* 2000;5(2).
18. Gaeta T, Fiorini M, Ender K, Bove J, Diaz J. Potential drug-drug interactions in elderly patients presenting with syncope. *J Environ Monit* 2002;22:159–162.
19. Goldberg RM, Mabee J, Chan L, Wong S. Drug-drug and drug disease interactions in the ED analysis of a high risk population. *Am J Emerg Med* 1996;14:44.

14

Responding to Toxicologic and Public Health Emergencies

Objectives
- Describe the risk associated with antidote use
- Describe effectiveness of an ED pharmacist (EDP) in toxicologic emergencies
- Review how to ensure adequate storage and access to antidotes in the ED
- Describe ED pharmacist activities, knowledge, and skills in toxicologic emergencies
- Describe safe and effective antidote use of N-acetylcysteine, calcium, glucagon, Digifab or Digibind, cyanide antidote, ethanol solution and fomepizole, flumazenil, methylene blue, and naloxone hydrochloride.
- Introduce public health emergencies and disaster preparedness
- Describe current role of public health and its evolution
- Compare and contrast public health and emergency medicine
- Describe public health and pharmaceutical care
- Explain role of the ED pharmacist in public health emergencies
- Review past and current roles of the ED pharmacist during response and recovery for the community and institution

In this chapter, we describe published reports of the EDPs role in toxicologic emergencies and in public health emergencies.

This chapter provides practical cases of types of error that can occur in the evaluation and management of various toxicologic scenarios and discusses the role of pharmacists in screening for risk of toxicologic emergencies, describing regulatory expectations with use and storage of antidotes, and providing tools to ensure safe and effective use of antidotes while attending initial acute stabilization at the bedside within the ED.

RISK ASSOCIATED WITH ANTIDOTE USE

Despite their life-saving potential and reputation of being innocuous, antidotes, if used in error, can have devastating consequences similar to other high risk medications. Brown and colleagues reported on three deaths resulting from hypocalcemia after administration of edetate disodium (Na_2EDTA). The deaths occurred in a 2-year-old girl who had an elevated blood lead level, a 5-year-old boy with autism, and a 53-year-old woman as part of naturopathic treatment. In all three cases, despite administration of calcium chloride or gluconate, the patients were unable to be resuscitated, and postmortem exams concluded that the deaths were attributable to hypocalcemia secondary to chelation therapy.[1] Authors concluded that the look-alike and sound-alike similarities in edetate disodium formulations may have been the cause of these deaths.[1] The use of Na_2EDTA is recommended as a second or third line agent for patients with hypercalcemia and is known to reduce calcium levels; however, other chelation formulations, such as calcium disodium versenate ($CaNa_2EDTA$), succimer, dimercaprol, and penicillamine are not associated with hypocalcemia and are currently the mainstay of therapy for chelation therapy in children with blood lead levels of ≥ 45 mcg/dL and for symptomatic adults. As per an audit of these charts, the varying formulations of EDTA that exist were written in the chart interchangeably, and it was suggested that Na_2EDTA may have been administered instead of safer chelators.[1] The authors concluded that healthcare providers and pharmacists should ensure that Na_2EDTA is never administered to children during chelation therapy and that a formulary review of Na_2EDTA and its need should be re-evaluated.[1]

In a case series of two paracetamol (acetaminophen) overdoses, a 73-year-old woman transferred to the intensive care unit for investigation and management of coma and suspected overdose had a paracetamol level of 410 mg/dL. Intravenous N-acetylcysteine (NAC) was prescribed; however, erroneously only 10% of the recommended intravenous dose was written for each of the infusion bags, i.e. 1200-mg loading dose instead of 12,000 mg, followed by 400 mg instead of 4,000 mg in the first infusion, followed by 800 mg instead of 8000 mg for the second infusion. The error was not detected until 40 hours after presentation. The correct dose finally did commence, and the patient recovered. In another case, a 28-year-old woman presented to the hospital within 30 minutes of ingestion of 35 grams of paracetamol and had a 4-hour level of 362 mg/dL. Intravenous NAC was started within 5 hours after ingestion.[2] With the INR and ALT at baseline being normal, the NAC infusion was discontinued after 20 hours. However, by 48 hours after ingestion, the patient INR increased to 3.4 and the ALT level rose to 9540 IU/L. Review of the medical chart revealed an error in dosing in which 10% of the normally recommended dose was administered (900 mg, 300 mg, and 600 mg as opposed to 9000 mg, 3000 mg, and 6000 mg of IV NAC). Standard doses were initiated 80 hours post ingestion, and the patient subsequently recovered. These cases illustrate the need for categorization of antidotes as high-alert medications, not for their inherent risk of toxicity, but for their mis-use as a cause for morbidity. Accordingly as for any high-alert medication, steps to minimize risk associated with their use must be taken.[2]

Recommended steps to minimize risk of other high-alert medications include 1) stock these agents in a limited number of areas, 2) store separately in the pharmacy, 3) provide in standard concentrations and when available have product formulation warning labels on the vials, 4) have additional drug preparation verification, 5) and require continual close monitoring.[3] Because of their infrequent use, less attention may be paid to the high-risk nature of the antidotes, and as a result, these precautions may not be taken. The EDP should put enhanced processes in place that ensure safe, effective use and continuity of antidotes while expediting their use within the ED.[3]

EFFECTIVENESS OF ED PHARMACISTS IN TOXICOLOGIC EMERGENCIES

Published reports describe pharmacists diversifying into hospitals to provide service in toxicology.[4] Poison control centers are directed and serviced by pharmacists. There are also published reports of pharmacists providing toxicology consultations, participating in the management of incidents involving hazardous materials, and responding to episodes of terrorism.[4–5]

Czajka et al. reports that pharmacists provide three basic services in conjunction with poisonings treated by the emergency department. First, they assist with obtaining the history and assessment of the toxicologic problem; second, they assist with recommending a plan for rational management; and third they provide poison prevention strategies to

parents of the victim in the case of accidental exposures in children.[4]

Czajka reported that 90% of the ED nurses and physicians strongly agreed that the pharmacist made suggestions for improving patient care, provided practical and useful information, exerted a beneficial effect on patient care, and understood his or her role and responsibility. Other descriptive reports have included similar accounts of pharmacists providing toxicologic support while stationed within the ED.[4]

ENSURING ADEQUATE QUANTITIES, STORAGE, AND ACCESSIBILITY OF ANTIDOTES FOR THE ED

First, the EDP must assure that antidotes are available and accessible to the emergency care staff when needed because under-stocking of antidotes has been reported as a problem throughout the United States.[6–9] Besides the clinical role in toxicologic emergencies, the pharmacist must ensure that the hospital pharmacy stock adequate amounts of poisoning antidotes in one immediately accessible location.[6] Reports have found that some antidotes were not stocked at all, some in insufficient quantities, and some antidotes were stored in disparate locations distant from the ED and often difficult to find. The EDP must ensure adequate antidote supplies and appropriate securing and accessibility. A consensus report released by poison control centers recommends a minimum storage of at least 16 antidotes in sufficient supply as seen in the Table 14-1.[10]

TABLE 14-1

Antidotes That Should Be Available and Stored by Hospital Pharmacies

- N-Acetylcysteine (NAC)(10 vials)
- Antivenin (1 vial)
- Atropine (150 mg)
- Calcium (200 mEq) (Chloride IV and Gluconate)
- Cyanide kit (2 kits)
- Deferoxamine (8.4 grams)
- Digifab (15 vials)
- Dimercaprol (280 mg)
- Ethanol solution(100% 181.4 ml absolute alcohol)
- Fomepizole (2.1 grams)
- Glucagon (50 mg)
- Methylene Blue (280 mg)
- Naloxone (30 mg)
- 2Pam (2 grams)
- Pyridoxine (10 grams)
- Na Bicarbonate (500 mEq)

Adapted from Dart RC, Goldfrank LR, Chyka PA, et al. Combined Evidence-Based Literature Analysis and Consensus Guideline for Stocking of Emergency Antidotes in the United States. *Ann Emerg Med* 2000;36(2):126–132.

Antidote	Recommended Par Level	Current Par Level	Storage Location
N-Acetylcysteine (NAC)	10 vials		
Antivenin	1 vial		
Atropine	150 mg		
Calcium (Chloride(IV) and Gluconate)	200 mEq		
Cyanide kit	2 kits		
Deferoxamine	8.4 grams		
Digifab	15 vials		
Dimercaprol	280 mg		
Ethanol solution(100%)	181.4 ml absolute alcohol		
Fomepizole	2.1 grams		
Glucagon	50 mg		
Methylene Blue	280 mg		
Naloxone	30 mg		
2Pam	2 grams		
Pyridoxine	10 grams		
Na Bicarbonate	500 mEq		

Figure 14-1. Antidote monthly inventory verification record.

We have assured these quantities are available using a monthly inventory sheet (Fig. 14-1) with the location, date of most recent expiration and amount that is expected to be on hand.

Monthly we conduct an antidote quantity check to assure we are in compliance with current guidelines. Several antidotes are stored in the ED, such as naloxone, flumazenil, glucagon, calcium and atropine, and sodium bicarbonate, because they are dual-purpose agents used during cardiac arrest and they may be needed in rapid response. The remaining antidotes require request from central pharmacy. Although this may be perceived as increasing the risk for delay to management, the EDP who responds to the toxicologic emergency expedites the acquisition of the antidote upon anticipation of its need during acute stabilization. Subsequently, the pharmacist has the opportunity to ensure optimization of management of the toxicologic emergency.

ED PHARMACIST ACTIVITIES, KNOWLEDGE, AND SKILLS IN TOXICOLOGIC EMERGENCIES

Our participation in managing toxicologic emergencies includes assisting with the assessment and confirming the likelihood of the suspected poison. The EDP is involved in the application of the knowledge of toxidromes; profiling the signs, symptoms, laboratory values, and diagnostics to confirm the toxicologic emergency and the correct indication for the antidote. The EDPs responsibility is to ensure appropri-

ate use of scarcely available, rarely used, and highly expensive antidotal therapies. EDPs are usually involved in the management of the complete antidote-medication use process, including the prescribing, emergent acquisition, procurement, administration, and monitoring. In addition, we assist with decontamination procedures. Often, we are consulted to apply toxicokinetics and toxicodynamics to determine the subsequent disposition of the patient and for how long until the toxin is to be eliminated. We also engage in public health considerations if an event requires reporting.

Mastery of the practicalities of the clinical use of these antidotes, how they are available (what dose strength and form), how to prepare them, and at what rate to administer them, their indication, contraindications, appropriate selection, precautions, dosing, and what to monitor for is essential knowledge that the EDP must provide at the bedside for the clinicians to provide optimal management and disposition in the emergency care setting. Furthermore, new antidotes are constantly emerging, and because these antidotes are usually recommended based on minimal data, it is essential to stay current and assist with initiating emerging antidotal therapies.

The EDP who is collaborating on a toxicology case should have proficiency in the most salient and essential features associated with the at the bedside use of antidotes and management of the associated toxidromes. This multidisciplinary collaboration between the emergency care providers can fill gaps in knowledge of the general emergency care physician and nurses on the nuances of the use of the antidotes and facilitates rapid decision making and implementation of antidote use at the bedside. The pharmacotherapist who can multitask kinesthetically enables successful optimization of care for toxicologic emergencies.

ASSURING SAFE AND EFFECTIVE ANTIDOTE USE IN THE ED

This review is based on a fusion of evidence-based medicine and practical observations and is not meant to be a full in-depth discussion on toxicologic management. This section presents the information that we have observed as to the logistical and operational considerations in using select antidotes and common misuses or problems with the antidotes. This section identifies clinical pearls that the EDP should be aware of when managing toxicologic emergencies. For a more comprehensive evidence-based review of antidotes and the associated toxidromes, we recommend the use of various references.[11-12]

In this section, we provide examples of 1) errors in diagnosis and antidote use occurring from attempting to rapidly manage the patient, 2) a cognitive process that the EDP conducts to rationalize the antidote use or recommend alternatives, and 3) possible interventions that can be made by the EDP during toxicologic emergencies. The EDP performs multiple cognitive tasks that include a review of the antidotes indication, contraindications, appropriate selection as it pertains to avoiding misuse due to diagnostic error or consideration for alternative formulations, at what dose to prepare and how to prepare, what potential toxicity may occur, and drug interactions that may be likely. In addition, the EDP provides reassurances to the patient during the episode and provides follows-up.

N-ACETYLCYSTEINE

N-acetylcysteine is indicated for symptomatic patients who ingested >150 mg/kg of acetaminophen, available in the oral, intravenous, and compounded formulations or if a serum acetaminophen blood level 4 hours from time of ingestion is plotted on the Rumack-Mathews nomogram and falls above the estimated toxicity line.

Peak-time efficiency routines that are performed by clinicians to manage the supply and demand for emergency care may obscure the correct diagnosis, resulting in overuse of the antidote and has further implications associated with risk of adverse events in the non-toxic patient. Errors occur in the assessment and interpretation of the acetaminophen level. Blood samples taken upon acute stabilization and without concern for time since ingestion results in erroneous interpretation of the serum level.

Overuse is caused by the imprecise and often inaccurate accounts of information on the severity of the ingestion; empiric administration of intravenous n-acetylcysteine is prescribed, even more so because of the availability and convenience of the intravenous form of n-acetylcysteine, and this may result in overuse and potential toxicity.

The EDP cognitively assesses if there are any contraindications associated with use of n-acetylcysteine. Other than prior known history of hypersensitivity to acetylcysteine resulting in anaphylaxis, of which prior knowledge of such an allergy history is unlikely, there are no absolute contraindications to its use. The selection of the optimal dosage form is often an area for the EDP to assist. The oral formulation is less tolerable and requires significantly more at-the-bedside nursing attention. Due to its putrid odor and difficult taste to mask, oral acetylcysteine is considered unpalatable, and patient compliance becomes an issue.[13] Many patients often have nausea and vomiting after the administration of oral acetylcysteine despite pretreatment with metoclopramide or ondansetron. This potential for delay in administration is of concern because of the importance of the therapeutic window of 8 to 10 hours from time of ingestion, when acetylcysteine is most effective in reducing risk of hepatotoxicity. These time delay risks may rationalize to some clinicians the use of a more expensive intravenous formulation despite its greater time to extemporaneous preparation.[13]

However, even more significant concerns for the intravenous formulation have been reported and include risk of anaphylaxis or anaphylactoid reactions. Patients with asthma or status epilepticus are at greater risk of these adverse events; these adverse events have only been reported with the intravenous formulation, not the oral preparation.[13]

Pharmacokinetics may also be an issue for the pharmacist to evaluate. Significant debate suggests that oral acetylcysteine, because it undergoes significant first-pass metabolism, reaches the liver where the intravenous formulation bypasses the liver. This suggests a theoretic benefit of the oral formulation over the intravenous formulation. In clinical studies, when the oral route is tolerated, either the oral or the intravenous dose form appears to be equally effective when given within 8–10 hours. Perry and Shannon compared a 52-hour intravenous acetylcysteine protocol to that of a historical control group who received conventional oral NAC (140 mg/kg load and then 70 mg/kg maintenance dose every 4 hours for 72 hours), with the mean time to treatment of 14 hours for the intravenous versus 10.4 hours for the oral treatment group, no hepatoxicity occurred in patients treated within 10 hours of ingestion for both groups, and similar rates of hepatotoxicity occurred when administration was delayed by 10–24 hours.[14] The small sample size, (IV-NAC, n=25 and oral-NAC =29) historical control, and 52-hour infusion duration does limit the absolute acceptance of these conclusions, and more study is needed. In response to these limitations, a meta analysis conducted by Buckley et al. reported that patients with high risk for hepatotoxicity outcomes were similar regardless of whether they were treated with oral or intravenous acetylcysteine. The shorter course of therapy and reduced hospitalization times rationalized this investigator's conclusion that the intravenous formulation is the preferred route.[15] Thus, the appropriate selection of the varying forms of acetylcysteine needs consideration of pharmacokinetics, drug interactions, risk of toxicity, resources available to procure, and thus, selection should be on a case-by-case basis.

To facilitate ease of use for the EDP to expedite weight-adjusted dosing and procurement we embedded within the CPOE system a tool for preparation and administration as seen in Figure 14-2A-C.[16]

Drug interactions are a concern with the oral formulation because of a delay in absorption. When given to a patient who may have ingested medications with anticholinergic properties, i.e., a concomitant tricyclic overdose, there is no simple sign to suggest that acetylcysteine is being appropriately absorbed until it is too late. Administration of oral

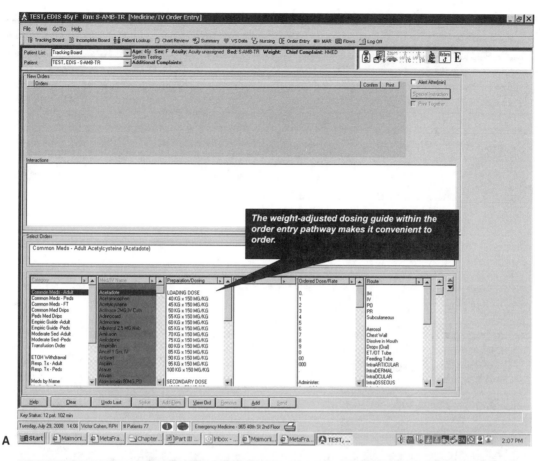

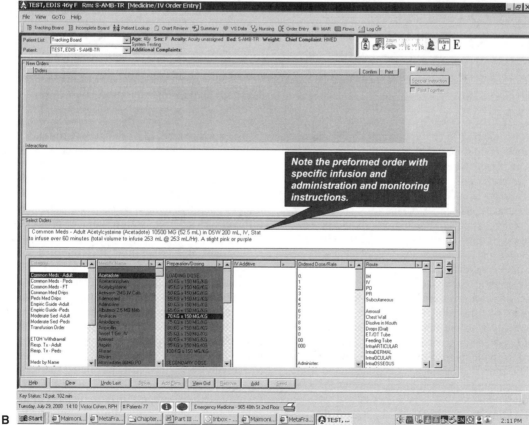

Figure 14–2. **A.** Acetadote loading dosing in HMED. **B.** Acetadote loading dosing and instructions. Courtesy of Allscripts®. *(continued)*

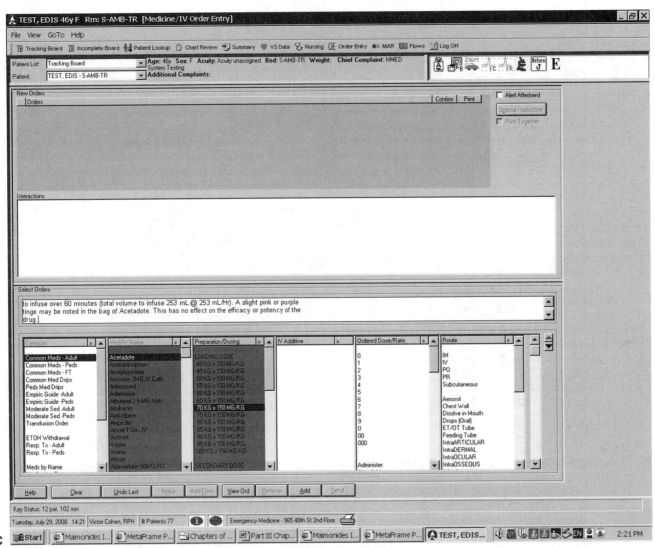

Figure 14-2. *(continued)* **C.** Continuation of instructions of Acetadote® loading dosing and instructions. Courtesy of Allscripts.

acetylcysteine with activated charcoal significantly reduced the binding to acetaminophen as reported in an in-vitro study.[13] Thus, in these cases, the intravenous dose of acetylcysteine may be preferred.

Side effects, such as anaphylactic reactions, have been reported with intravenous acetylcysteine in 3–6% of acetaminophen-poisoned patients.[13] Precautions should be taken and consideration for this negative outcome should be made with the EP because it is not commonly associated with antidotes.[17–19] Anaphylactoid reactions may occur within 30 minutes of infusing the loading dose. Sunman et al. reported that anaphylactoid reactions were higher in patients who received iatrogenic overdoses of acetylcysteine (73%), compared with patients who did not receive overdoses (up to 3%). Rates of hypotension were also higher in the n-acetylcysteine overdose patients than those who did not have an overdose.[20] The rate of infusion has been attributed to adverse events such as anaphylactoid reactions when given over 15 versus 60 minutes, for example (18% vs. 14%, respectively).[13] Although not statistically significant, these results are clinically significant and rationalizes the approach we have taken of initial infusion to be administered over at least 1 hour.

To expedite care, EPs are likely to initiate empiric use of acetylcysteine when suspicion of acetaminophen overdose is high but not confirmed. Data to support this strategy is lacking and may introduce unexpected morbidity and should be avoided. Several investigators found an increased rate of anaphylactoid reactions in patients treated with intravenous acetylcysteine whose pretreatment serum acetaminophen level were below the Rumack-Mathews nomograms' treatment line at 4 hours defined as <150 micrograms/dL. In one study, 42% (13) of patients with anaphylactoid reactions had acetaminophen levels below the treatment line, and the investigators suggested that these patients when treated within 8 hours have a greater likelihood of an anaphylactoid reaction to acetylcysteine.[21,22] Other reports have suggested a correlation between low serum acetaminophen levels and adverse events to acetylcysteine and have speculated that toxic serum levels may be autoprotective against acetylcysteine-induced toxicity. Others suggest that toxic acetaminophen levels functionally inhibit neutrophils, lymphocytes, and thrombocytes perhaps due to the cyclooxygenase and subsequent prostaglandin inhibition.[23–24] Dalhoff postulated that acetaminophen inhibits the function of basophils and mast cells, resulting in decreased anaphylactoid reactions to acetylcysteine with toxic acetaminophen levels. [22]

Status epilepticus has been reported in two children treated for acetaminophen overdose, one who developed intracranial hypertension due to a 10-fold cumulative overdose of intravenous n-acetylcysteine and the other who also developed cortical blindness but fully recovered her vision after 18 months.[25,26] Neither child had hyponatremia, a predisposing factor for seizures. Hyponatremia had been a concern with the original protocol for infusion because it would provide a significant amount of excess free water increasing the risk of hyponatremia-induced seizures. In one case, a 3-year-old girl, with acetaminophen overdose, received the recommended dose of intravenous acetylcysteine, and the child serum sodium level dropped from 141 to 118 mmol/L after 9 hours of intravenous acetylcysteine.[26] These authors subsequently developed a modified treatment protocol for pediatric patients who weigh less than 40 kg to avoid and minimize the risk of hyponatremia and hypervolemia in young children.

The EDP can immediately aid in the emergency care of patient with acetaminophen overdose by quantifying all sources of acetaminophen to ascertain the risk for hepatotoxicity. For example, it has been reported that if a patient has taken >150 mg/kg, it automatically places the patient at risk for hepatotoxicity, and hence a recommendation to start a regimen of n-acetylcysteine should be made once confirmation with a positive toxic level is reported.

MITIGATING HEALTHCARE-ASSOCIATED MEDICATION ERRORS (HAMES)

We have simplified the process of prescribing acetylcysteine. The intravenous formulation is part of the acetaminophen toxicity preformed order set, as previously demonstrated. The lack of bidirectional interface between CPOE systems in the ED and inpatient setting prevents the order from being transferred to the inpatient CPOE system. Because of these healthcare-associated system-based issues, the intravenous acetylcysteine order has to be re-entered by the admitting team, increasing the risk for error. The EDP must assure appropriate continuity of care and transition.

Another factor increasing the risk for medication error exists because of cost containment associated with the use of intravenous n-acetylcysteine. As reported by Lavonas et al., the treatment of a 70-kg patient for 20 hours costs the pharmacy $416 for Acetadote, $57 for Mucomyst, and $32 for generic acetylcysteine.[27] From a cost minimization perspective, the use of the oral and generic acetylcysteine are preferred over the Acetadote, even despite the perceived reduction in length of stay, which is not always realized and may not be preferred as insurers will certainly reduce the payment based on actual care given. If the pharmacy and therapeutic committee does not approve intravenous n-acetylcysteine for routine use because it is cost prohibitive, then it will not be made available on the current inpatient CPOE system. Non-formulary agents may be prescribed; however, a type-in order is needed to be created. Often, this order is incorrectly composed. The dosing of the oral formulation may be erroneously substituted for the intravenous regimen and the diluents are incorrect. Most often, the EDP will be consulted to enter the order for the clinicians.

The EDP also will consult with the poison control center for further assistance in evaluation and management and closely monitor the patient throughout the stay in the ED and at transfer to assure the continuity of care is optimized. This enhanced monitoring includes follow up on the inpatient setting. In so doing, we have discovered errors in management.

ERRORS IN CONTINUITY

Because patients inevitably transition to an admitting team, the admitting team may not know what has already been done for the patient, and they may initiate the traditional oral n-acetylcysteine because they may not be as adept at using the intravenous form. Some clinicians may use the intravenous form erroneously, duplicating the loading dose, instead of continuing with the more appropriate maintenance doses. Furthermore, because of boarding and overcrowding, timely re-evaluation may not be completed and inappropriate dosing, administration, or procurement with the intravenous formulation may not be discovered for some time, increasing the risk for morbidity.

ERRORS IN LABORATORY INTERPRETATION

Erroneously, the acetaminophen level may be used by clinicians to gauge toxicity instead of the liver enzymes. This is a common error in which subsequent acetaminophen blood levels are drawn and are beginning to go below the nomogram. This suggests to the admitting resident that the patient is not toxic and he or she discontinues the full course of n-acetylcysteine. We often intervene at these points.

CALCIUM

Calcium, as an antidote, is indicated for calcium channel blocker overdose. Prescribing calcium is often confusing because the recommended dose is not evidence-based, but based on customary approach. Although calcium salts are indicated to reverse the hypotensive and bradycardic effects of calcium channel blocker overdoses, its reported effects have been mostly in increasing cardiac output by increasing inotropy and has little if no effects on heart rate and conduction.[28]

In numerous case reports, in addition to other adjuvants such as normal saline, glucagon, pressor agents, and hyperglycemia-euglycemia insulin therapy (HEIT), large doses of calcium salt is part of the mainstay of therapy for calcium.

There are no absolute contraindications of calcium salts as part of management of calcium channel blocker toxicity, with the exception of a masquerading digoxin overdose. Then, calcium salts should be avoided.

MITIGATING MANUFACTURE-ASSOCIATED MEDICATION ERRORS (MAMES)

There are no clear guidelines as to what salt of calcium to use, and this is a source for error. Selection of the appropriate calcium salt is frequently raised as the CaCl salt is associated with pain on injection and so the calcium gluconate salt is recommended as a substitute when given peripherally. However, errors in prescribing are a frequent occurrence as the one gram of calcium chloride that is required to be delivered (using 10 mL of the available 10% calcium chloride solution) equates to delivery of 3 grams of calcium gluconate (30 mL of a 10% calcium gluconate solution). EPs will prescribe one vial or 10 mL of the calcium gluconate or 1 gram of calcium gluconate to be administered. The ED pharmacist must intervene and assure appropriate dosing, or less-than-expected effect will occur.

Clinical pearls and dosing are provided in the antidote clinical use guide (see Appendix B: Antidote Clinical Guide). The calcium infusions are to be administered at 0.2–0.4 mL/kg/hr of a 10% CaCl solution or 1.4 g/hr in a 70-kg patient. To avoid hypercalcemia, the serum calcium level should be monitored at baseline every 30 minutes initially and then every 2 hours.

Alternatively, 1 gram of calcium chloride or 3 grams of calcium gluconate may be administered every 10–20 minutes for 3–4 doses, each given as a bolus over 5 minutes or by infusion if mixed in 50 mL of D5w or normal saline.

The metabolic activation of the gluconate salt has been a cause for concern over the therapeutic equivalence with the chloride salt. In one letter to the editor concerning this issue, the author reports that the availability of ionized calcium may be limited with calcium gluconate because of chelation, until it is hepatically metabolized.[29] In those with hemodynamic instability and poor liver perfusion, hepatic activation may be impaired, and thus, the gluconate salt may not work effectively. This may rationalize why recommended calcium salt in cardiac arrest is the chloride salt. Despite this consideration, one study failed to show a difference in ionized calcium and hemodynamic effects in the anhepatic stage of liver transplantation in 15 patients randomized to the chloride or the gluconate salt.[30] Based on this information differences in efficacy between calcium salts do not appear to be significant when therapeutically equivalent doses are selected. However, the desired endpoint of the calcium salts should be monitored and other adjuvants should be instituted.

Toxicity associated with large doses of calcium salts are rare but may result in calciphylaxis or acute hypercalcemia. Calciphylaxis is an extremely rare complication of therapeutic intravenous calcium infusion that can result in severe vasoconstrictive complications with manifestations of ischemic necrosis of the skin, fat, and muscle of the lower extremities. In one case, reported by Sim et al., of acute hypercalcemia[31] no baseline calcium level was obtained and the extent of verapamil overdose was in question, yet aggressive management was initiated to reverse the hemodynamic effects of a 61-year-old woman who developed bradycardia with a heart rate of 40 beats per minute and systolic blood pressure of 60 mmHg. With no baseline calcium level and refractory to initial resuscitative efforts, such as 2 L of normal saline, 1 mg of atropine, the emergency care clinicians attempted resuscitation and added 5 grams of calcium gluconate, 3 grams of calcium chloride, and 5 mg of glucagon with only marginal response, and the clinicians preceded to intubate and initiate high output transcutaneous pacing resulting in a systolic blood pressure maintained at 140 mm Hg. The toxicology consultant recommended an intravenous drip of calcium chloride 4 grams/hour (patient weight was 85 kg). At 4 hours since time of presentation to the ED and after admission to the MICU, the calcium level drawn was 31.2 mg/dL (normal range 10.5 mg/dL). In response, the calcium chloride infusion was reduced to 2 grams/hour, and saline was increased to 500 mL/hour. A repeat calcium level checked at 8 hours later was 32.3 mg/dL, and the calcium chloride intravenous infusion was stopped. Over the next 6 hours, despite the patient's normal blood pressure and heart rate urine output diminished, a repeat calcium level was 23.4 mg/dL, and the patient became anuric. Hemodialysis was consulted, and subsequent hemodialysis therapy reduced the calcium level to 8.3 mg/dL; however, the patient remained anuric, developed elevated hepatic transaminases, pancreatic enzymes, and cardiac markers all despite normal hemodynamics without pressors and pacing. The patient's clinical course worsened gradually, and the patient died 17 days after admission. Upon autopsy, the diagnosis was acute tubular necrosis, acute ischemic ileitis, massive liver necrosis, and multiple infarcts of the spleen all secondary to calciphylaxis confirmed on pathology postmortem.[31] Based on this case, the author recommended several important points when using large doses of calcium salts 1) high dose intravenous calcium infusion must be used judiciously and with close monitoring in treating calcium channel blocker overdose, which includes drawing baseline calcium levels free and total, 2) acute severe hypercalcemia can provoke vasoconstrictive complications; and 3) hemodialysis should be considered early as part of treatment of hypercalcemia to achieve normocalcemia as quickly as possible.[31] ED pharmacists must attend to these considerations either at the bedside or perhaps via protocols used within the ED at the time of management.

GLUCAGON

Glucagon is indicated in calcium channel blocker and beta blocker overdose available as 1 mg lyophilized powder for injection usually with a 1-mL accompanying diluent. With the exception of prior knowledge of hypersensitivity to glucagon, there are no contraindications for its use.

Glucagon is supposed to reverse the myocardial depressing effects; however, its beneficial effects are consistently unsatisfying as a reversal agent, and other therapies must be initiated. There are no published human controlled trials with the use of glucagon in BB or CCA overdose, and although there are successful case reports suggesting improved heart rate and blood pressure, there are also cases of reported failures.

Initial dosing of 50 mcg/kg infused over 1–2 minutes is recommended or 3–5 mg in a 70-kg patient, and higher doses can be given if the initial boluses are not effective, up to a maximum of 10 mg.[32] A continuous infusion of 2–5 mg/hour should be infused up to 10 mg/hour in 5% dextrose and tapered as the patient improves. The available 1-mg vial procurement is arduous because 3–5 vials need to be diluted for just one bolus. Because of the 8–18 minute half life of glucagon, rapid onset within one minute, and short duration of 15 minutes if an effect is seen, a continuous infusion should be initiated A delay in therapy can occur because of the dosage strength available because 10 vials are needed to prepare a 10-mg infusion bag and that requires time to procure. Often, this amount of glucagon is not stored in the ED.[32]

Toxicity with glucagon includes, in our observations, any doses above 3 mg and is associated with significant and rapidly developing nausea and vomiting that often precludes the upward titration or subsequent increase in bolus dosing. Yet, guidelines suggest up to 10 mg by bolus administration may be safely administered; instead, alternative adjuncts should be used.

With administration of glucagon, we must monitor blood glucose as hyperglycemia may occur, exacerbated by the lack of insulin release due to the calcium channel blocker effects.[28] However, the increase in glucose may be beneficial if high dose insulin therapy is initiated because it may improve cardiac function.

PROCUREMENT ERRORS

During emergency care, procuring the glucagon continuous infusion is often confused and done in error. The compatible intravenous diluent is nebulous as precipitate has been reported when used with saline, thus dextrose 5% in water is preferred and should be used to procure the infusion.[16]

CONTINUITY OF CARE ISSUES

We have used a glucagon 5–10 mg in 50 mL dextrose in water solution. This infusion will only last 2–5 hours, depending on the titrated dose. It is likely that a repeat infusion will need to be procured because glucagon competes with the long-lasting effects of extended release beta blocker and calcium channel blockers. Upon transition to the intensive care units, this must be communicated. Notification to the purchasing pharmacist is required because significant hours of glucagon therapy may be required. In one patient, up to 411 mg over 41 hours was infused after a propranolol overdose, suggesting a need to prepare in advance.[75]

DIGIFAB OR DIGIBIND

DigiFab or Digibind is a digoxin Fab fragment available as a ~40 mg/vial of lyophilized powder indicated for the patient with 1) digoxin-induced dysrhythmia either brady or tachycardia, 2) acute digoxin overdose and hyperkalemia >5.5 mEq/L, and 3) cardiovascular collapse associated with an overdose.[33] Sole elevation of a digoxin level does not constitute an indication for Digibind, yet clinicians will immediately conclude digoxin toxicity even in the face of an asymptomatic patient. EPs may assess the serum digoxin level without consideration of the post-dose distribution of up to 6 hours after the last dose taken. Thus, a patient who presents at 12 noon may have consumed their early morning dose of digoxin, and by 12 noon serum levels may still be elevated but nontoxic. The novice may presume due to nonspecific clinical manifestations that the patient is digoxin-toxic and empirically start digoxin Fab fragment.

Conversely, the symptomatic patient with a therapeutic digoxin level may not prompt the clinician to suspect digoxin toxicity despite symptoms. This underscores the importance to obtain serum electrolytes and consider any electrolyte abnormalities as a means to exacerbating a digoxin overdose

state. There are no absolute contraindications to the use of DigiFab or Digibind in suspected digoxin overdose.

There are minimal pharmacotherapeutic differences amongst the Fab products. The Molecular weight of Digibind (38 mg, Glaxo Wellcome Inc.) and DigiFab (40 mg, Protherics Inc.) are the same, and a single vial of either will bind 0.5 mg of digoxin in vivo. As such, clinical claims, dosing, recommendations, and administration of each are identical.[34] Within 30 minutes, improvements in signs and symptoms should be seen and within 4 hours complete reversal. Repeat dosing at 25–50% may be needed in patients who remain symptomatic. Dosing in an acute overdose situation with unknown ingestion is empirically based (10 vials); however, in a patient with acute-on-chronic overdose, as seen in the elderly population, dose determination should be based on the serum digoxin level using total body weight and dividing by 100.

Digibind is frequently overused and inappropriately prescribed. For example, we have intervened on behalf of elderly patients who are mildly symptomatic on chronic doses of digoxin prescribed 10 vials where 2–3 vials would be more appropriate. When infusing Digibind, a 0.22 micron filter must be used.

Monitoring digoxin levels post Digibind will produce falsely elevated levels making total levels meaningless; free digoxin levels should be obtained. Positive interference with digoxin immunoassays occurs, thus, ultrafiltration must be used to accurately obtain free digoxin concentrations in the presence of therapeutic Fab products. In the patient with renal failure, free digoxin levels may not return to normal for up to 7 days.

Continuity of care issues are important because Digibind may exacerbate congestive heart failure and or atrial fibrillation; it is imperative to consult with cardiology prior to instituting Digibind to prepare for this risk. Furthermore, ECG should be monitored along with various electrolytes.

CYANIDE ANTIDOTE

A hypoxic patient who does not initially appear cyanotic presenting to the ED must be clinically screened and managed for the risk of cyanide toxicity. In most cases, treatment will be based on the presentation and not identification of the etiology. An occupational history, travel history, and recent ingestions are less obvious causes than smoke inhalation and accidental poisonings, and the EDP must consult and help research these issues rapidly. The cyanide antidote may be prescribed empirically,[35] and the EDP must again multitask to rationalize its use and prevent inappropriate overuse. Thus, mastery of these elements of knowledge is essential to expedite optimal safe and effective care.

The cyanide antidote kit (formerly known as the Lilly kit) has three components, 1) amyl nitrite pearls, 2) sodium nitrite solution for injection, and 3) sodium thiosulfate solution for injection. The combination ultimately works by freeing up ferric iron from the heme protein to improve oxygen binding and subsequent cellular respirations as cellular hypoxia is the pathologic cause of the manifestations that initially presents.[35] Alternatively Cyanokit (hydroxocobalamin, also vitamin B12a) is available as a 5 gram lyophilized powder.

It works through binding cyanide to form cyanocobalamin and thus eliminating cyanide via the kidneys.[35]

The cyanide kit is indicated for the management of accidental and intentional cyanide poisoning, and more recently components of the cyanide kit such as sodium thiosulfate are recommended for use empirically in smoke inhalation. Smoke inhalation secondary to a fire within a closed location may contain a mixture of hydrogen cyanide from combustion of plastic and other common household materials.

The evidence-based pharmacotherapy to support the use of the cyanide kit versus hydroxocobalamin is a dilemma because the evidence to use either sodium thiosulfate or hydroxocobalamin empirically is incomplete. There is a lack of objective data for empiric use of sodium thiosulfate. Experience with hydroxocobalamin comes from its use in France and other countries, and there are retrospective and prospective clinical studies available, but no prospective, controlled clinical trial efficacy data in humans for either agent and no comparable data exist. Safety benefits of hydroxocobalamin exist in smoke inhalation cases and other suspected cyanide-poisoned patients in the out-of-hospital setting because there is no risk of life-threatening hypotension or methemoglobinemia as that seen when administering nitrite-containing compounds such as sodium nitrite. Another advantage of the hydroxocobalamin is that it can be administered in cyanide poisoning even when there is concomitant carbon monoxide poisoning suspected, a contraindication for the nitrite component of the cyanide kit. Furthermore, sodium thiosulfate appears to work too slow alone to work as a cyanide antidote for emergency use.[17] Thus the EDP must ascertain which cyanide antidote kit would be available, if not both, and which should be used to expedite emergency care. Cost for each antidote kit favors that of the three component cyanide antidote kit at a cost for two kits of $549.12, where as just one vial of hydroxocobalamin costs ~$600.00, and two doses of 5 grams are recommended.

Components of the cyanide kit that are contraindicated for use empirically include sodium nitrite due to the risk of hypotension, and methemoglobinemia that may exacerbate a carbon monoxide-induced hypoxemia. Dosing and administration procedures include initiating Amyl nitrite pearls for 30 seconds of each minute, alternating the inhalant and 100% oxygen with new pearls used every 3 minutes to form a mild methemoglobinemia 2–5%, but only if intravenous access is delayed. If venous access is available, there is no need for the pearls, An ampoule of sodium nitrite is given slowly at 5 mL/minute (300 mg/10 mL) to produce a methemoglobin of 20–30%, 50 minutes after administration. Sodium thiosulfate is administered IV over 10–20 minutes. Repeat dosing within 30 minutes using half the initial doses have been recommended in patients with recurrent symptoms. Hydroxocobalamin (5 grams) should be administered over 30 minutes and repeated once. It should be diluted with 100 mL of normal saline.

Toxicity of concern occurs with sodium nitrite hypotension, and formation of methemoglobin that exacerbates a carbon monoxide-induced hypoxemia makes its less desirable for empiric use, especially outside the facility.

Drug interactions are uncommon but most notable avoid mixing hydroxocobalamin and sodium thiosulfate because the two will inactivate chemically so separate intravenous lines should be used for administration.

INTRAVENOUS ETHANOL SOLUTION VERSUS FOMEPIZOLE

Intravenous ethanol solution or fomepizole are indicated for methanol or ethylene glycol poisoning. Toxic alcohol exposure may present with an initial altered mental status of unknown etiology, and only positive identification mainly by history of ingestion raises suspicion. Emergency care is initiated with ABCs IV-O2–monitor and substrates, such as thiamine, dextrose, and naloxone, as the coma cocktail initiated, to rule out other causes and to prevent a Wernicke's encephalopathy. Laboratory studies may reveal an increased osmol gap and wide anion gap acidosis given that other causes are excluded. Treatment should ensue and not wait for a confirmed methanol level. The EDP, in addition to assisting with emergency care and acquisition and procurement of each antidote, should attempt to identify the extent of ingestion. Of note, cleaning products often have small concentrations of a toxic alcohol in addition to ethanol. The EDP should estimate the ingestion by multiplying the percent of methanol in solution by the estimated volume ingested; with that said, often there is also a similar percent of ethanol that may actually prove to be protective against the manifestations of toxic alcohols. Thus rapid identification of the source of toxic alcohol is an essential activity that will determine subsequent management.

The administration of both fomepizole (4-methylpyrazole) and ethanol have been used successfully in the treatment of methanol and ethylene glycol intoxication. They work to reduce the production of toxic metabolites such as formic acid and other toxic alcohol metabolites. Fomepizole non-competitively inhibits alcohol dehydrogenase (ADH) whereas ethanol competes with methanol for ADH yet ethanol has a 10–20 greater affinity for the enzyme essentially blocking methanol from binding.

The primary advantage of fomepizole over ethanol is avoidance of further CNS depression and unnecessary inebriation; however, that advantage only exists if the patient is not already intubated. In addition, fewer laboratory studies are needed.

Fomepizole has increased affinity to ADH, 8000 times more than ethanol, and fomepizole has been marketed as having the potential to reduce the need for hemodialysis; however, current data does not support this contention.

The cost of fomepizole at $1,000.00/gram is a cause for concern for pharmacy departments. This may rationalize why compliance with current recommendations to stock fomepizole is currently suboptimal in cases of toxic alcohol poisoning. Mycyk et al. demonstrated that when given a choice of which ADH inhibitor to use hospitals were more likely to administer ethanol more frequently than fomepizole.[36]

The EDP can intervene and support the use of the less expensive, yet more labor intensive, ethanol solution for injection. In fact, a consensus panel recommends that either ethanol solution 100% or fomepizole should be kept in stock at sufficient quantities. From continuity perspective if the ED pharmacist provides this cost avoidance intervention, which is significant (~$6,000.00), then achieving the goal of therapy must be assured. To achieve a positive therapeutic outcome, a level of 100–150 mg/dL is needed to inhibit methanol metabolism to formic acid or other toxic alcohol metabolites. Subsequent dialysis should be performed safely. Furthermore the glucose level should also be monitored otherwise hypoglycemia may arise as ethanol inhibits glycogenolysis.

A barrier to successful management of toxic alcohol overdose is negotiating the need for dialysis to a novice renal fellow physician. They may not see the need for renal dialysis initially because anion gap acidosis is absent early after overdose, and an osmol gap is typically absent later after overdose, potentially delaying the recognition of toxicity and need for dialysis. The inexperience with toxic alcohols is a potential barrier to expediting care; however, with assertive discussion with the attending, this barrier can be overcome.

Implementing the use of the ethanol solution is not an easy process, and it is labor intensive. Before committing to this activity, relinquish other pharmacy-specific responsibilities or ensure that coverage is available to manage other tasks within the ED.

Dosing and procurement of fomepizole is an advantage over an ethanol drip (see Appendix B: Antidote Dosing Guide). Unfamiliarity with its use is expected, yet this error in dosing can have significant cost implications. The EDP should oversee its procurement and assure appropriate use.

Depending on the available solution in stock, ethanol 10% in D5w should be prepared with a bolus of 10 mL/kg, followed by a maintenance rate of 1.6 mL/kg/hr. We stock the 5% ethanol in a 1 liter of D5W; thus, the ED pharmacist must calculate the appropriate rate based on the available stock solution.

As recommended by numerous dosing handbooks, a 10% ethanol solution is recommended at a rate of 10 mL/kg bolus. A total of 700 mL should be infused, which equals a total of 70 grams of ethanol. But, if only a 5% solution is available, then only 35 grams will be administered with this same dose (10 mL/kg); thus, the ED pharmacist must double the dose of the bolus, i.e., 20 mL/kg to correctly achieve the recommended level desired of 100–150 mg/dL level. A similar recalculation is needed for the maintenance infusion and dose titration every hour. The ethanol level should be monitored frequently to the desired level of 100–150 mg/dL.

With the exception of anaphylaxis to pyrazoles, there are no absolute contraindications to the use of fomepizole. Rare side effects with fomepizole have occurred such as bradycardia, tachycardia, hypotension and pruritus. Hypertriglyceridemia in 30% of healthy subjects have been reported, and nausea in 11% of patients studied according to the manufacturer. Dizziness and headache were among the most frequent neurologic effects, and in one 6 year-old girl vertical nystagmus developed and resolved with out complication and no further treatment with fomepizole.

The goal of fomepizole therapy is prevention of neurologic dysfunction, permanent blindness, or death, and permanent parkinsonian syndrome. These complications are all related more to the degree of the acidosis than the absolute methanol level.

Drug interactions with fomepizole include the concomitant use of ethanol because they both compete with ADH and reduce the elimination of both drugs. The patient should be observed for 12–18 hours post ingestion despite being asymptomatic because the toxic metabolite may take some time to be eliminated.

FLUMAZENIL

Flumazenil (Romazicon), a benzodiazepine antagonist, is indicated in pure benzodiazepine overdose setting. For example, during a conscious sedation procedure, using midazolam in an elderly, thin COPD female given too much may result in sudden respiratory depression and loss of consciousness. The morbidity of an invasive intubation outweighs that of risks of flumazenil use in this unique clinical setting. This is a rare event in the ED because there are far more confounders that precludes flumazenil use.

Relative contraindications to its use include hypersensitivity to benzodiazepine, the risk of seizure associated with antagonism of benzodiazepine receptor in chronic benzodiazepine users, or the risk of co-ingestions such as tricyclics that pose a neurotoxic risk in the overdose setting, or because of its lack of dose-response relationship and predictability. These are justifications for the EDP to hold the use of flumazenil.

The risk-benefit of benzodiazepine withdrawal and subsequent management may prove to be worse for the patient and the emergency care staff than managing the otherwise placid benzodiazepine overdose. Because of these well-published problems, the use of flumazenil has gone out of favor within the emergency department. In a 12-month period, we ordered 60 vials of flumazenil throughout the hospital demonstrating its lack of use relative to the use of benzodiazepines. Even an evidence-based consensus guide for stocking of emergency antidotes in the US could not come up with a consensus for flumazenil to be stocked.[10]

Yet the novice physician who reviews various general references or refers to the Pharmacopeia handbook or MicroMedex in the event of a quick review while managing a suspected benzodiazepine overdose may attempt the use of flumazenil. This is done erroneously because of the assumption that flumazenil works as predictably as naloxone.

The EDP should intervene to either justify its use or avoid its use. Rationalizing to not use this treatment can best be done by suggesting that there is a risk of seizures induced by withdrawal or a co-ingestion may precipitate a seizure. Flumazenil has a 60-minute duration of action so it can induce sustained morbidity. Thus, it is essential for the EDP to rationalize holding flumazenil, and one way is to attempt to identify other agents that were ingested.

METHYLENE BLUE

Methylene Blue (Urolene) one of the more unique antidotes is indicated for the management of methemoglobinemia, presumptively if unstable, and if stable but with methemoglobin levels of >20% with signs of global hypoxia.

At its worst, a patient with methemoglobinemia presents with altered mental status and central cyanosis (blue tinge), which may appear more grey and ashen depending on the skin tone of the patient. The patient will have reduced oxygen saturation (82–95%) but still may present unresponsive with hyperdynamic vital signs secondary to global hypoxia.

Even after intubation and securing of the airway, suspicion may arise as blood samples are obtained; they will appear brown-black in color. To the experienced EP and toxicologist, this, coupled with the initial clinical presentation, would raise a red flag. The EDP can rapidly identify through investigation of the patient's medication use and initial presentation, that methemoglobinemia is likely. This can expedite the quality of care.

Methylene blue works by accelerating our own endogenous processes for removing methemoglobin by converting ferric to ferrous in the 6th coordination site of the heme molecule of hemoglobin, which allows for improved oxygen binding. It is when exogenous consumption of nitrates, or anesthetic agents (benzocaine, lidocaine, and prilocaine) or other reducing agents overwhelms this endogenous process that clinically important methemoglobinemia occurs.

The blue appearance of methylene blue does concern nursing; administration of a blue intravenous bolus is not a daily routine. Furthermore, because of stocking the 1 mL ampoules, procurement may take a significant time. The EDP rapidly procures methylene blue, aids in counseling the staff on appropriate use, and assures the ED nurse as to the need and instruction on safety of administration. As the urine turns blue with its administration, the ED clinical staff becomes even more concerned. Reassurance by the EDP helps to allay the fear of administering the blue solution and the resultant blue urine.

The EDP can further assist the EP by avoiding solely relying on the oxygen saturation as a specific desired endpoint for improvement. A slight improvement or resolution of cyanosis or "improved color" should be noted and improvements in symptoms suggestive of resolution of global ischemia should be a sign of improvement.

Dosing is rather simple, 1–2 mg/kg (or 0.1–0.2 mL/kg of a 1% solution). In a 70-kg patient, administer 7 mL using 7 ampoules, each containing 1 mL of solution administered over 5 minutes (in the real world setting far more rapidly), followed by a 15–30 mL flush to reduce local pain on injection. If unresponsive with the first dose (defined as central cyanosis continues after 1 hour), it is recommended to administer a second dose.

From a continuity of care perspective, the rate of elimination of the source of methemoglobinemia may be protracted, and as such, the EDP must assure that the intensive care pharmacist is aware of management that was initiated and that treatment may need to be continued. Furthermore because there may be limited stock available, the pharmacy purchaser must be notified to order more methylene blue and or have another means to obtain it.

The maximal dose administered is 7 mg/kg; however, paradoxical reports of methemoglobinemia induced by methylene blue may occur.

NALOXONE

Naloxone hydrochloride is indicated for opioid intoxication and is a part of the coma cocktail in the patient with an altered mental status of unknown etiology. Naloxone is routinely administered by emergency care providers. Naloxone is also often administered by pre-hospital care personnel because it aids in the confirmation of suspected opioid intoxication even before presenting to the ED. The true therapeutic outcome with naloxone in complex multi-drug overdoses is not routinely achieved, and despite its use, patients may require intubation.

Given as a 2-mg intravenous push naloxone has an immediate onset and rather short duration of 15–20 minutes. To reduce the risk of withdrawal and loss of analgesia, the use of a diluted dose of naloxone 0.4 mg is recommended in chronic pain patients to reverse respiratory depression. However, this dosing is not commonly used because the initial history of the patient may not be known. The EDP may assist with researching the patient's medical history to ascertain their opioid use and can caution clinicians on the risk of withdrawal and potential for loss of analgesia.

Indication and justification for use of naloxone infusion is another area in which the EDP can intervene and impact the quality of care within the ED. The EDP often provide guidance to emergency clinicians as to the decision of when to initiate a naloxone continuous infusion. The novice emergency physician may start an infusion on any opioid-intoxicated patient, regardless of severity of intoxication. The seasoned clinician who has experience with the effects of naloxone and had to manage through the subsequent agitated, withdrawing opioid-intoxicated patient who became combative and required significant nursing attention may avoid such treatment while in the ED. The naloxone infusion may affect the overall care process for other patients, and this is why we are often reluctant to start a continuous naloxone infusion.

The EDP can expedite the procurement of the infusion, such as in the methadone-intoxicated patient in whom expected duration of intoxication is prolonged due to the extensive half life of methadone. The dosing and procurement of naloxone is provided in the antidote dosing and procurement tool.

EMERGING ANTIDOTES

Poison control center personnel when consulted on a case may not be witness to the severity of the overdose and may recommend antidotes for which clinicians are not familiar, as in the case of the use of an emerging antidote, **high-dose insulin–euglycemia** (HIE) for CCA or BB overdose. HIE requires the administration of a high dose bolus of insulin at 1 unit/kg (70 kg patient is given 70 units of regular insulin) with a bolus of 25 grams of dextrose, followed by a continuous infusion of insulin, at a rate of ~0.5 unit/kg/hr, in addition to continuous infusion of dextrose 5% and supplemental potassium.[28] The goal of HIE is to provide an exogenous source of glucose and to assure glucose utilization by the myocytes while maintaining euglycemia to correct the drug-induced cardiogenic shock. Its current use is indicated in most cases as rescue therapy.

HIE has the theoretic advantage of maintaining myocyte energy production by providing an exogenous source of glucose and insulin, making available glucose for uptake and subsequent transformation to adenosine triphosphate (ATP), the energy source of the cell. This is essential because during drug-induced shock, the heart shifts its preferences of its primary energy substrate from free fatty acids to carbohydrates.[28] Cardiac cells are deficient in glucose uptake because calcium channel blockers and beta blockers both inhibit insulin release, preventing glucose utilization by the myocyte. HIE has been successfully utilized in a canine model, at improving contractility, coronary blood flow, and survival when added to epinephrine, calcium, and glucagon versus these agents alone.

HIE has demonstrated success in human cases, such as increased blood pressure and contractility within 15–60 minutes after initiated. However, no randomized controlled clinical trials have been conducted. Problems with current data for its use include: dosing regimens have varied; not all patients received a bolus and the bolus dose varied; or the duration of infusion varied. Adverse effects, although infrequent, have been reported, such as hypoglycemia, and resulted in discontinuation of therapy. Hypokalemia has been reported along with other electrolytes abnormalities. Thus intensive monitoring is required to initiate HIE therapy. For example, insulin infusion should be titrated every 30 minutes to achieve the desired effect on contractility or blood pressure. Euglycemia defined as 100–250 mg/dl is the target of the intravenous dextrose bolus and subsequent dextrose infusion of 0.5 g/kg/hr given via a central line; and this is titrated every 20–30 minutes until the blood glucose is stable. The potassium level must be monitored. These multiple interventions and management all create the perfect storm in an overcrowded ED and provides ample opportunity for the EDP to intervene and expedite.

In summary, the EDP has a vital role in managing the safe and effective use of antidotes in the emergency care setting and must assure adequate supply and accessibility. Assuring safe and effective use of antidotes is another step taken in successful achievement of a safe medication use system in the ED.

PUBLIC HEALTH EMERGENCIES AND DISASTER PREPAREDNESS

The intentional release of anthrax resulted in 21 confirmed cases, 11 cutaneous and 10 inhalational, and another 30,000 victims potentially exposed requiring postexposure prophylaxis including ciprofloxacin or doxycycline.[37] Three thousand causalities resulted from the 9/11 World Trade Center disaster. Most recently, the devastation associated with Hurricane Katrina has displaced many families. However, these events all pale in comparison to the 1923 influenza pandemic, which accounted for approximately 500,000 casualties in the U.S. With the current risk of another pandemic on the rise and reports of inadequate responses by federal agencies, the need for improved readiness and preparedness has gained significant attention. In attempts to fortify the public health system, the Joint Commission has added emergency management standards EC4.11–4.18[38] (Table 14-2) that require organizations to address emergency preparedness and institutional readiness as it pertains to pharmaceutical assets.

CURRENT ROLE OF PUBLIC HEALTH AND ITS EVOLUTION

The current public health infrastructure concentrates on preventing adverse health outcomes and reducing risk for disease with the health of the population as the center of attention.[39] Public health interventions are usually designed for long-term effects spanning months to years.[39] The underlying theme in public health is health promotion and disease prevention, emphasizing efforts to reduce the amount of disease, morbidity, and mortality within the general population.[39] The current public health system is designed to track acute and chronic illnesses and anticipate future threats, such as from influenza A H5N1, currently called avian flu. Public health also includes the surveillance of disease patterns and trends essential to gaining understanding of treatment and prevention for populations and individuals. The identification of risk factors for illness and injury is used to plan strategic population-wide interventions, establishing this link between an exposure and disease outcome allows health care professionals to intervene to reduce the prevalence and morbidity and mortality of a disease.[39]

PUBLIC HEALTH AND EMERGENCY MEDICINE

In contrast to the public health focus being the population, each individual is the focus in emergency medicine. In the ED, most interventions are implemented for immediate effect. Despite these differences, the health of the population is the common theme across these fields. For example, the ED guarantees accessible health care and services for the general and uninsured populations. As the safety net for healthcare, the ED provides acute and urgent care to patients in rural and urban settings. The ED is typically located at the center of numerous epidemics including infectious diseases, violence, and substance abuse. It is a logical place for public health and emergency medicine to partner to protect and improve the health of the population.

PUBLIC HEALTH AND PHARMACEUTICAL CARE

The role of pharmacists in national defense extends back to the 1960s. Pharmacists were viewed as medication experts who could assist in emergency medical treatment of patients, train the public in medical self help, and coordinate preparedness measures by establishing standby operational plans.[40] Hepler and Strand in 1990s defined pharmaceutical care as the provision of drug therapy to achieve outcomes that improve a patient's quality of life—these outcomes are: 1) cure of a disease, 2) elimination or reduction of symptoms, 3) arresting or slowing of a disease process, and 4) preventing a disease or symptoms.[41] Furthermore the American Society of Health-System Pharmacy 2015 Initiatives include goal 6, which entails increasing the extent to which pharmacy departments in health systems engage in public health initiatives on behalf of their communities.[42] The public health, objective 6.5 requires 90% of pharmacy departments to have formal, up-to-date emergency preparedness programs integrated with their health systems and their communities preparedness and response programs.[42] Furthermore, as public health emergencies may result in massive surges of patients to facilities for treatment or prophylaxis, pharmacists in addition to other

TABLE 14-2

Pharmacy Department Emergency Management Elements of Performance

Pharmacy Department Specific Emergency Management Elements of Performance

EC4.11 Elements of performance

9   The organization keeps a documented inventory of the assets and resources it has on-site that would be needed during an emergency (at a minimum, personal protective equipment, water, fuel, staffing, medical (CAH, HAP: surgical) and pharmaceuticals resources and assets.
Note: the inventory is evaluated at least annually as part of EP11.

10   The organization establishes methods for monitoring quantities of assets and resources during an emergency.

11   The objectives, scope, performance, and effectiveness of the organization's emergency management planning efforts are evaluated at least annually.

Elements of Performance for EC.4.14

1   The organization plans for: obtaining supplies that will be required at the onset of emergency response (medical, pharmaceutical and non-medical);

2   replenishing medical supplies and equipment that will be required throughout the response and recovery, including personal protective equipment where required;

3   replenishing pharmaceutical supplies that will be required throughout response and recovery, including access to and distribution of caches (stockpiled by the organization or its affiliates, local, state or federal sources) to which the organization has access;

7   potential sharing of resources and assets (e.g., personnel, beds, transportation, linens, fuel, PPE, medical equipment and supplies, etc.) with other health care organizations within the community that could potentially be shared in an emergency response;

8   **potential sharing of resources and assets with health care organizations outside of the community in the event of a regional or prolonged disaster;**

11   transporting pertinent information, including essential clinical and medication-related information, for patients to an alternative care site or sites when the environment cannot support care, treatment, and services.

Elements of Performance for EC.4.15

3   **The organization identifies process that will be required for managing hazardous materials and waste once emergency measures are initiated.**

4   (CAH,HAP) The plan identifies means for radioactive, biological, and chemical isolation and decontamination.

Elements of Performance for EC.4.18

2   **clinical services for vulnerable populations served by the organization, including patients who are pediatric, geriatric, disabled, or have serious chronic conditions or addictions;**

4   **the mental health service needs of its patients;**

6   **The organization plans for documenting and tracking patients' clinical information.**

Elements of Performance for EC.4.20

1   The [organization] tests its Emergency Operations Plan twice a year, either in response to an actual emergency or in a planned exercise.

10   resource mobilization and allocation, including responders, equipment, supplies, personal protective equipment, and transportation.

16   Completed exercises are critiqued through a multi-disciplinary process that includes administration, clinical (CAH, HAP: (including physicians)), and support staff.

**Table includes elements that mandate direct pharmacy involvement. Other elements may involve pharmacy as part of the organizational process of emergency management but are not reflected here

± A comprehensive list of EM standards are found in the Joint Commission Emergency Management Standards *http://www.iroquois.org/cmt/cf/documents/JCAHO%20EM%20Standards%20Jan.%2008.doc - - Cached*

healthcare providers have emerged as important collaborating partners to manage use of pharmaceutical assets during response and recovery.[43]

ROLE OF ED PHARMACIST IN PUBLIC HEALTH EMERGENCIES

Overcrowded emergency departments place a significant demand on the cognition of the physician and nurse. They will manage this demand by performing routine peak time efficient tasks. These strategies in coping with the surge may prevent early screening and identification of a unique presentation that may indicate the start of a pandemic such as anthrax, the early identification of contaminated heparin, or cyanide-laced Tylenol products. Although there are few accounts of EDP involvement in public health activities, EDPs and their specialized knowledge in emergency medicine, toxicology, hazmat, infectious diseases, health information, and preventive care training make them ideal healthcare professionals to bridge the gaps between emergency medicine, public health, and pharmacy to create the common thread needed. Providing screening while in the ED through prospective review assures surveillance that may not be seen by the healthcare staff because they manage each patient; the EDP can take a step back and profile the entire ED patient population. The EDP can provide notification and education to the ED and pharmacy staff of health alerts transmitted through the internet by the CDC or FDA.

There are numerous accounts of pharmacists or public health services pharmacy teams responding to disasters[43–45]; however, there are only few published reports of the role of the EDP during response and recovery of a disaster, assuring emergency preparedness and institutional readiness.[44–45] We describe the past and current roles the EDP has played during response and recovery within the medical institution, tools in assuring the department of pharmacy's preparedness and compliance with current Joint Commission standards, and the daily active surveillance provided by the EDP that may assist in early identification, notification, and education associated with a public health emergency.

PAST AND CURRENT ROLES OF THE ED PHARMACIST DURING RESPONSE AND RECOVERY FOR THE COMMUNITY AND INSTITUTION

As a member of the Pharmacy and Therapeutics committee, the EDP served as the informational expert for the needs for purchasing pharmaceutical assets to assure community and institutional preparedness. During the anthrax release, the EDP provided presentations to the Pharmacy and Therapeutics Committee on the probability and likelihood of various hazards and whether to stockpile medications for these types of emergencies and to what extent. As a result, the Pharmacy and Therapeutic Committee agreed to stockpile medications needed for episodes of terrorism.[43]

The strategy we adopted was to assure, at minimum, that the medical center will maintain its viability by assuring employees and family members that the medical center will prepare for them. Subsequently, each unit of the institution requested in-services on the hazards and the institutional preparedness.

Through word of mouth, requests came from the medical centers public relations officers for information regarding the risk of anthrax. As the EDP became more known for lecturing on this topic, he was asked to provide expert health information and the pharmacological management on anthrax to various news media networks stations (CNN, New York 1, Fox 5), all of which were being targeted at the time through the mail, and many were concerned.

During this same time, the EDP also provided support to the CDC through health fairs conducted at the Madison postal facility in Manhattan, where a team of healthcare professionals (pharmacists, nurses, physicians, pharmacy interns) assisted in tracking use of ciprofloxacin and counseling patients to assure compliance and screening for adverse events.

During such emergencies, healthcare providers often take on roles that may be nontraditional with little preparation. This is the cornerstone for preparation for public health emergencies—be ready for anything.

ED PHARMACISTS OBTAIN SPECIALIZED ON-THE-JOB TRAINING

The EDP was a provider and instructor in advanced hazardous material life support (AHLS) training provided by the Arizona Emergency Medicine Research center,[46] which he received as part of on-the-job training activities. Post 9/11 and during the anthrax release, the ED pharmacist was also invited and attended training at Fort Hamilton barracks by the United States Army Medical Research Institute for Infectious Diseases (USAMRID) for citywide preparedness and has been certified in the National Incident Management System. Furthermore, as part of the Hazmat decontamination team, he was trained by various disaster specialist programs held by the institution.

INSTITUTIONAL TRANSFORMATION AND IMPLEMENTATION OF HOSPITAL EMERGENCY INCIDENT COMMAND SYSTEM (HEICS)

Prior to the 9/11 World Trade Center disaster and the anthrax scare, the medical center's disaster plan was fragmented, and there was no one unifying command, which resulted in inefficiencies, redundancies, and waste. The EDP was included as part of a multidisciplinary team of healthcare professionals from the institution on the newly formed emergency management committee lead by a consultant whose mission was to transform the medical center from the current disaster response plan that had no unifying command to an all-hazards approach including a HEICS that included one unifying command.

The EDP was included as part of training the hospital leadership in understanding that emergency management principles including that hospitals cannot perform in isolation, that past plans are inadequate for current and future disasters; and because the institution cannot plan for everything, we need to plan for anything.

The training highlighted lessons learned from past disasters, such as the Firefighting resource of California Organized for Potential Emergencies (FIRESCOPE) [47] findings that included a lack of common organization in terminology and communications, lack of capability to expand and contract, poor on-scene and interagency communication, inadequate joint planning and inadequate resource management. Efforts to address these findings resulted in the development of the original incident command system model. Over time, this has evolved to the "all risk" or "all hazards system" for use in a variety of incident types including nonemergency incidents.

The Joint Commission's emergency management standards, which have adopted this all hazards approach for hospitals, requires institutions to conduct a hazard vulnerability analysis, ensure community wide integration and interoperability, ensure cooperative planning amongst organizations, initiate staff development activities, and assure alternative care sites. In addition, preparation includes four phases of a disaster such as: 1) mitigation, 2) preparedness, 3) response, and 4) recovery. This further rationalized the adoption of what is now termed HEICS. HEICS is a crisis management tool; it is the national standard for response by police, fire department and emergency medical services, and now hospitals. HEICS allows for a consistent management organization, standard terminology, an all hazards approach that is flexible and adaptable, organized documentation, seamless integration, prioritization of duties, and minimal disruption. It works because the system is based on common management skills that leaders know, trust, and use, such as planning, directing, organizing, coordinating, communicating, delegating, and evaluating. HEICS uses basic management principles such as management by objective, which shifts the focus on the event, allows for a manageable span of control, and assures clear responsibility and accountability. HEICS includes several components such as a table of organization, management by objective plan, job action sheets, forms, and a glossary. Included in HEICS is an organizational hierarchy that begins with the incident commander, a command staff officer, section chiefs, branch directors, supervisors, and unit leaders in that order. The organizational leadership included the incident commander, the command staff that includes a liaison officer, safety and security officer, public information officer, and the section chiefs including logistics, planning, finance, and operations, all report back to the incident commander up the chain of command.

As part of HEICS, an emergency operations center (EOC) is established as a means to move the emergency out of the emergency department. The EOC provides a central location for communications, decisions makers, and internal and external activities to occur. The move to an incident command structure placed the pharmacy department unit leader under the operations chief.

During a HEICS response, the pharmacy unit leader would be expected to respond to the emergency operations center depending on the HEICS level announced as per the emergency operation plan activation protocol. There are four levels of activation authorized by the highest ranking administrator on duty. Announcements are made upon initial activation, escalation, and de-escalation. A job action sheet is provided for each member of the incident command including the pharmacy unit leader and includes a list of general activities.

The job action sheet includes a concise mission statement, prioritized job responsibilities that are immediate, intermediate and extended, and describes reporting relationships during emergency operations. Thus as a member of the emergency management committee, the EDP assisted in the transformation of the institution into the all hazards approach to public health emergencies.

Currently, the EDP maintains this role and assists in addressing issues associated with Joint Commission changes in emergency management standards. The EDP is part of the Hazmat decontamination team and is alerted during any HEICS activation through the paging system. Day-to-day, the EDP collects health alerts and advisories and updates staff on potential emerging health concerns. The EDPs play a significant role in assuring that Hazmat decontamination equipment is maintained and ready for use and available when needed. The integration of the pharmacy unit leader within the HEICS organization representing the pharmacy department assures that the pharmacy department's plan for response is integrated with the institutional plan, and this allows for compliance with standards and goals set forth by ASHP 2015 initiative and the Joint Commission. The pharmacy unit leader will be relied upon to assure the pharmacy department is prepared to respond, as such a policy and procedure is needed to guide the pharmacy unit leader to respond effectively during a disaster and achieve the expected objectives delegated by the incident commander based on the specific event.

PHARMACY DEPARTMENT-SPECIFIC TOOLS FOR MANAGING PUBLIC HEALTH EMERGENCIES

Prior to the institutional transformation to HEICS and based on new Joint Commission standards post-9/11, the anthrax episode, and the realization that the pharmacy had to be self-sufficient for a 72-hour period in the event of a disaster, the EDP in collaboration with the pharmacy department developed an incident command structure that we later titled the pharmacy emergency response team (PERT) as depicted in the flow diagram in Figure 14-3.[43]

The pharmacy unit leader would assume the administrator role of the pharmacy emergency response team. This unit-specific incident command structure allowed for a flexible tiered response focused on the hazard material released. The EDP, based on past experience and specialty, took on the Hazmat role. Furthermore, as many incidents may initiate within the ED, the fortuitous presence within the ED setting permits the EDP to be aware of events or possible public health issues far in advance of the pharmacy department. The EDP would notify and keep the pharmacy department on alert.

The PERT was organized on the principles of an incident command structure with the mission of assuring an appropriate pharmaceutical response; the department would be able to mobilize, procure, distribute, and track assets to manage the surge that may occur during a public health emergency while still maintaining normal operations to serve the community's need, despite the event.

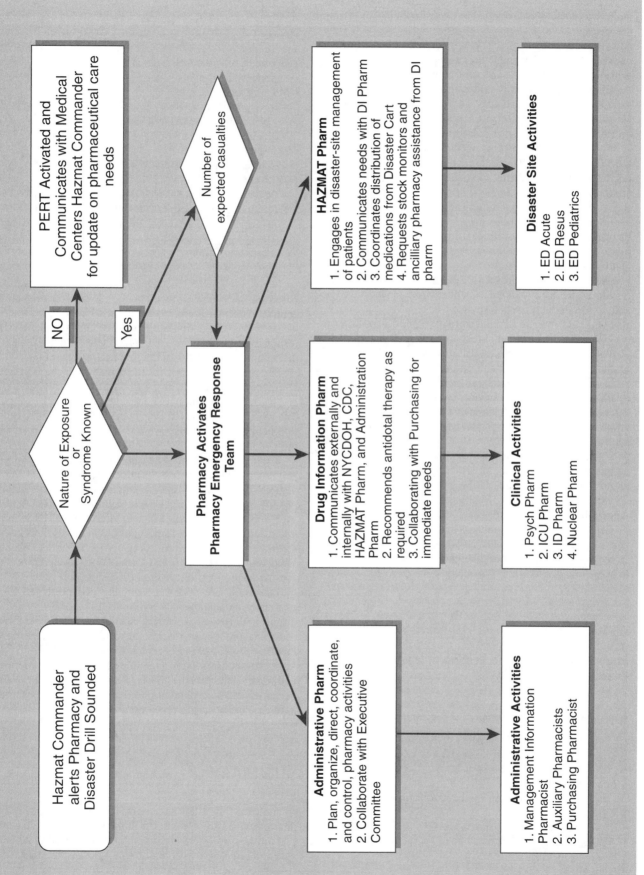

Figure 14–3. Disaster needs analysis algorithm.

Accompanying this department-specific incident command was a tool we developed to expedite the needs during the disaster. We developed a disaster needs analysis flow and form for the pharmacist who would be answering the phone 24 hours a day and 7 days a week. The disaster needs analysis flow would require any pharmacists who answer the phone to immediately ascertain the problem, the exposure, the number of casualties, and the projected amount of pharmaceuticals on hand and needed to be purchase based on suspected number of casualties.

Furthermore, this process would automatically activate the PERT. As important as preparedness were the steps in response during the event, for which few staff pharmacists are trained. The EDPs developed procedures to respond to a suspected hazardous exposure (Table 14-3).

To execute the mission of PERT, which is to assure pharmaceutical assets were delivered and managed appropriately, we developed procedures for disaster response (Table 14-4).

The EDP also developed a PERT manual that includes a response grid for any pharmacist at anytime to use and to be able to provide a rational response.

The PERT manual for bioterrorism (Table 14-5) instructs the pharmacist on the initial response required and the lead pharmacist's responsibilities. The manual provides sections on the likely infectious agents and treatment.

In accord with current Joint Commission standards, the PERT manual contains an accounting of pharmaceutical assets and instructs the pharmacist to inquire on estimated number of patient's to proactively estimate the purchasing needs.

Furthermore, the grid instructs the lead pharmacists to assign staff for procuring, distributing, tracking the appropriate inventory, and designating a pharmacist on site to respond and communicate any additional needs (See Appendix B: Dosing Guides and Tables).

Because there is a likelihood that during disaster phone and internet lines may be unavailable, a paper manual is stored that contains the most likely suspected toxin in an easy to view manner that helps to identify the expected toxicity based on the exposure. A clinical pathway for the pharmaceutical care management of the most likely exposures, the triage, and re-evaluation of the patient during the emergency response is also included. All to facilitate the management of the disaster while still maintaining routine operations.

The recommendations for these pathways come from the Department of Health, the United States Army Chemical and Radiological handbook, and CDC.gov website. Much of this work was completed due to the lack of organized institutional response as there were few standards on emergency preparedness at the time.

Recent environment of care standards now require organizations to have a process in which they document the inventory of the assets and resources on site that may be needed during an emergency, including pharmaceutical assets, a method for monitoring the quantities of these assets and resources during an emergency, and capabilities and response efforts if no support is likely for 96 hours. We have addressed these issues in the form of a policy and procedure (see Appendix A: Policies and Procedures).

The assets are reviewed annually and presented to the pharmacy and therapeutics committee for approval of any additions or deletions. An emergency response tracking form is used to record receipt, returns, and distribution of pharmaceutical assets and method of replenishment (Fig 14-4).

A contact list is made available of local, state, and federal authorities. The disaster policy of prime vendors have been reviewed and incorporated into this policy and procedure to assure delivery during response and recovery.

TABLE 14-4

Disaster Antidote Procurement Guidelines

- Disaster assessment and needs analysis
  - Know your inventory
- Mobilize antidotes
  - Have preformed labels, disease fact sheets, drug fact sheets, vials, ready to be mobilized and distributed in mass quantities
- Distribute antidotes
  - Contact list, patient profile
- Track antidotes
  - Prepare for shipment, deploy staff to manage National Pharmaceutical Stockpile (NPS), donations, create networks for acquisition of antidotes, prepare for on demand inventory

TABLE 14-3

Steps in Responding to Technologic Hazardous Exposures

Goal: Maintain normal function of department

- Conduct a disaster needs analysis
  - Is the nature of exposure known
  - How many victims are expected
- Activate PERT
  - Initiate a command and control in the pharmacy
  - Develop action plan
- Deploy pharmacist intelligence as needed
- Prepare antidotal distribution
- Prepare to mobilize stockpile
- Prepare to track stockpile
- Prepare to purchase and receive more stock

SUMMARY

In summary, the EDP has a vital role in managing the safe and effective use of antidotes in the emergency care setting and must assure adequate supply and accessibility. Assuring safe and effective use of antidotes is another step to successful achievement of a safe medication use system in the ED. Toxicology knowledge and skills from postgraduate training and emergency care considerations obtained from residency

TABLE 14-5

Biologic Exposure Response Protocol

Incident	Description	Initial Pharmacy Response	Responsibility of Lead Pharmacist	Follow Up
Exposure to Biological Casualties	The Medical Center receives one or more patients exposed to a biological agent, and the Pharmacy is notified with a request of Post Exposure prophylaxis or Treatment	▶ Conduct a pharmaceutical needs analysis. ▶▶ Identify the infectious agent. ▶▶ Identify the antimicrobial agents indicated. ▶▶ Identify the amount of antimicrobial on-hand for amount in stock. ▶▶ Determine number of patients requiring treatment and post-exposure prophylaxis. ▶▶ Estimate if more antimicrobial agents are needed than that on-hand and establish emergency contacts for purchasing more antimicrobials.	1. Upon initial notification, complete pharmaceutical needs analysis, and brief pharmacy staff of situation. 2. Assign staff to prepare emergency antidote cart and to fill bins with needed antimicrobials. 3. Assign staff to deliver antimicrobial agents to site of distribution. **Collaborate with incident commander** 4. If requested, initiate a point of distribution site 5. Assign staff to track inventory at site of distribution and restock as needed. 6. Assign staff to assist with communications and drug information calls and to disseminate fact sheets, and home use info of postexposure prophylaxis.	1. Notify emergency contacts if not already done. 2. Debrief staff at termination of public health emergency. 3. Document all antimicrobials distributed for accounting purposes.

Courtesy of Maimonides Medical Center Pharmacy Department.

Bulk Pharmaceutical Asset Distributed/Returned/Received Recording Form							
Date/Time	Item#	Item Description	Quantity Distributed Received Returned	Organization Receiving/ Person (Print) Receiving	Contact Information	Estimated Cost	Method of Replenishment Undeclared Return Financial Compensation
7/3/08, 5PM	N123456	Maalox 30 ml unit dose 25 /pack	1 case (2 dozen) Distributed** Received Returned	Methodist Jon Doe	718-283-7205	$27.00	U R** F
			Distributed Received Returned				U R F
			Distributed Received Returned				U R F
			Distributed Received Returned				U R F
			Distributed Received Returned				U R F

Figure 14–4. Bulk pharmaceutical asset distributed/returned/received form.

training through specialized certification courses contribute to the EDP as an educator and informer to the public and the community. Regulatory standards mandate that pharmaceutical assets be available and maintained in response to a public health emergency. The ED is likely the location to manage the initial crisis of public health emergencies. The EDP can support this response and ensure that pharmaceutical assets are delivered in a timely manner, tracked, replaced, and appropriately used.

References

1. Brown MJ, Willis T, Omalu B, Leiker R. Deaths resulting from hypercalcemia after administration of edentate disodium: 2003–2005. *Pediatrics* 2006;118:e534–e536.
2. Little M, Murray L, McCoubrie D, Daly F. A potentially fatal prescribing error in the treatment of paracetamol poisoning. *MJA* 2005;183(10):535–536.
3. Golembiewski J, Wheeler P. High-alert medications in the perioperative setting. *J Peri-Anesthesia Nursing* 2007;22(6):435–437.
4. Czajka PA, Skoutakis VA, Wood GC, Autian J. Clinical toxicology consultation by pharmacists. *Am J Hosp Pharm* 1979;36:1087–1089.
5. Levy DB, Barone JA, Raia JJ, York JM, Vogel DP. Pharmacist participation in the management of incidents involving hazardous materials. *Am J Hosp Pharm* 1987;44:549–556.
6. Chyka PA, Conner HG. Availability of antidotes in rural and urban Tennessee. *Am J Hosp Pharm* 1994;51:1346–48.
7. Dart RC, Stark Y, Fulton B et al. Insufficient stocking of poisoning antidotes in hospital pharmacies. *JAMA* 1996;276:1508–15–10.
8. Woolf AD, Crisanthus K. Onsite availability of selected antidotes: results of a survey of Massachusetts hospitals. *Am J Emerg Med* 1997;15:62–66.
9. Pettit HE, McKinney PE, Achusim LE, Lindsey C. Toxicology cart for stocking sufficient supplies of poisoning antidotes. *Am J Health-Syst Pharm* 1999:56:2537–2539.
10. Dart RC, Goldfrank LR, Chyka PA, et al. Combined evidence-based literature analysis and consensus guideline for stocking of emergency antidotes in the United States. *Ann Emerg Med* 2000;36(2):126–132.
11. Goldfrank LR, Flomenbaum NE, Lewin NA, et al. *Goldfrank's Toxicological Emergencies, 7th Edition*. New York: McGraw Hill.
12. Medscape e-medicine from WebMD, Toxicology. http://www.emedicine.com/emerg/index.shtml. Accessed December 2008.
13. Kanter MZ. Comparison of oral and IV acetylcysteine in the treatment of acetaminophen poisoning. *Am J Health-Syst Pharm* 2006;63:1821–1827.
14. Perry HE, Shannon MW. Efficacy of oral versus intravenous N-acetylcysteine in acetaminophen overdose: results of an open-label clinical trial. *J Pediatr* 1998;132:149–52.
15. Buckley NA, Whyte IM, O'Connel DL, et al. Oral or intravenous N–acetylcysteine: Which is the treatment of choice for acetaminophen poisoning? *J Clin Toxicol* 1999;37: 759–67.
16. Gahart BL, Nazareno AR. *Acetylcysteine in 2007 Intravenous Medications, Twenty-Third Edition*. St Louis, MO: Mosby-Elsevier.
17. Mant TG, Tempowski JH, Volans GN, et al Adverse reactions to acetylcysteine and effects of overdose. *Br Med J* 1984;289;217–219.
18. Kerr F, Dawson A, Whyte IM, et al. The Australian Clinical Toxicology Investigators Collaboration randomized trial of different loading infusion rates of N-acetylcysteine. *Ann Emerg Med* 2005;45:402–8.
19. Lynch RM, Robertson R. Anaphylactoid reactions to intravenous n-acetylcysteine; A prospective case controlled study. *Accident Emerg Nursing* 2004;12:10–5.
20. Sunman W, Hughes AD, Sever PS. Anaphylactoid response to intravenous acetylcysteine. *Lancet* 1992;339:1231–2, Letter.
21. Rumack BH, Peterson RC, Koch GG, et al. Acetaminophen overdose: 662 cases with evaluation of oral acetylcysteine treatment. *Arch Intern Med* 1981;141:380–5.
22. Schmidt LE, Dalhoff K. Risk factors in the development of adverse reactions to n- acetylcysteine in patients with paracetamol poisonings. *Br J Clin Pharmacol* 2001;51;87–91.
23. Panush RS. Effects of certain antirheumatic drugs on normal human peripheral blood lymphocytes. Inhibition of mitogen- and antigen-stimulated incorporation of tritiated thymidine. *Arthritis Rheum* 1976;19:907–917.
24. Shalabi EA. Acetaminophen inhibits the human polymorphonuclear leukocyte function in vitro. *Immunopharmacology* 1992;24:37–46.
25. Bailey B, Blais R, Letarte A. Status epilepticus after a massive intravenous N-acetylcysteine overdose leading to intracranial hypertension and death. *Ann Emerg Med* 2004;44;401–06.
26. Hershkowitz E, Shorer Z, Levitas A, et al. Status epilepticus following intravenous N-acetylcysteine therapy. *Israel J Med Sci* 1996;32:1102–1104.
27. Lavonos EJ, Beuhler MC, Ford MD, et al. Intravenous administration of N-acetylcysteine: oral and parenteral formulations are both acceptable. *Ann Emerg Med* 2005;45:223–224, Letter.
28. Kerns W. Management of beta-adrenergic blocker and calcium channel antagonist toxicity. *Emerg Med Clin North Am* 2007;25:309–311.
29. Davey M, Caldicott D. Calcium salts in management of hyperkalemia. *Emerg Med J* 2002;19: 92–93.
30. Martin TJ, Kang Y, Robertson KM, Virji MA, Marquez JM. *Anesthesiology* 1990;73(1):62–65.
31. Sim MT, Stevenson FT. A fatal case of iatrogenic hypercalcemia after calcium channel blocker overdose. *J Med Toxicol*.2008;4(1)25–29.
32. Howland MA. Antidotes in Depth. In: Golfrank LR, Flomenbaum NE, Lewin NA, et al. *Goldfrank's Toxicological Emergencies, 7th Edition*. New York: McGraw Hill.
33. Hack JB, Lewin NA. Cardiac Glycosides. In: Golfrank LR, Flomenbaum NE, Lewin NA, et al. *Goldfrank's Toxicological Emergencies, 7th Edition*. New York: McGraw Hill.
34. McMillin GA, Owen WE, Lambert TL, et al. Comparable effects of DIGIBIND and DigiFab in thirteen Digoxin Immunoassays. *Clin Chem* 2002;48(9):1580–83.
35. Hall AH, Dart R, Bogdan G. Sodium thiosulfate or hydroxocobalamin for the empiric treatment of cyanide poisoning? *Ann Emerg Med* 2007;49(6):806–813.
36. Mycyk MB, Deslauriers C, Metz J, et al. Compliance with poison center fomepizole recommendations is suboptimal in cases of toxic alcohol poisoning. *Am J Therapeut* 2006; 13(6)485–489.
37. Investigation of bioterrorism-related anthrax and adverse events from antimicrobial prophylaxis. *MMWR* 2001;50(44):973–976. http://www.cdc.gov/mmwr/preview/mmwrhtml/mm5044a1.htm
38. Comprehensive Accreditation Manual for Hospitals (CAMH) Update 2, May 2003: The Official Handbook. http://www1.va.gov/emshg/docs/JCAHO_EC_Stds_2004.pdf. Accessed July 1, 2009.
39. Hirshon JM, Morris DM. Emergency medicine and the health of the public: the critical role of emergency departments in US public health. *Emerg Med Clin North Am* 2006;24(4):815–9.
40. Health mobilization. APhA policy. *J Am Pharm Assoc* 1966;NS6: 80–6.
41. CD Hepler, LM Strand. Opportunities and responsibilities in pharmaceutical care. *Am J Health-Syst Pharm* 1990;47:533–543.

42. American Society of Health-System Pharmacists. http://www.ashp.org/s_ashp/docs/files/2015_Goals_Objectives_0407.pdf

43. Cohen V. Organization of a health-system pharmacy team to respond to episodes of terrorism. *Am J Health-Syst Pharm* 2003;60(12);1257–63.

44. Velazquez L, Dallas S, Rose L, et al. A PHS pharmacist team's response to Hurricaine Katrina. *Am J Health-Syst Pharm* 2006;63:1332–1335.

45. Young D. Pharmacists play vital roles in Katrina response. *Am J Health-Syst Pharm* 2005;62:2202,2204,2209,2216.

46. The University of Arizona, Advance HAZMAT Life Support, http://www.ahls.org/ahls/ecs/courses/courses.html. Accessed December 2008.

47. Firefighting Resources of California Organized for Potential Emergencies http://www.firescope.org/. Accessed December 2008.

15

Emergency Care Pharmacotherapy of the Critically Ill: Tools to Expedite Care

Objectives

- Review the role of emergency department (ED) in treating critically ill/resuscitation patients
- Describe sepsis outcomes that support importance of early treatment in the ED
- Describe the levels of management of the critically ill in the ED
- Identify potential high-risk areas in the management of critically ill patients
- Describe the gap in critical care management and the need for the ED clinical pharmacist
- Discuss tools and safeguards developed by ED clinical pharmacy service to reduce risk
- Review ED clinical pharmacist responsibilities in the management of critical care patients
- Describe safe and effective management of medications during resuscitation

ROLE OF THE EMERGENCY DEPARTMENT IN TREATING CRITICALLY ILL PATIENTS

Over the past decade there has been an increasing number of critically ill patients treated in the emergency department throughout the United States.[1] Twenty-Five percent of admitted patients from the ED are considered critically ill.[2] Fromm and colleagues revealed that about 186 days of the year are focused on treating critically patients in the urban ED setting.[3] The length of stay for critically ill patients was on average 6 hours in the ED and is longer than in the past.[4] Emergency departments play an integral role in managing critically ill patients.

SEPSIS OUTCOMES THAT SUPPORT IMPORTANCE OF EARLY TREATMENT

The role of the ED in stabilizing and significantly improving outcomes in critically ill patients must be emphasized, as studies concluded that patients with severe sepsis and septic shock who receive early goal-directed therapy (EGDT) in the ED have improved outcomes.[5] Rivers and colleagues concluded that there is an absolute reduction of 16% in hospital mortality after EGDT of critically ill patients with sepsis or septic shock in the ED.[6] Other studies have also concluded that a significant reversal of physiologic derangement could occur during the patients' ED stay.[7] All of these factors support a vital role of ED management in providing intensive care toward critically ill patients.

LEVELS OF MANAGEMENT OF CRITICALLY ILL PATIENTS

Critical care has become so important in emergency medicine that there is a movement toward sub-specialization and certification of emergency medicine physicians. Management of the critically ill patient in the ED occurs on many different levels, from transport of the patient to the ED by EMS to the resuscitation and stabilization procedures provided by the ED.

POTENTIAL HIGH-RISK AREAS IN THE MANAGEMENT OF CRITICALLY ILL PATIENTS

There are several high risk situations prone to error during management of critically ill patients at all levels during the transition into and out of the ED environment.

From initial entry incorrect triaging may occur, management dilemmas associated with insufficient information for patient evaluation, complex drug administration that is aggressive and time dependent, extensive procedures for stabilization, resuscitation, and transfers require procedures to avert risk.[5]

CRITICAL CARE PHARMACIST AND THE GAP IN CRITICAL CARE MANAGEMENT IN THE ED

Critical care pharmacists have evolved and are considered to be essential team members and essential intensive care practitioners within intensive care units.[8–10] No data describes the role of the critical care pharmacist providing initial management of critically ill patients within the ED, and yet as described, significant pharmacotherapeutic interventions are likely to be started in the ED. The ED clinical pharmacy services must take on this role to ensure optimal emergency care pharmacotherapy for the critically ill patient until the patient is transferred.

Management of critically ill patients in the ED may often include a host of pharmaceutical interventions, including vasopressors, vasodilators, sedatives, paralytics, antibiotics, thrombolytics, anticoagulants, and acid suppressing agents. Although there are systems in place to limit the potential for medication error in the ED, such as electronic medical records and CPOE systems, automated dispensing machines that control access to medications, SMART infusion pumps that standardize concentrations and restrict maximum and minimum drip rates, and multi-disciplinary efforts to assure quality prescribing through decision support, there is still inherent risk for error in the overall execution of these activities.

Many critical care medications are administered according to the weight of the individual patient, and this is usually based on estimations as weighted beds are often too big to store within the ED setting, which increases the risk for over- and under-dosing. Furthermore, EPs and nurses may not be able to focus their cognitive skills when dealing with the nuances and idiosyncrasies associated with the use of the critical care pharmacotherapy. Thus, there is ample opportunity for the EDP to enhance and assure safe and effective management of the critically ill patient.

TOOLS AND SAFEGUARDS DEVELOPED BY ED CLINICAL PHARMACY SERVICE

To facilitate the optimal implementation of pharmacotherapy of the critical care patient while in the ED, our clinical pharmacy service developed easy-to-use drug dosing sheets (see Appendix B: Guide to Management of Critical Care Drug Infusions in the ED) that simplify drip rate calculations, thus limiting the potential for medication error; this tool corresponds to SMART pump technology and preformed order sets for the order entry system.

In addition, the clinical effects of each pharmaceutical intervention are included to assist the pharmacist with bedside titration.

ED PHARMACIST RESPONSIBILITIES AND THE CRITICAL CARE PATIENT

The EDP is often consulted by nursing to assist in procuring critical care drug infusions in resuscitation that require close monitoring and titration according to the patients hemodynamic profile because this close observation by an ED nurse may place an increased strain on an already undersupplied resource within the ED. Although critical care activities by the ED pharmacist are shared with those of critical care pharmacists, the ED pharmacists may engage in other unique activities (Table 15-1) in the care of the critical care patient.

TABLE 15-1

ED Pharmacist Role and Activities During Emergency Care for the Critically Ill Patient

1. Assess the problem clinically and ascertain the correctness of the therapy.
2. Access drug information to assess risks and appropriateness of therapy (i.e. MicroMedex® or ncemi.org®).
3. Rapidly procure medicated intravenous infusions.
4. Assist the nurse with preparing the critical care infusion drugs for administration.
5. Prime intravenous tubing.
6. Setup the infusion pump.
7. Calculate the appropriate intravenous drip rate to confirm the rate set on the infusion pump.
8. Prepare the cardiac monitor to titrate the drip so vital signs can be monitored continuously, and check that all vital signs are being read appropriately.
9. Titrate the intravenous drips for hypotensive, hypertensive emergencies, tachycardia, and sedation.
10. Assure the blood pressure cuff is functional and appropriate, and take periodic manual blood pressures.
11. Prepare, with management consideration, for adverse consequences, for example, prepare for fluid boluses, have epinephrine, atropine, lidocaine ready to use if the patient becomes unstable.
12. Be prepared to differentiate rapid intubation medications. We use etomidate and succinylcholine as the preferred intubation drugs of choice.
13. Recommend to nursing to initiate the sedation before paralysis as this is not always taken into consideration.
14. Be prepared to differentiate agents for sedation that don't affect intracranial pressure, such as propofol.
15. Quantify the Ramsey Sedation Scale and Riker Sedation-Agitation Scale
16. Quantify the indication/contraindication for thrombolysis

SAFE AND EFFECTIVE MEDICATIONS DURING RESUSCITATION

The EDP is also called to assist and support the emergency care team in procedures performed to stabilize the critically ill patients. Intubation, line insertion, implementation of advanced cardiac life support (ACLS) or pediatric advanced life support (PALS) protocols, dose recommendations, and procurement are all examples of these procedures, and the pharmacotherapist may also support the resuscitation team as a recorder and dispenser of emergency medications. Those familiar with emergency equipment may assist in providing basic life support, such as cardiopulmonary resuscitation (CPR), bagging the patient, or serve as an extra in retrieving emergency equipment as needed.

PRIMARY SURVEY

The initial emergency department evaluation includes the primary survey in which the emergency physician conducts the following tasks. First, the EP assesses if the patient needs resuscitation. To be successful, it must be started early, thus, it must be evaluated first. If the patient requires resuscitation, the ED team acts in parallel form to perform assessment-treatment-procedures (ATP) all at once and includes the immediate approach, as listed in the Table 15-2. The goal is to perform all therapies that are essential to allow safe transport to an inpatient bed. This is in contrast to first admitting the patient and then transporting to an inpatient bed for stabilization.

AIRWAY/BREATHING MANAGEMENT AND EMERGENCY CARE PHARMACOTHERAPY

Often, there is no clear etiology to the patient demise and need for resuscitation; however, if the patient is not yet intubated in the field, the emergency physician (EP) assesses if there is a need for intubation, i.e., airway and breathing (AB). Because the history at the time may not be fully known, the team must spring into action to intubate. The pharmacotherapist must be prepared with medication on hand, with the expected dose to be administered, if possible a drug label prepared, and a recording of the timing and administration.

TABLE 15-2

Early Evaluation and Management of Resuscitation

1. Evaluate ABCs (Airway, Breathing, Circulation).
2. Initiate peripheral intravenous lines and start normal saline 0.9%.
3. Start oxygen using nasal canula, non-rebreather mask and dial up to 100% FIO2.
4. Place the patient on a monitor (blood pressure cuff, pulse oximeter).
5. Assess vital signs, and conduct primary survey.

SAFE AND EFFECTIVE MEDICATION USE DURING MECHANICAL INTUBATION

The patient, depending on the problem, may receive various pretreatments explained by the nemonic LOAD that is abbreviated for Lidocaine, Opioids, Atropine, and Defasciculation when rapid sequence intubation is indicated.[11]

In most adult cases, the patient needs sedation and paralysis to facilitate rapid endotracheal intubation, and we use etomidate (0.03 mg/kg, available in a 2 mg/1 mL vial, total 10 mL) for sedation and succinylcholine (1–1.5 mg/kg, available as 20 mg/mL vial in 10 mL) for paralysis. A safe dose routinely used (for a 70-kg patient) is 10–20 mg of etomidate administered by intravenous push before paralysis, and succinylcholine 70–100 mg as an initial dose. Almost 90% of intubations will receive this combination. Although etomidate has become the mainstay for emergent sedation during intubations, a hotly debated issue is its potential for inducing adrenal suppression in septic shock patients. Although there is no evidence to suggest the need to substitute at this time, the EDP can alert the EP to this issue, survey a patient who may have a history of adrenal issues, and recommend alternative agents. Furthermore, the EDP must assure continuity by communicating the risk to the critical care pharmacotherapist.

Infrequently, rocuronium is requested for paralysis in similar doses (1–2 mg/kg) because it has a similar onset of action within 1 minute; however, with a threefold greater duration of action, 30–60 minutes as compared to that of succinylcholine. The two agents do differ as succinylcholine is a depolarizing agent and rocuronium is a non-depolarizing agent; this difference has little significance during resuscitation other than succinylcholine will induce muscle fasciculations within 10–15 seconds and cause muscle paralysis within 1 minute. The importance of fasciculation is seen in patients who cannot have their intracranial pressure raised.

However ideal, this short duration of succinylcholine may cause the patient to spontaneously breathe on his or her own within 5 minutes, thus requiring additional dosing or the use of longer-acting paralytic agents, such as vecuronium and pancuronium. These non-depolarizing agents have a 1.5–2 minute onset and a 1–2 hour duration of action; the advantage of pancuronium is that it does not need to be mixed because it is already in solution form; vecuronium does require reconstitution with normal saline or sterile water for injection. We use 10 mL because there is 10 mg in the vial to create a 1:1 solution for ease of dose preparation. The paralytics are stored in a red bin in a self-locking refrigerator to prevent accidental errors with look-alike and sound-a-like medications. For example, intravenous diltiazem also kept in the refrigerator has a similar appearance and can be accidentally selected instead of a paralytic.

Although paralytics are associated with significant side effects, such as muscle fasciculation, hyperkalemia, bradycardia, trismus, and malignant hyperthermia, we rarely see these effects with a one-time dose initial ED resuscitation.

Hyperkalemia is more of a concern in the trauma or burn patient. Clinicians should opt for rocuronium to avoid any risk because the potassium can increase by as high as 5–10 mEq/L. However, even in these high risk patients, it may take 2–7 days after and with continued administration, of succinylcholine for potassium to elevate so manifestation of hyperkalemia may not occur immediately, unless the patient had an existing elevated potassium.[11] In the medically ill patient, the extent of hyperkalemia that occurs initially is an increase in serum potassium of <1 mEq/L and is not significant clinically unless the patient has pre-existing hyperkalemia, as seen in patients with renal failure.[11] It is prudent to monitor the ECG at that time because this can result in life-threatening dysrhythmia and cardiac arrest.

Succinylcholine is avoided in patients who cannot have their intracranial pressure (ICP) raised, i.e., those with intracranial bleeds, meningitis, head trauma, because these patients are at risk of increased cerebral edema. Any further increase in intracranial pressure can be catastrophic, resulting in exacerbating brain cell death. Although a defasciculating dose of vecuronium (1–2 mg IV push) may be used to prevent the increased ICP by preventing muscle fasciculations, we alternatively use rocuronium to avoid any risk because this method may be more expeditious. It is difficult to time the administration and be assured that vecuronium will take effect before the administration of the succinylcholine to prevent fasciculations.

During the resuscitation, most orders are verbal (orally given), and this is a potential source for medication error. Nurses are occupied with line placements, and physicians are occupied with intubations and patient assessment. The EDP, during resuscitation, must be attentive, aware, courageous to question, but also open-minded to accept instruction. The EDP can be invaluable if he or she conforms to the team approach but leads when needed.

If peripheral intravenous access is not obtained, intraosseous or central line administration may be used. During the resuscitative measure and after initial sedation and paralysis, the pharmacist helps with intubation by providing the Sellick's maneuver also known as Cricoid pressure (only to be done if trained in advanced cardiac life support).

Sellick's maneuver is performed using 10 lb of pressure placed to the cricoids cartilage; it compresses the esophagus and prevents the patient from passive regurgitation of gastric contents because once paralysis commences the patient is at risk of aspiration because they have no gag-reflex.[11] A side effect of Sellick's maneuver is vomiting when applied too early.[11]

Another maneuver the pharmacist may be asked to do is the BURP (Backward, Upward, Rightward, Pressure); this is done when the glottis aperture is not readily visible.[11] The hand is placed on the thyroid cartilage followed by application of the BURP to help bring the glottis into view by the intubator, which significantly improves visibility of the glottis during laryngoscopy.[11]

The EDP should know that the endotracheal tube should be placed at the 23 cm marker for males and 21 cm for females because this will avoid the tube penetrating too deep into the right stem bronchus.[11] The EDP can also assist as the intubator removes the stylet; the EDP using a 10-mL syringe will inflate the endotracheal cuff with 10 mL of air. If the EDP is not assisting with intubation, the EDP should be continuously monitoring the cardiac rhythm, blood pressure, and oxygen saturation. Conformation of endotracheal tube

(ETT) placement is essential as the ETT may have inadvertently been placed in the esophagus. The stomach will appear rising and falling, a cause for morbidity if not quickly corrected. We confirm appropriate placement clinically, by pulse oximetry, end tidal CO2 detection, and auscultation of clear and equal breath sounds over the lung fields with absence of breath sounds over the epigastrium and symmetrical chest rising during ventilation and fogging (condensation of ETT).[11] Pulse oximetry drop after intubation is a clear problem because the ETT may be in the esophagus; this needs re-evaluation. Because pulse-oximetry alone cannot be used to confirm adequate placement, we also use end tidal CO2 detector.

Colorimetric end tidal carbon dioxide detection is a small disposable device that connects between the bag and the ETT.[11] When the device detects end tidal CO2, it changes color from purple to yellow; absence of this color change indicates wrong placement.

POST-INTUBATION COMPLICATIONS

Post-intubation, the ETT must be taped or tied to ensure it does not move; this requires multiple hands to maneuver and still hold the ETT in place. Adverse events may occur due to improper tube placement. Bradycardia may ensue due to esophageal intubation, hypertension may occur due to inadequate sedation, and hypotension may occur due to tension pneumothorax, a decreased venous return, a cardiac cause, or due to the induction agents used.[11] The EDP must monitor the vital signs continuously to alert the clinicians and be prepared to respond accordingly.

EMERGENCY CARE PHARMACOTHERAPY OF SEDATION AND PARALYSIS

The EDP should prepare for long-term sedation and paralysis using benzodiazepines and boluses of vecuronium or pancuronium. For continued sedation, lorazepam (0.1 mg /kg) is given initially. EPs will start with 2 mg and continue repeating this dose until adequate sedation; however, we often start a midazolam drip prepared as a 50 mg/50 mL normal saline solution and run it starting at 1 mg/hour and titrate up to 10–30 mg/hour. The EDP assists the ED team in titrating down the midazolam drip by considering level of organ function, depth of sedation using the modified Ramsey scale, and management of agitation using the Riker sedation and agitation scale.

Measures to assess adequacy of sedation are not commonly employed. Ramsay scale should be considered to avoid over-sedation; however, the EP is usually on to the next patient. Only if the patient awakens or is combative, agitated, or bucks the ETT will the nurse alert the EP. The EDP can employ the Ramsay scale to assure adequate sedation. It is important to note that sedatives and paralytics do not provide analgesia; this is a common misconception. Thus, if the patient is hyperdynamic, it may indicate that the patient is experiencing discomfort or pain. The patient should receive a dose of morphine at 0.1–0.2 mg/kg IV push over several minutes or fentanyl 50–100 mcg by IV bolus dosing.

CIRCULATION MANAGEMENT AND EMERGENCY CARE PHARMACOTHERAPY

Emergency physicians (EPs) are trained in recognizing and managing the undifferentiated patient in cardiac and respiratory arrest; they are experts in the pathophysiology of cardiac arrest and principles of resuscitation.[12] The highest potential survival rate from cardiac arrest is achieved if early warning signs are detected, emergency medical services (EMS) is activated, basic life support is initiated immediately, rapid defibrillation if needed, and advanced cardiovascular life support (ACLS), which includes definitive airway management and intravenous medications, are instituted.[12]

To make an impact, the EDP must master the pharmacotherapeutic interventions used during this time to deliver these medications quickly during the emergency and to intercept a potential error that will constitute a risk with the intervention. The EDP must have the courage to recommend an alternative approach. This is a complex cognitive task because of the patient's morbid condition, unknown etiology, and lack of alternative therapeutic choices. Intervening during cardiac arrest is a highly specialized activity.

Despite all pharmacotherapy available, the most important intervention is basic life support (BLS)/CPR. Obviously, the quality of CPR provided by clinicians varies and requires immediate audio feedback during the event to assure appropriateness. With timely and appropriate CPR, successful intervention can be made with ACLS. If ACLS measures are started within 8 minutes, successful resuscitation occurs in 27% of patients, and if CPR is started within 4 minutes and ACLS within 8 minutes, the rate of successful resuscitation is 43%.[12]

Algorithms have been developed by multidisciplinary emergency cardiac care groups to identify essential cardiac rhythms that, if present, require immediate action to be taken. In the unresponsive patient found in the field, EMS will initially provide BLS and ACLS. Despite this, the patient still may arrive with no pulse. While paramedics are providing CPR, the emergency team needs to spring into action. EMS will usually have the patient on a cardiac monitor to evaluate the current cardiac rhythm. The emergency care team transfers the patient to a hospital bed, and in parallel form, starts the airway-breathing-circulation (ABCs)-IV-O2-monitor intervention while chest compression continues. If the patient has already been intubated in the field, the respiratory therapist is available to place the patient on a mechanical ventilator.

The pharmacist can assist in all BLS and ACLS procedures. The pharmacist should know the ACLS algorithms for cardiac resuscitation and have already mastered the medications needed for immediate treatment. Although this event appears chaotic (and it is), there are limited numbers of interventions so if the ED pharmacist plans correctly, he or she will be prepared to respond and succeed in the team approach to saving a life in the ED.

PULSELESS/UNRESPONSIVE PATIENT AND EMERGENCY CARE PHARMACOTHERAPY

In the event of an unresponsive patient who is not breathing on their own and has no pulse, a cardiac rhythm should be assessed, and a determination of what rhythm the patient is in must be made.

The EDP must be familiar with the nuances of the cardiac monitor and the types of life-threatening rhythms that exist. Reading and recognizing ominous but treatable identifiable cardiac rhythms that may occur is a distinguishing feature of EDP's specialization from other pharmacists.

VENTRICULAR FIBRILLATION/ VENTRICULAR TACHYCARDIA

In parallel manner, all resuscitative procedures are being completed by the code team without prompting, including chest compressions. EPs assess for two relatively easily identifiable cardiac rhythms: ventricular fibrillation/ventricular tachycardia or asystole/pulseless electrical activity as part of a primary survey. The EP will emergently call out for medications. The novice EPs leading the resuscitation team will need prompting or proactive recommendations by seasoned EDPs and nurses because they are sometimes not fully equipped to lead a code in contrast to experienced ED residents and attending.

Ventricular Fibrillation/Ventricular Tachycardia
Epinephrine
Vasopressin
Amiodarone
Lidocaine
Magnesium
Procainamide

For the pulseless, unresponsive, non-breathing patient, the EDP must have ready to administer epinephrine and/or vasopressin because either may be requested. EDPs may have a code cart available that stores these medications, in addition to other supplies. Depending on the construct of the ED, the code cart, which is labor intensive to prepare, can be avoided with advanced preparation for the code by the EDP. Avoiding use of the code cart is a potential cost-saving activity.

EPINEPHRINE OR VASOPRESSIN

Epinephrine is available as a 1-mg prefilled syringe (1:10,000 or 0.1 mg/mL), and the preparation of the syringe needs to be mastered because it is unique in comparison to how a normal syringe is used. Epinephrine primarily is indicated for the preservation of the myocardium and cerebrum until measures are instituted to achieve return of spontaneous circulation (*return of a pulse*). Epinephrine has been associated with improving success rates of defibrillation as it lowers the defibrillation threshold.

In addition to procuring, dispensing, and administering epinephrine, a pharmacist records the time and dose on a resuscitation form (Fig. 15-1). The form is devised with the ACLS protocol in mind and the sequence of medications that are required to be administered. If the EDP is preparing

DEFIBRILLATIONS/CARDIOVERSIONS ☐ **AED Used** ☐ **Powerheart Used** ☐ **Number of shocks**

TIME						
JOULES						

MEDICATIONS ADMINISTERED

I.V. PUSH (available strength)	USUAL IVP DOSE	TIME	DOSE	TIME	DOSE	TIME	DOSE	TIME	DOSE	TIME	DOSE	TIME	DOSE
Epinephrine HCL (Adrenalin) 1:10,000 1mg = 10ml	1mg (1:10,000) IVP												
Atropine Sulfate 1mg = 10 ml	0.5mg - 1mg IVP (0.04mg/kg)												
Lidocaine (Xylocaine) 2% 100mg = 5ml	50mg - 100mg IVP (1-1.5mg/kg) Total = 3mg/kg												
Adenosine (Adenocard) 6mg = 2ml	6mg IVP (proximal port admin. only) 6mg- 12mg- 12mg												
Magnesium Sulfate 50% 1gm = 2ml	1 -2gm IVP												
Procainamide (Pronestyl) 1gm = 10ml	Loading dose (1gm/50ml D5W) 20-30mg/min infuson up to 17mg/kg												
Sodium Bicarbonate 7.5% 44.6mEq = 50ml	1mEq/kg IVP followed by 0.5mEq/kg q 10 min												
Calcium Chloride 10% 1gm = 10 ml	2 - 4 mg/kg IVP												
Vasopressin (Pitressin) 20 unit = 1ml	40 units IVP												
Amiodarone (Cordarone) 150mg = 3ml	150mg IVP X 1 (repeat X 2 PRN)												

I.V. DRIPS

	TIME / INFUSION RATE			
Lidocaine (Xylocaine) 1gm/250ml D5W 2 - 4 mg/min				
Dopamine (Inotropin) 400mg/250ml D5W (Max 20mcg/kg/min) Titrate to SBP greater than 90 (MAP greater than 60)				
Norepinephrine (Levophed): 8mg/250ml D5W Titrate to SBP greater than 90 (MAP greater than 60)				
Procainamide (Pronestyl): 1gm/250ml D5W 1 - 4mg/min				
Dobutamine (Dobutrex): 250mg/250ml D5W 2 - 5mcg/kg/min				
Amiodarone (Cordarone): 900mg/500ml D5W 1mg/min				

ABG'S

TIME	pH	pCO₂	pO₂	HCO₃	O₂SAT

IV SOLUTIONS & OTHER
DRIPS 1. _____
2. _____

COMMENTS: _____

INVASIVE PROCEDURE: ☐ NO ☐ YES-TYPE (i.e., chest tube, central line, etc.): _____
Pt cooled with hypothermia blanket post code? ☐ NO ☐ YES *(ED or ICU ONLY)

Figure 15–1. CPR recording sheet.

the medications and assisting with procedures, the EDP may relegate recording to an intern, resident, or an extra nurse. But, timing and accuracy of recording are essential to reviewing performance improvement and quality assurance.

Pharmacists may not feel it is their role to participate in a cardiac arrest code. The EDP should be expected to be at the bedside. Our policy and procedure for the code team includes the pharmacist and delineates their role (see Appendix A: Policies and Procedures).

If the patient is pulseless and ventricular fibrillation or ventricular tachycardia is identified, then vasopressin 40 units may be prescribed. The procurement will cause delay, for example, two vials of 20 units/mL needs to be drawn into a syringe and administered as a single dose. Alternatively, epinephrine may be given as a 1 mg dose and then repeated every 3–5 minutes using a prefilled syringe.

ANTIARRHYTHMIC DRUGS

Antiarrhythmics such as amiodarone, lidocaine, and procainamide increase the ability of defibrillation to work by reducing the fibrillation threshold. For ventricular fibrillation or pulseless ventricular tachycardia after defibrillation with 360 joules using a biphasic current, amiodarone available as a 150 mg/3 mL should be administered at a dose of 300 mg IV push. Alternatively lidocaine available as a 20 mg/mL in 5-mL prefilled syringe should be given at a dose of 1.5 mg/kg, usually 100 mg is given. Excessive amiodarone may cause nausea, vomiting, bradycardia and hypotension. The EDP must be prepared to assist with managing these complications. Excessive dosing of lidocaine may cause myoclonus. Benzodiazepines may be started to reduce these movements.[12] The same initial antiarrhythmic with countershocks should be continued to avoid risk of proarrhythmia due to multiple antiarrhythmics used. The EDP procures, dispenses, and records the timing of each antiarrhythmic administered while monitoring the cardiac rhythm for any change.

Magnesium should be administered when hypomagnesemic states are likely, such as in chronic alcoholics and wasting syndrome, because it stabilizes the cardiac cell membrane. Procainamide is rarely used in this setting despite it being available; its method of administration is too cumbersome. Both amiodarone and lidocaine require subsequent intravenous infusion to be initiated to prevent recurrence. Lidocaine is available as a premix, whereas amiodarone requires procuring in a glass bottle, making it difficult to prepare in an expedited manner, so the pharmacist at the bedside can facilitate the procurement and ordering.

■ Case Study

Resuscitation Errors Do Occur

When verbally prescribed by the EP, amiodarone was mistaken for amrinone by the nurse. This error occurred because a nurse used old dosing guides and read the dosing rate to be started off the amrinone dosing chart. The nurse labeled the bag amrinone despite actually using amiodarone vials. Despite these errors, once amiodarone was started, the patient became severely hypotensive and bradycardic, which caused the EP to hold the amio-

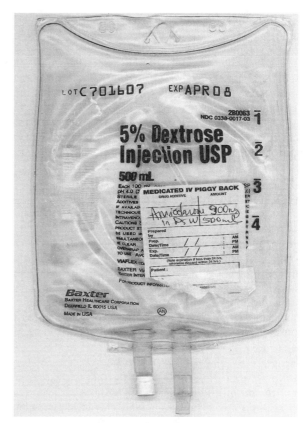

Figure 15–2. Amiodarone procured in an intravenous bag.

darone. The intravenous infusion was procured using a bag instead of a bottle (Fig. 15-2), and no filter was used.

Upon review, it was identified that the patient was in atrial fibrillation as opposed to ventricular tachycardia, a less ominous life-threatening dysrhythmia that likely did not require such aggressive management. It is important for the EDP to confirm the presence of disease when dispensing high-risk medication during high risk emergent situations. This safeguard will assure that the errors in drug ordering and delivery process are averted.

ASYSTOLE

Bradycardia leading to asystole (flat-line on a cardiac monitor) may be due to cardiac causes, hypoxia, stroke, medications such as beta blockers, calcium channel blockers, or opiates.[12] The EP will call for atropine and epinephrine both at 1 mg repeated every 3–5 minutes. Atropine is given at a maximum of 0.04 mg/kg, which means in a 70-kg patient, no more than 3 doses of 1 mg should be given because there will be no further benefit of atropine. More frequent doses may cause anticholinergic toxicity. The mechanism of effect of atropine practically speaking is the equivalent of taking the foot off the brake of a car. Atropine inhibits the vagus nerve. The vagus nerve innervates the atrioventricular (AV) node, which regulates the delivery of impulses to the ventricle. Removal of this regulatory control is like removing your foot off the brake of a car. Thus atropine may result in increasing the heart rate and resolving the bradyasystolic rhythm. Transcutaneous pacing (low voltage electrical activity) is used in conjunction with these medications.

Asystole has a poor prognosis in geriatric patients; the care team considers if the patient has a Do Not Resuscitate and Do Not Intubate (DNR/DNI) order. Persistent asystole should be an indicator to the EDP to assess 1) quality of resuscitation being conducted, 2) whether this is an atypical clinical presentation of fine ventricular fibrillation masquerading as asystole (so check a second lead that may reveal a fine ventricular fibrillation or confirm the asystole); or 3) lack of response and indicator to support cease-efforts protocol to be started.[12]

PULSELESS ELECTRICAL ACTIVITY (PROGNOSIS 1–4% SURVIVE)[12]

Pulseless electrical activity (PEA) occurs when electrical activity is identified on the cardiac monitor; however, this rhythm is associated with no true mechanical pumping of the ventricular chamber, in other words, a rhythm without a pulse. EPs will go through a differential of causes that pharmacists must also recall to expedite treatment. The 5Hs and 5Ts mnemonic is a way to remember the possible causes and allows one to prepare for what is needed if PEA is identified.

5Hs

The 5Hs include hypovolemia, hypoxia, hydrogen ions–acidosis, hyper- or hypokalemia (and other electrolyte abnormalities) and profound hypoglycemia and hypothermia.[12] Treatment of PEA begins immediately as some interventions are already instituted such as intubation for hypoxia, IV crystalloids for hypovolemia. A compression bag is used to increase the rate of delivery of the fluids, and the pharmacist may assist with procuring the intravenous fluids. Emergency care pharmacotherapy for the 5Hs is sodium bicarbonate for acidosis or potassium chloride for hypokalemia. Hyperkalemia is treated with the combination of sodium bicarbonate, glucose and insulin, calcium chloride/gluconate administered to induce a transcellular shift of potassium into the cell while also stabilizing the cardiac membrane from further ventricular ectopy. Dextrose 50% is given with thiamine if the patient was found to be hypoglycemic.

PEA

For the 5Hs:
Saline
Oxygen
Sodium Bicarbonate
Dextrose 50%
Insulin
Potassium Chloride
Calcium Chloride
Calcium Gluconate
Magnesium Sulfate

HYPOKALEMIA

When cardiac arrest is the result of an electrolyte abnormality, it does create a problem because it is likely that treatment is needed before laboratory values are obtained; a strong familiarity with electrolyte-related EKG signs is an essential skill for pharmacists responding to a cardiac arrest. Intravenous potassium replacement is indicated in patients with severe losses <2.5 mEq/L, but this is likely not to be known and instead will initially manifest as weakness, fatigue, paralysis, respiratory difficulty, constipation, or leg cramps. Most importantly, the ECG changes that need to be screened for are a **U wave, T wave flattening**, and ventricular arrhythmias, especially while on digoxin,. The EDP must relate initial presentation to the possible causes, such as, the initial unstable sign of hypokalemia in the ED may be pulseless electrical activity or asystole.[13]

Dosing of potassium is empiric when indicated in emergent conditions and should include 10–20 mEq/hour given with continuous ECG monitoring. Peripheral administration of potassium is usually the mainstay in the ED but a central line is preferred.[13]

HYPERKALEMIA

The EDP can focus on certain issues familiar to pharmacotherapy training and deduce that the patient is having hyperkalemia-induced cardiac arrest by identifying the patient's past history. Chronic renal failure, recent chemotherapy and tumor lysis syndrome, rhabdomyolysis, and drug-induced causes such as potassium-sparing diuretics, ACE inhibitors, NSAIDS, potassium supplements, succinylcholine, heparin, and beta blockers are all risks for hyperkalemia.[13]

The EDP at the bedside should not be an idle observer instead he or she should be ready to take instruction and initiate fact finding activity that can aid in the assessment of the cause of the patient's event.

The initial presenting rhythm maybe PEA, but before this rhythm develops, early screening of the ECGs can detect abnormalities such as *peaked T waves (tenting), flattened P waves, prolonged PR interval (first degree heart block), widened QRS complex, and deepening S waves and merging S and T waves*. If left untreated, a sine wave, idioventricular rhythms, and asystolic cardiac arrest may develop.

Pharmacotherapy for hyperkalemia is usually severity dependent; based on the level, but during a cardiac arrest, is unknown so standard treatment must be used empirically to shift the potassium into cells. Initially, calcium chloride 10%, 500 to 1000 mg or 5–10 mL intravenously over 2–5 minutes should be administered to immediately reduce the effects of potassium at the myocardial cell membrane and lower the risk of ventricular fibrillation.[13] Calcium chloride is available as a prefilled syringe or in a vial. There is no need to substitute with calcium gluconate because the pain secondary to calcium chloride injection is not relevant in an unresponsive patient. Furthermore, use of calcium gluconate is often under dosed in terms of elemental calcium as it is only 30% of that of calcium chloride and not able to afford as much protection. Often calcium gluconate is incorrectly prescribed. Administer sodium bicarbonate 50 mEq intravenously over 5 minutes.

The combination of glucose and insulin is prescribed to help shift potassium into the cell. Routinely glucose in the form of 25 grams of dextrose 50% 50 mL is administered with 10 units of regular insulin each individually. Some suggest mixing the two and giving them at the same time, yet during this event, that is a rare occurrence and nurses usually push each as soon as they are obtained.

Nebulized albuterol (10–20 mg) over 15 minutes although effective is not commonly administered. The EP may request its use because it has been shown to reduce potassium levels.

Since these measures are temporary, they are likely to be repeated as potassium may rebound so a re-evaluation is required within 1 hour.

HYPERMAGNESEMIA

Magnesium is required for sodium, potassium, and calcium movement across the cell and to stabilize excitable membranes. Severe hypermagnesemia is associated with bradycardia, cardiac arrhythmias, and cardiorespiratory arrest. Fortunately, treatment of hyperkalemia with calcium chloride also corrects for lethal arrhythmias due to hypermagnesemia. Dialysis is recommended once stable.

HYPOMAGNESEMIA

Torsades de pointe is the classic rhythm associated with severe hypomagnesemia along with an altered mental status, tremors, and fasciculation. MgSO4 (1–2 gram over 5 minutes) is requested by the EP. The duration of infusion may be up to 60 minutes but in practice it is usually given by intravenous bolus.[13] Calcium is usually given empirically during cardiac arrest as hypomagnesemic states are often associated with hypocalcemic states.

HYPERCALCEMIA

Due to the shortened refractory period, arrhythmias can occur secondary to hypercalcemia. It can worsen digitalis toxicity and may induce hypokalemia, both of which make the patient more susceptible to arrhythmias. *The ECG signs may be of shortened QT interval, with prolonged PR and QRS waves.* Complete heart block may develop and progress to cardiac arrest with levels of calcium above 15 mg/dL.[13] The immediate use of saline fluids at rates of 300–500 mL/hr will enhance calcium excretion in the urine. This should occur until diuresis with a urine output of 200–300 mL/hr.[13] Then, the saline infusion may be reduced to 100–200 mL/hr. The EP may call for emergent hemodialysis to rapidly decrease serum calcium especially in renal patients or CHF patients. EDTA (10–50 mg/kg) over 4 hours may be used in extreme conditions.[13]

THE Ts OF PULSELESS ELECTRICAL ACTIVITY

The 4Ts of PEA include 1) "tablets of toxins" associated with accidental or intentional overdose, 2) tamponade, 3) tension pneumothorax, (maybe iatrogenic) and 4) thrombosis with pulmonary or cardiac origin.

Toxins

Common toxins may ultimately present to the ED with PEA and include beta blockers, calcium channel blockers, and tricyclic antidepressants. In undifferentiated toxin-related causes of PEA, the EDP should be prepared to aid in identifying and confirming the toxin through profiling the history, clinical manifestations, and probing the caregivers of the patient's medication history and drug use. Alongside the patient's initial clinical presentation, often this history and fact finding leads to a strong presumptive etiology and diagnosis helping to direct the management as illustrated in the case study below.

PEA

For the 5 Ts:
Calcium Chloride
Calcium Gluconate
High Dose Insulin and Dextrose therapy
Glucagon
Saline
Sodium Bicarbonate
Thrombolytics

 Case Study

ED Pharmacist Deduces Possible Toxin

A 40-year-old woman with a history of migraines presents to the ED with initial vital signs of bradycardia and hypotension. The patient claimed to have taken her usual calcium supplements. She reported dizziness and had a witnessed syncopal episode; the ambulance transported her to the ED. Immediately the ED physician and pharmacotherapist assisting on the case suspected either beta blocker (BB) or calcium channel antagonist (CCA) overdose. This was based on the initial presenting vital signs and the history of migraine pain described. Migraines sufferers may be prescribed propranolol or verapamil as prophylaxis. Management for either CCA or BB was initiated. Subsequently, the husband arrived and confirmed our suspicion. The patient accidentally selected verapamil rather than the calcium supplements. The error occurred because both medications were stored in the same vial. The vial was an oversized vial with multiple sections and separate chambers (Fig. 15-3). Verapamil has a similar appearance to that of calcium supplements (Fig. 15-4). The patient was resuscitated and after a lengthy stay in the ICU, she recovered. This case could have progressed to a PEA but knowledge of the toxins initial presenting toxidrome and management by the emergency care team improved the overall quality of care for the patient and avoided a delay in correctly making the diagnosis and proper management.

TAMPONADE/TENSION PNEUMOTHORAX

The pharmacotherapist may assist, at the EP's request, with procedures for relieving tamponade and tension pneumoth-

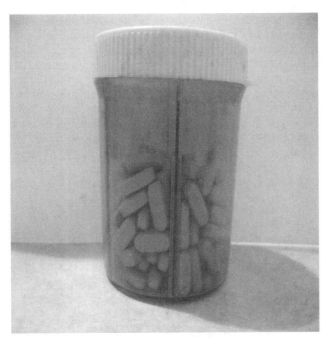

Figure 15–3. Oversized medication vial with multiple (6) sections.

orax. A chest tube is needed to be placed and/or a needle aspiration to relieve the tension pneumothorax. Pharmacists should be aware that the presenting sign of tension pneumothorax may be something as benign as shortness of breath. Furthermore, pneumonia may be a cause of pneumothorax, and pneumothorax may resolve itself unless a tension pneumothorax occurs. When this occurs, complications include an obstructive shock. That is, the cardiopulmonary circuit is being obstructed from filling the ventricle and permitting normal contraction. Within minutes, coronary blood flow may be obstructed and evolve into a PEA. The surgical team is consulted to place a chest tube and relieve the pneumothorax. The EDP must assist in the management of the shock state, titrating appropriate vasopressors, usually norepinephrine or phenylephrine. Intubation in these cases may be catastrophic because the positive pressure ventilation can further obstruct the cardiopulmonary blood flow. The EDP must be ready with epinephrine and atropine because the patient may become pulseless at anytime.

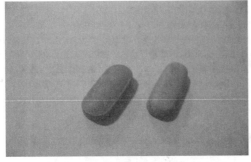

Figure 15–4. Similarities in calcium supplement and verapamil tablet.

THROMBOSIS

Thrombolytics differ in doses for acute coronary syndrome, pulmonary embolism, and stroke; close attention is required by the pharmacotherapist to assist with appropriate implementation. Dosing errors are common in all situations.

CARDIAC ARREST AND PULMONARY EMBOLISM (PE)

Kurkciyan et al. reported that of 1246 cardiac arrest victims over an 8-year period, 60 patients were found to have pulmonary embolism. The initial identifiable rhythm was PEA in 63% of the study population with confirmed PE, and 32% in asystole, whereas only 3% were found in ventricular fibrillation. Among the 60 cases of PE, the investigators identified that dyspnea, syncope, and chest pain were the most common reported symptoms before the cardiac arrest event. The authors identified 21 patients who were treated with thrombolytic therapy and compared with 21 patients who did not receive thrombolytic therapy. Although there were only three survivors, two in the thrombolytic group and one in the non-thrombolytic group, there was a statistical significant increase in the number of patients in the thrombolytic group who had a return of spontaneous circulation compared to that of the non-thrombolytic group, 17/21(81%) versus 9/21(43%), supporting the use of thrombolytic therapy in suspected cases of PE during cardiac arrest with an identifiable rhythm.[14] No cases of cerebral bleed occurred with thrombolytic therapy despite administration of a double bolus of 50 mg given 15 minutes apart. However, bleeding complication was exacerbated by resuscitative efforts and may have been exaggerated by thrombolysis, as two patients suffered a ruptured liver, and one other case had mediastinal bleeding. Currently, there is no evidence supporting this bolus dosing in PE, and recommendations of the Fifth American College of Chest Physicians Consensus Conference are to administer either 100 mg of alteplase over 2 hours or a bolus of streptokinase 250,000 units followed by 100,000 units/hour over 24 hours.

ROLE OF THE ED PHARMACIST AND EXPEDITING DELIVERY OF THROMBOLYSIS

To expedite the use of thrombolytic therapy, a thrombolytic kit is stored in a locked cabinet available in the ED at the bedside during the resuscitative efforts. The kit includes a policy and procedure for use in stoke and acute myocardial infarction, dosing guide for various thrombolytics, and subsequent management pathway (Fig. 15-5). An rt-PA-indication/contraindication scoring form is included with the National Institute of Health Stroke Scale for assessment to assist the EP and the neurology fellow.

The relevance of contraindications in this life-threatening situation is less significant than that of other emergent situations, such as a patient with ST-elevation MI. A systematic and proactive assessment of risk and benefit is needed during PEA. The EDP should take on this role and assist the EP in confirming that there are no contraindications. Conversely a rationale for the use should be made as throm-

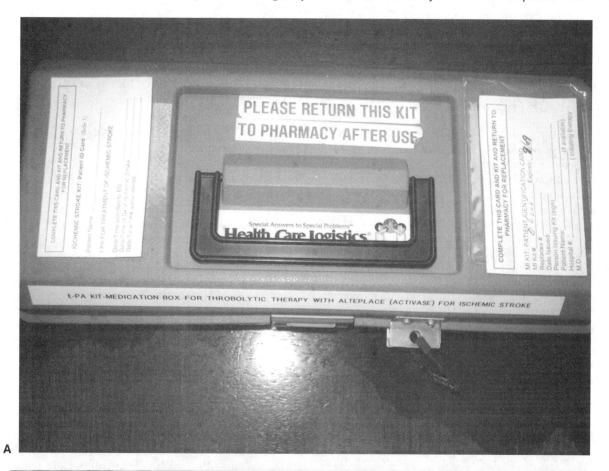

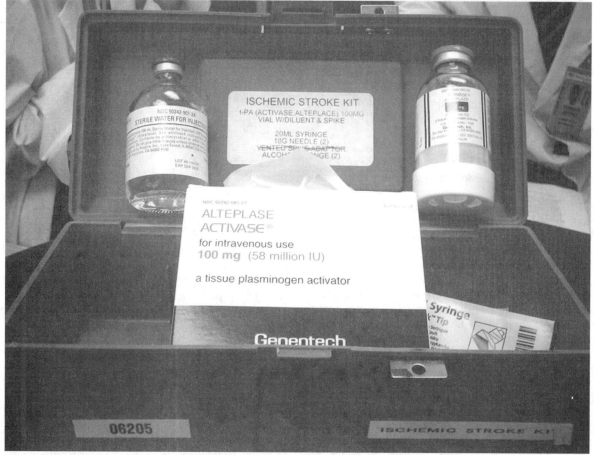

Figure 15–5. **A.** Thrombolytic kit. **B.** Note the drug evaluation cards for quality assurance of thrombolysis.

bolytics are costly, and arbitrarily administering thrombolytic therapy in PEA in suspected futile cases would be inappropriate.

ED PHARMACIST INTERVENTIONS DURING DELIVERY OF THROMBOLYSIS

Incorrect dosing regimens for thrombolysis have been reported and may adversely impact success for initial management of acute coronary syndrome (ACS), stroke, and pulmonary embolism (PE) and the EDP must be at the bedside to confirm the weight-adjusted dosing and administration.

Streptokinase is much less expensive than that of alteplase so it is used more often to reduce costs. Streptokinase does pose a risk of anaphylaxis, and many clinicians are wary of its use. However, routinely the physician will accept whatever is available if the pharmacotherapist is present with it, as a means to avoid delays.

Streptokinase (Streptase) is available as a 1.5 million unit vial, often a cause for confusion on how to calculate the appropriate dosing. The EDP must verify the dosing and administration. Streptokinase procurement requires that the vial be reconstituted with 5 mL to obtain dosage strength *of 250,000 unit/mL;* the solution should be swirled gently, not shaken, and it may appear slightly yellow. A bolus dose for PE is 250,000 units given over 30 minutes so diluting 1 mL of constituted streptokinase in 50 mL of D5W or NS is appropriate for the initial bolus. Then, the remaining vial may be diluted with 500 mL of either D5W or NS, attaching the intravenous bag to an infusion pump line, as an infusion pump must be used to avoid risk of infusing the dose to rapidly. At the outset, the EDP must ensure that the nurse has obtained a dedicated line for thrombolytic therapy and that an infusion pump device is available for thrombolytic therapy. The maintenance rate of infusion for PE is 100,000 units/hour given for 24 hours, thus, the infusion pump should be running at the appropriate rate and should be checked. Because the total dose required exceeds that of the contents of the vial of streptokinase, a second bag must be prescribed and procured. The need for the second bag of the remaining dose should be anticipated to avoid delay. The clinicians assure frequent monitoring for bleeding using various diagnostic approaches, such as ultrasound, and special precautions are taken to avoid inducing a bleed.

For PE, alteplase is given as 100 mg over 2 hours then followed by heparin. Alteplase (100 mg vial of lyophilized powder) is accompanied with 100-mL vial of diluent. Alteplase is compatible in both D5W and NS; however, using the vial provided by the manufacturer of 100 ml of sterile water for injection will be all that is needed. The vial has a loop for hanging it on to an IV pole. Similar to streptokinase, alteplase must be placed on an infusion pump, and because the 100 mg needs to infused over 2 hours, the infusion rate should be set to 50 mL/hour, not 100 mL/hour; this a common cause for error in administration. Also, it would be wise to program the infusion pump to alarm when approaching near the end of the infusion because at the end of the infusion, the line should be flushed with 20–30 mL of saline to ensure the entire dose is administered.

Epinephrine should be given for the duration of PEA, and if the heart rate is slow atropine may be given at similar doses as those discussed earlier until thrombolytic therapy is completed. We rarely see the use of thrombolytics during PEA cardiac arrest, perhaps due to compressions administered, and futility associated with the patient's age. These agents are not routine in emergency care resuscitation, but pharmacists must be prepared to suggest and manage these therapies if called for by the EP.

CARDIAC ARREST AND CORONARY THROMBOSIS

Sample policies and procedures for the use of thrombolysis for acute stroke and acute myocardial infarction are seen in Appendix A: Policies and Procedures.

Thrombolytic therapy should be instituted if there is strong suspicion of acute coronary thrombosis. First, fifteen milligrams of alteplase is initially administered as an IV bolus over 1 minute by the physician. The physician should be at the bedside; then, 0.75 mg/kg, up to a maximum of 50 mg, is administered over 30 minutes (rate of infusion is set at double the normal rate/hour to deliver the appropriate dose within 30 minutes). Routinely, the volume to be infused is set to alarm the nurse to initiate the remaining amount of rt-PA over the next hour, i.e., 0.5 mg/kg up to 35 mg is administered over the next 60 minutes. Subsequently, the intravenous line should be flushed with saline after the infusion.

PERI-INFUSION COMPLICATIONS

An unexpected case of angioedema occurred while a patient was receiving rtPA for stroke. The patient had a past history of angioedema to captopril and there may be a pharmacologic relationship between the two classes of medications that would increase the subsequent risk for angioedema. This would be an unexpected event during use of thrombolysis and could undermine the safe and effective use of thrombolysis in the ED. Thus the EDP should prepare to detect any peri-infusion reactions, i.e., evidence of bleeding. A bleeding protocol has also been developed for nurses to follow and is kept in the thrombolysis kit.

Thrombolytics in cardiac arrest may be "a last ditch effort" of survival for the patient. Thrombolytic errors may occur and may affect the outcome. An EDP can put processes in place to assure quality of thrombolysis and give this intervention the best chance to succeed by continuously monitoring thrombolysis use. The thrombolytic kit includes a medication use evaluation card for follow up for continued performance improvement.

OTHER COMMON RESUSCITATIVE SITUATIONS

Shock

Another common acute resuscitation situation pharmacists may encounter in the ED is the patient who presents with undifferentiated shock. Shock is a state in which the oxygen and metabolic demands of the body are not being met. This decompensated state leads to multiple system organ failure and inevitable death.[15]

Several pitfalls in the management of shock include 1) failure to recognize early signs of shock before hypotension develops, 2) failure to provide early ventilator support to the hemodynamically compromised patient, 3) inadequate fluid resuscitation of the volume-depleted patient before initiating vasopressors/dilators, 4) delay in administration of empiric broad spectrum antibiotics in septic shock, 5) failure to continuously monitor hemodynamic parameters as a guide to titration of fluid therapy and vasopressor/dilator therapy, 6) improper selection of vasoactive agent, and 7) reliance on the pulse oximeter as an index of oxygen saturation (SaO2) during periods of hypoperfusion, severe hypoxemia, or when various anemias exist.[15] The EDP is invaluable in preventing that these pitfalls do not occur during this critical event.

The core goal of pharmacotherapy for shock patients is optimizing delivery of oxygen to vital organs. Often the pharmacotherapy of decompensated shock begins before any conclusive etiology is identified and is based more on initial presenting vital signs and mental status.

For example, intravenous fluids are immediately initiated for hypovolemia secondary to either hemorrhage or dehydration. This is a minimal risk intervention that can achieve the immediate goal of inadequate oxygenation while providing time for evaluation.

In the elderly, we see multiple etiologies that cause the decompensated shock-like state, and thus we have developed a mnemonic to help with early consideration of the cause of shock. The mnemonic "NOCHD" can be used to remember the various classes of shock (Fig. 15-6).

Neurogenic shock most often associated with a spinal cord injury disrupts sympathetic outflow resulting in bradycardia and hypotension. Obstructive shock describes the obstruction to blood flow that is occurring through the heart and lungs and is caused by tension pneumothorax, pericardial tamponade, constrictive pericarditis, a massive pulmonary embolus, severe pulmonary hypertension, and severe valvular stenosis. Cardiogenic shock is caused by pump failure, valvular disorder, cardiac arrhythmias, and hypovolemia which has already been described.

Distributive shock is due to sepsis, anaphylaxis, and/or drug overdose. Each of these shock-like states requires extensive evaluation and management; however, certain signs and elements of the past medical history are invaluable to increase the index of suspicion, and some of the interventions are of

- # N-eurogenic

- # O-bstructive

- # C-ardiogenic

- # H-ypovolemic

- # D-istributive

Figure 15–6. NOCHD mnemonic used to help remember general causes of shock.

low risk and high reward that they can be initiated without full diagnostic confirmation (IV normal saline fluids).

ED PHARMACIST INTERVENTIONS DURING DELIVERY OF CARE FOR SHOCK PATIENTS

The EDP at the bedside can assist with stabilization and can probe the paramedics or family members (did the patient sustain any trauma or was there any evidence of trauma?), the patient's medical records (did the patient have any allergies to medication or food?), nursing home notes (was the patient febrile, what source for infection exists?), prior admissions to the hospital (does the patient have cardiopulmonary disorder, such as atrial fibrillation PUD/UGIB/anemia?), prior medication profiles (is the patient taking beta blockers, calcium channel blocker, digitalis, diuretics, NSAIDS, Coumadin?),[15] and current medication from the ambulance call record to gain at least an improved hypothesis as to the most plausible etiology. This entire information gathering helps to avoid over-use, under-use, and inappropriate interventions while still stabilizing the patient.

SAFE AND EFFECTIVE MEDICATION USE DURING ACUTE STABILIZATION

Physical examination is essential to guide management, and the use of a right heart catheterization would be optimal to assess the physiological derangements that are occurring to direct the EP to the most likely cause of the shock-like state.[15] Parameters such as central venous pressure, pulmonary artery occlusion pressure, systemic vascular resistance, and cardiac output/index should be assessed. However, during acute stabilization of shock in the ED, these monitoring techniques are not routinely available.

The two major goals of resuscitative efforts includes oxygen saturation of at least 90%, and mean arterial blood pressure of 70–80 mmHg because it is a function of vital organ perfusion pressure. The mean arterial blood pressure may be calculated $\{MAP = DBP + 1/3(SBP-DBP)\}$. Most modern day EDs have cardiac monitors that provide this information along with the systolic and diastolic blood pressures, heart rate, and oxygen saturation, and most PDA medical calculators provide these immediate calculations. Devices such as the personal digital assistant (PDA) have medical calculator applications to enable the clinician to conduct immediate calculations of important vital parameters.

The EDP must be trained to use these monitors to allow for continued effective titration of vasoactive agents and prevent pitfalls of not achieving these desired endpoints. Clinically early signs of decreased oxygenation and perfusion may be detected through assessment of the patient mental status, screening for cyanosis, delay in capillary refill, skin mottling, blood returning from their rectum or from the nasogastric tube.[15] In addition these clinical findings can help increase suspicion toward the most likely etiology.

Management of hypovolemic shock includes nonpharmacological approaches such as intravenous fluids with crystalloids and transfusion of blood products in the suspected dehydrated or hemorrhagic patient for hypovolemic shock. Elderly patients may have less cardiac reserve so they may only need several hundred milliliters of crystalloids to stabilize; this is in contrast to the younger patient who may need large amounts of fluids to resuscitate. Two bags of normal saline are infused via two 18-gauge needles at a wide open rate initially.[15]

Transfusion of blood products is frequently used in patients with a below normal hematocrit and hemoglobin, and furosemide 20 mg IV push is given prior to avoid fluid overload. Studies have shown the impact of furosemide on preventing increases in pulmonary artery wedge pressure and other important cardiovascular parameters suggesting its role prior to transfusion, yet most studies are of small sample size and several have produced equivocal results. We have not observed any adverse effect associated with furosemide in its use prior to transfusion. Transfusion is administered and verified by two nurses to ensure no error occurs because it is a high-risk intervention.

In neurogenic shock, most commonly related to spinal cord injury and loss of sympathetic tone, norepinephrine or phenylephrine is indicated among other interventions, i.e., steroids.

During obstructive shock, surgical intervention is needed, such as pericardiocentesis, or needle decompression for cardiac tamponade or tension pneumothorax. Intravenous fluids may be initiated until the procedure is completed.

For cardiogenic shock, despite the lack of strong evidence supporting one vasopressor over another, the ACC/AHA consensus committee has recommended the use of dobutamine if the SBP is >90 mmHg, dopamine if SBP is <90 mmHg, and norepinephrine if hypotension is severe or refractory to dopamine infusions. If unresponsive to vasopressors, an intra-aortic balloon pump is considered but not routinely employed in the ED. Patients in cardiogenic shock are assessed by the cardiac interventional team for assessment and transfer.

Dobutamine is available as a 250 mg/250 mL bag, and dopamine is available as a 400 mg/250 mL premix bag; each is given at a consistent at rate of 1 mcg/kg/minute up to a maximum 20 mcg/kg/minute. Dobutamine is rarely ever implemented as patients with SBP of >90 mmHg are not viewed as hemodynamically unstable, as their MAP appears to be >70 mmHg, and because clinicians may not have all the information at the time to differentiate the etiology.

Dopamine is frequently initiated because patients with a SBP <90 mmHg is more of a trigger for hemodynamic instability. Dopamine is titrated to response; however, it is routinely started at 10 mcg/kg/minute, not the 5 mcg/kg/minute as usually recommended, and is titrated to greater than the maximum recommended dose of 25–30 mcg/kg/minute despite the lack of data supporting any additional effectiveness at these doses. The major limiting side effect of dopamine is tachycardia and the risk to exacerbating ventricular dysrhythmias. The patient who may be volume depleted is at risk of exacerbating a myocardial infarction and rationalizes the use of alternative pressor agents that do not increase heart rate such as norepinephrine and /or phenylephrine.

Norepinephrine is prepared as 4 or 8 mg/250 mL bag or 500 mL (nursing often consults pharmacy on how to use these drips and physicians will consult to assist in titration of these drips). Norepinephrine is given at a rate of 0.05 mcg/kg/minute to 2 mcg/kg/minute, and instituted only if the patient is refractory to dopamine or if there is intolerance to dopamine due to the tachycardia.

In distributive shock due to sepsis or anaphylaxis, the shock state is due to loss of vasomotor tone. Both norepinephrine and phenylephrine are options. Phenylephrine is prepared as a 100 mg in 250 mL bag and titrated at rate of *0.01 mcg/kg/minute to 0.5 mcg/kg/minute*, to goal. Both norepinephrine and phenylephrine do not increase heart rate, but they do potentially reduce cardiac output because they increase systematic vascular resistance SBP, DBP, MAP, and PCWP.

We compare the hemodynamic effects of each vasopressor, based on their effects on hemodynamic parameters as published in clinical trials and use this tool at the bedside to ensure the desired endpoint is achieved (see Appendix B: Guide to Management of Critical Care Drug Infusions in the ED). Often, we are limited to HR, SBP, DBP, MAP, and perhaps central venous pressure that reflects the ability of the heart to pump blood into the arterial system. The benefit of such a tool is to be able to anticipate the effects of the vasopressor while titrating and assuring no unexpected outcomes.

SUMMARY

Integrating critical care skills into the EDP practice is important to assure safe and effective medication use of the critically ill patient. Monitoring may not be as intensive, the ED clinical staff may not be as familiar with the critical care pharmacotherapy, and the shear number of interventions to provide quality resuscitation may be overwhelming. It requires a team approach and pharmacotherapists must be a part of that team. However, to add value, pharmacists must gain experience to master the nuances of critical care pharmacotherapy implemented in the ED. They must master evidence-based critical care pharmacotherapy to understand the current expectations of safe and effective drug use in the critical care patient and fill the gaps that may otherwise hinder optimal implementation of quality critical care. This skill is gained only through multiple experience and observations while in the ED.

References

1. Rivers EP, Nguyen HB, Huang DT, et al. Critical Care and emergency medicine. *Curr Opin Crit Care* 2002;6:600–606.
2. Nelson M, Waldrop RD, Jones J, et al. Critical care provided in an urban emergency department. *Am J Emerg Med* 1998;16: 56–59.
3. Fromm RE, Gibbs LR, McCallum EGB, et al. Critical care in the emergency department: A time based study. *Crit Care Med* 1993;21:970–976.
4. Svenson J, Besinger B, Stapczynski JS. Critical Care or medical and surgical patients in the ED: Length of stay and initiation of intensive procedures. *Am J Emerg Med* 1997;15:654–657.
5. Goldstein RS. Management of the critically ill patient in the emergency department: Focus on safety issues. *Crit Care Clin* 2005;21:81–89.
6. Rivers E, Nguyen B, Havstad S, et al. Early goal directed therapy in the treatment of severe sepsis and septic shock. *N Engl J Med* 2001;345:1368–1377.

7. Nguyen HB, Rivers EP, Havstad S, et al. Critical care in the emergency department: A physiologic assessment and outcome evaluation. *Ann Emerg Med* 2000;7:1354–61.

8. Papadopoulous J, Rebuck JA, Lober C, et al. The critical care pharmacist: An essential intensive care practitioner. *Pharmacotherapy* 2002;22(11):1484–1488.

9. Horn E, Jacobi J. The critical care pharmacist: Evolution of an essential team member. *Crit Care Med* 2006;34(3): 46–51.

10. Kane SL, Weber RJ, Dasta JF. The impact of critical care pharmacists on enhancing patient outcomes. *Intensive Care Med* 2003;29:691–698.

11. Mahadevan SV, Sovndal S. Airway Management. In: Mahadevan SV, Garmel GM. *An Introduction to Clinical Emergency Medicine.* UK: Cambridge University Press.

12. Leschke RR. Cardiopulmonary and Cerebral Resuscitation. In: Mahadevan SV, Garmel GM. *An Introduction to Clinical Emergency Medicine.* UK: Cambridge University Press.

13. American Heart Association Guidelines for Cardiopulmonary Resuscitation and Emergency Cardiac Care. Part 10.1: Life threatening electrolyte abnormalities. *Circulation* 2005;112(24);IV-121–IV-125. Available at http://circ.ahajournals.org/cgi/reprint/112/24_suppl/IV-121 accessed December 2008

14. Kurkciyan I, Meron G, Sterz F, et al. Pulmonary embolism as cause of cardiac arrest. *Arch Intern Med* 2000;160: 1529–1535.

15. Sigilito RJ, Deblieux PMC. Shock. In: Mahadevan SV, Garmel GM. *An Introduction to Clinical Emergency Medicine.* UK: Cambridge University Press.

16

Clinical Decisions and Instructional Support System: Clinical Pharmacy Service and Informatics

Objectives

- Review implementation of clinical decision support system and instructional support to ensure knowledge translation.
- Discuss what emergency department pharmacists (EDPs) should know concerning clinical decision support systems (CDSS) implementation.
- Describe the clinician's evolving role in information technology.
- Review examples of transition from protocol order sets using paper to electronic medical records.
- Demonstrate instructional support to streamline nursing administration.

IMPLEMENTATION OF CDSS AND INSTRUCTIONAL SUPPORT TO ENSURE KNOWLEDGE TRANSLATION

Information technology has been widely recognized as a key element supporting the process of knowledge translation. Increasing awareness that clinicians, policy makers, and patients do not consistently use knowledge generated by research ("The knowledge to action gap") has made the need to assure translation of research increasingly urgent.[1] The use of information and communication technologies has been termed "technology-enabled knowledge translation (KT)."[2] Clinical decision support system (CDSS) have been defined as systems "designed to aid directly in clinical decision making, in which characteristics of individual patients are used to generate patient-specific assessments or recommendations

that are then presented to the clinicians for consideration."[3] Emergency departments (EDs) are implementing emergency department information systems (EDIS) to streamline operations and provide clinical decision support. The ED clinical pharmacist can play a significant role in the selection of the optimal EDIS and participate in preparation, implementation, and maintenance of CDSS to optimize the utility of the EDIS while assuring optimal use of pharmacotherapy.

WHAT SHOULD ED PHARMACISTS KNOW CONCERNING CDSS IMPLEMENTATION?

Despite the concentrated efforts of Colleges of Pharmacy to emphasize the need for pharmacists to be repositories of knowledge, a new role has evolved that includes pharmacists becoming managers of information. Pharmacists now must know how to incorporate this information into the clinical arena. Pharmacists interested in the ED setting, and for that matter any hospital setting, may be involved in managing or supervising information technology as it pertains to the unique needs of the unit. To provide support, pharmacists need to understand factors associated with successful implementation of computerized physician order entry (CPOE)/CDSS in the ED, and they need to know which systems have been shown to improve practice, barriers to successful implementation, and factors associated with failure. Furthermore, pharmacists must be aware of new types of errors that can arise with use of a CDSS and how to recommend successful implementation in the ED setting.

We review the literature on the role of the EDP in assisting with implementation of CPOE/CDSS, provide our experience in implementing new decision and instructional order sets and describe the role the pharmacist plays in ensuring the integrity of the CDSS and EDIS while important pharmaceutical care quality indicators are incorporated.

FACTORS FOR SUCCESSFUL DEPLOYMENT OF CDSS

Evidence related to deployment of CDSS provides insight into key factors for successful implementation. Garg et al. undertook a systematic review of articles evaluating the effect of a CDSS compared with care provided in its absence on practitioner performance and patient outcomes.[4] This review included studies through September 2004 and identified 100 studies meeting their inclusion criteria. They identified that in 64% of studies practitioner performance improved. Two factors were identified as being associated with CDSS success that contributed to improved practitioner performance. The first factor was related to the system: users were automatically prompted to use the system, as compared with other systems in which users had to actively initiate the system. The second factor was that the authors evaluating the CDSS were the developers of the same system. Wears and Berg pointed out that less than 50% of systems showed improvement when authors were not system developers.[5]

Bates et al. synthesized 8 years of observations in the deployment of a variety of CDSSs to characterize common factors that contributed to success of these systems (Table 16-1).[6]

BARRIERS TO SUCCESSFUL DEPLOYMENT OF CDSS

Several factors influence failure of CDSS, such as 1) clinicians did not support it, 2) lack of effective output and time to influence clinical decisions, 3) lack of effective output to convince clinician to change their behavior, 4) output was convincing, but the clinician was unable to alter his or her practice, and 5) clinical performance was already optimal.[7]

MEDICATION ERRORS ASSOCIATED WITH CPOE

Not all is perfect with CPOE/CDSS, as errors may arise from its use as well. Koppel et al. identified 24 different types of medication error risk facilitated by the CPOE system and classified them into two categories.[8] The first category was information errors generated by fragmentation of data and failure of integration with other hospital information systems, and the second was human-machine interface flaws, reflecting machine rules that do not correspond to work organization or usual behaviors.[8] The author cautioned that the implementation process for CPOE systems must carefully consider and address these potential sources of error.

CDSS IMPROVE CLINICAL PRACTICE

Despite the error risk of CPOE/CDSS, Kawamoto et al. reported that 68% of trials showed CDSS does improve clinical practice,[3] thus it is likely that institutions will inevitably be required to implement some form of decision support. Kawamoto et al. highlighted four factors that were independent predictors of improved clinical practice. They included 1) automatic provision of decision support as part of the clinician workflow, 2) provisions of recommendations rather than assessments, 3) provision of support at the time and location of decision making, and 4) computer-based decision support.[3]

RECOMMENDATIONS FOR SUCCESSFUL IMPLEMENTATION OF CPOE/CDSS

Handler et al., reporting from the Academic Emergency Medicine consensus conference relating to CPOE and on-

---

TABLE 16-1

Key Factors in the Successful Deployment of CDSS

1. Speed is everything (users value speed as the highest priority).
2. Anticipate need and deliver in real time (provide information when clinician needs it, even when they don't anticipate needing it).
3. Fit into user's workflow (integrate decision support tools into clinicians workflow).
4. Little things can make a big difference (application usability is essential and influences success of implementation).
5. Recognize that physicians will strongly resist stopping (physicians resist suggestions not to order a medication if a viable alternative is not provided).
6. Changing direction is easier than stopping (physician behavior does change and can be influenced if viable alternative is provided).
7. Simple intervention works best (single screen format is best suited for clinical guidelines).
8. Ask for additional information only when really needed (success of implementation of CDSS is inversely proportional to the number of extra data elements needed).
9. Monitor impact; get feedback and respond (audit use and compliance with decision support and modify alerts to optimize workflow).
10. Manage and maintain knowledge system (update system to reflect current knowledge, utilization patterns, and workflow processes).

Adapted from Bates DW, Kuperman GJ, Wang S, et al. Ten Commandments for effective clinical decision support making the practice of evidence based medicine a reality. *J Am Med Inform Assoc* 2003;10:523-530.

line decision support, outlined a variety of recommendations for successful implementation of these tools specific to the ED. These include seamless integration of CPOE and CDSS tools, systems, and workflow. The CPOE system should provide integral error and drug interaction checks, facilitate calculation of appropriate dosages and selective use of alerts only for issues of greatest clinical significance, and should be customized on an institutional basis.[9]

In addition, educational and continuous professional development programs should provide trainees and practicing emergency care clinicians with the skills to utilize information technology (IT) and CDSS tools in their delivery of clinical care. In this era of vast information resources, clinicians are increasingly required to be expert information managers, rather than repositories of expert information.[10–11]

ED PHARMACIST AND IMPLEMENTATION OF CDSS

Factors to successful implementation of CDSS, both those associated with improved clinical practice and those associated with barriers to success were considered by our multi-disciplinary team to develop various CDSS that enabled successful achievements of quality indicators including quality indicators for acute myocardial infarction and pneumonia (AMI-1-8a and PN-1-7). The multidisciplinary group also considered The Joint Commission's (TJC) national patient safety goals for *anticoagulation*, and best practice standards, such as the *surviving sepsis campaign* in developing the CDSS.[12]

We have designed the decision support system to enhance implementation of the institutional-specific antimicrobial guidelines as described earlier. Monthly updates are conducted by the ED clinical pharmacy services. The EDP attends the antibiotic surveillance committee meetings to assure that the current local protocol for antimicrobial use is still valid and up to date.

Protocol orders have been designed for common urgent or emergent care visits to the ED. The EDIS coordinator was responsible for the actual coding process on Allscripts, and the EDP provided assistance with review of the evidence-based guidelines, protocol development, and preferred drugs of choice. For example, CDSS protocol order sets for altered mental status (Fig. 16-1), abdominal pain (Fig. 16-2), ischemic chest pain (Fig. 16-3), acute ischemic stroke (Fig. 16-4), sepsis (Fig. 16-5), pneumonia (Fig. 16-6), empiric antimicrobial guide (Fig. 16-7), hyperkalemia (Fig. 16-8),

(text continues on page 156)

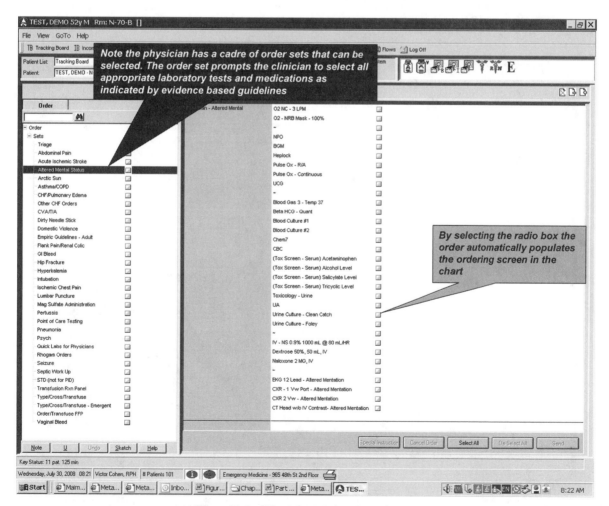

Figure 16–1. Altered mental status order set.

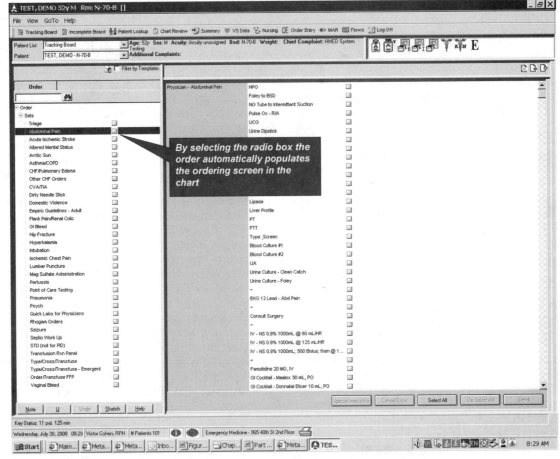

Figure 16–2. Abdominal pain order set.

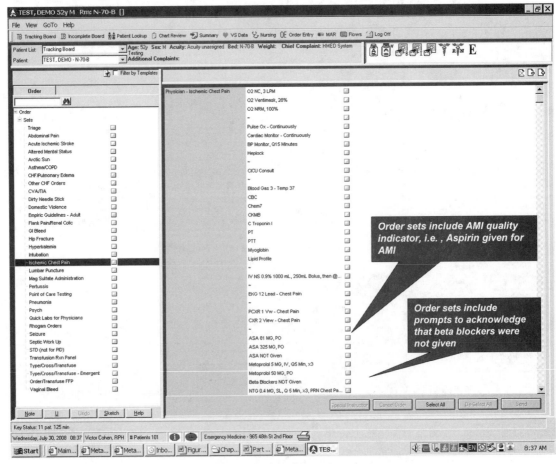

Figure 16–3. Ischemic chest pain order set.

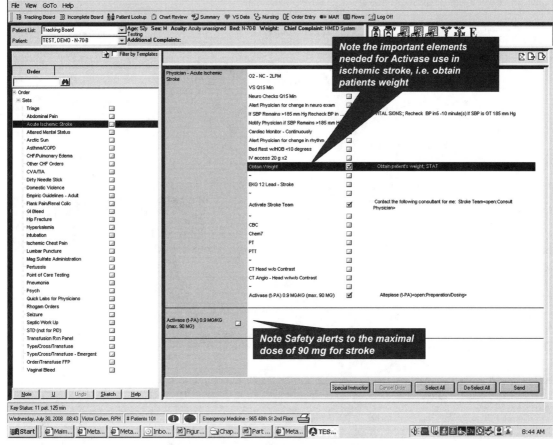

Figure 16–4. Acute ischemic stroke order set.

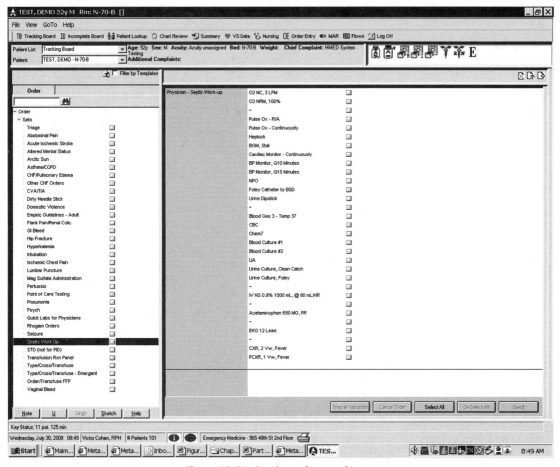

Figure 16–5. Septic work-up order set.

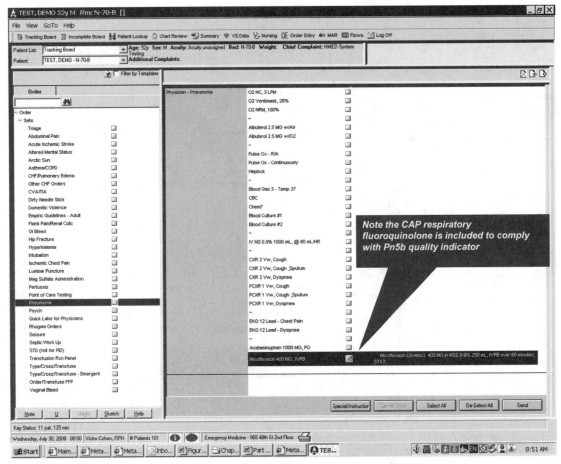

Figure 16–6. Pneumonia order set.

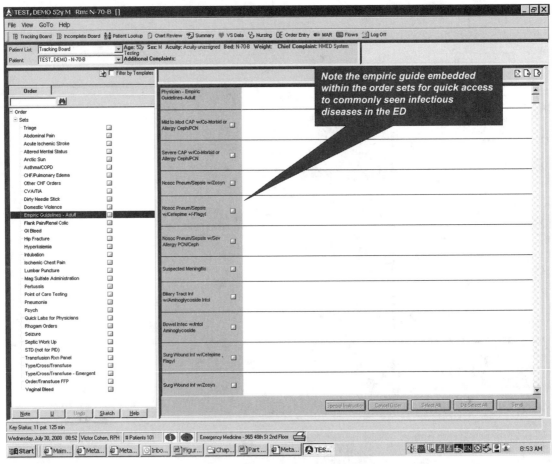

Figure 16–7. Empiric antibiotic guide.

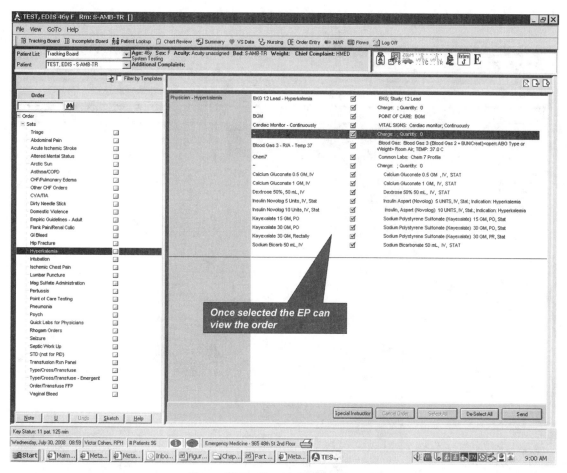

Figure 16-8. Hyperkalemia order set.

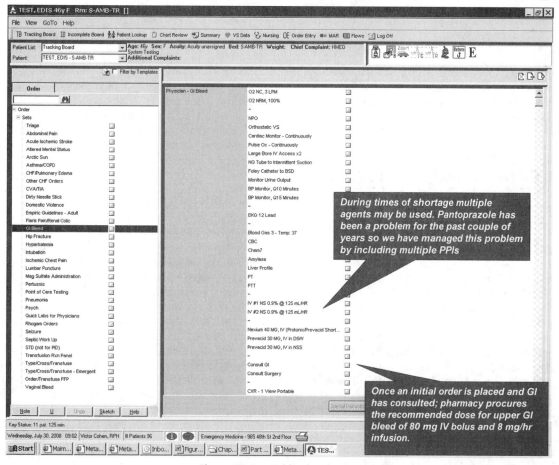

Figure 16-9. GI bleed order set.

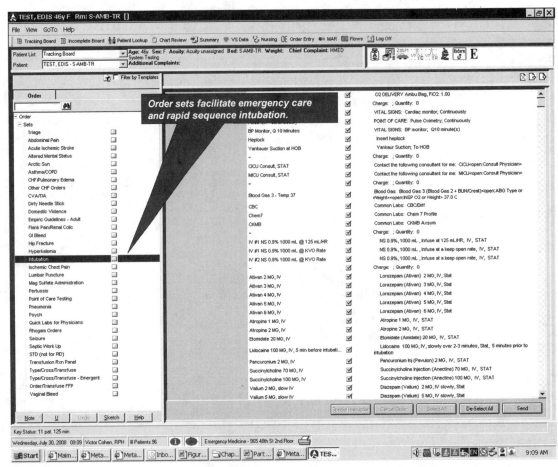

Figure 16–10. Intubation order set.

gastrointestinal (GI) bleed (Fig. 16-9), and intubation (Fig. 16-10) are samples that have been developed. Instructional order sets for weight-adjusted dosing heparin have been implemented (see Fig. 16-11A,B).

TRANSITIONING FROM PROTOCOL ORDER SETS USING PAPER TO ELECTRONIC MEDICAL RECORDS

ISCHEMIC CHEST PAIN ORDER SET

A description of our experience with transitioning from paper to CDSS and implementation of the order set may prove useful to those who are responsible for maintaining these order sets. We present our experiences first with implementation of the ischemic chest pain protocol and then with the heparin weight-adjusted nomogram.

A sample electronic CDSS protocol order set for ischemic chest pain is illustrated in Figure 16-3. These protocols are available in real time at point of clinical decision making and have gone through thorough peer review and approval by a multidisciplinary team of clinicians including medicine, nursing, and the ED clinical pharmacy service using up-to-date evidence-based medicine.

When the ED clinical pharmacy service was first initiated in 1998, we had a paper system in place. The door-to-needle times for acute coronary syndrome ST elevation myocardial infarction (STEMI) patients were not optimal, and patients who required various adjunctive medications (i.e., aspirin, beta blockers) did not always receive the indicated medication without explanation provided as to why, despite the correct indication. Through leadership of the Vice Chairman of the Department of Emergency Medicine, we set out to improve the implementation of the American College of Cardiology-American Heart Association guidelines for the management of chest pain in the ED.

We joined a multidisciplinary team of clinicians to discuss optimal management of chest pain and designed a simple easy-to-use protocol order form. A sample paper protocol order sheet is seen in Figure 16-12.[12]

The protocol order set included the medication regimen indicated, any clinically relevant contraindications, i.e., allergy to medications, and warnings to the physician if significant hypotension was seen upon presentation as possible contraindications. The protocol order set served as a reminder to the physicians and permitted the clinician to document rationale for not giving a routinely indicated medication. The nurse was then able to execute these orders by signing off as to whether the drug was given.

With the introduction of the electronic medical record (EMR), we adopted this same approach of protocol orders.

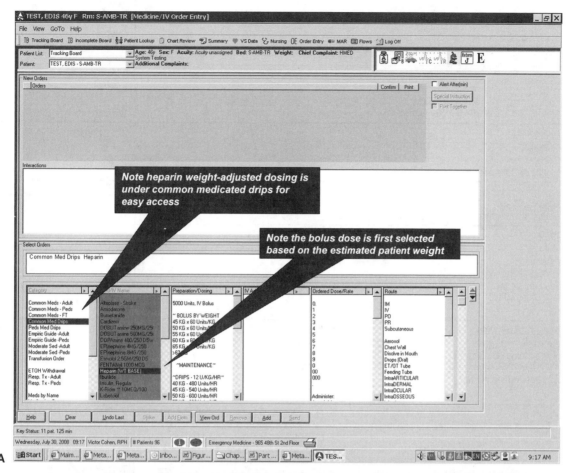

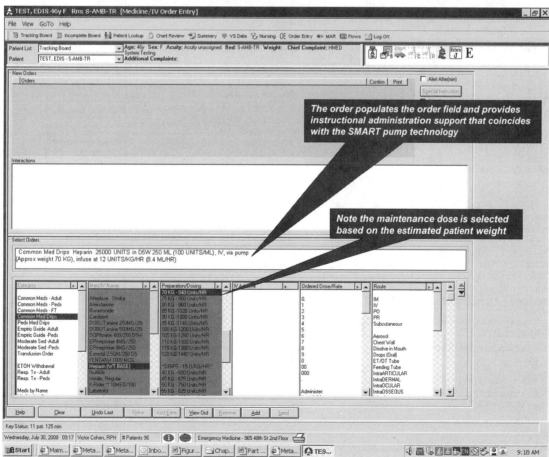

Figure 16–11. A: Computerized physician order entry selection for weight-adjusted Heparin. **B:** Heparin administration instructional order set.

			Nursing
Oxygen ☐ NC@3L/min ☐ other			**Oxygen** Time:
IV Access ☐ Hep-Lock ☐ NS @10 CC/hr ☐ rPA/tPA/SK Access Protocol			IV Access Fluid Time:
ECG Monitoring ☐ 12 Lead ECG ☐ Continuous Cardiac Monitor ☐ Continuous Pulse Oximeter	☐ ECG Posterior Leads ☐ Auto BP q___minutes ☐ Notify Physician as per protocol		ECG Monitoring Time:
Labs ☐ Initial CK-MB ☐ Repeat CK-MB q8hrs	☐ Initial Troponin ☐ Repeat Troponin q8hrs		Labs: Time:
Nitroglycerin ☐ SL 0.4 mg ☐ Nitropaste ___ ☐ NTG Drip @20 mcg/min ☐ Titrate Drip up in 10 mcg until no pain or 　SBP < 100 mmHg	Nitrates Contraindicated: ☐ Took Viagra (Sildenafil) within last 24 hours		Nitrates Time:
Aspirin/Thienopyridines ☐ Already taken or given ☐ Aspirin 162 mg po stat ☐ Aspirin 325 mg po stat ☐ Clpidogrel 300 mg po stat	ASA Contraindications ☐ Allergy ☐ Active GI Bleed ☐ Recent ICH		Antiplatelet Time:
Beta Blockers ☐ Metoprolol, 5 mg IVP q5minutes × 3 and then 　50 mg po now and q12h ☐ Criteria not met	Beta-Blocker Contraindication ☐ Active Asthma/COPD ☐ SBP < 90 mmHg　☐ CHF ☐ 3rd degree AV block		Antiischemic Therapy Time:
STEMI Reperfusion ☐ Criteria Not Met ☐ tPA Front load protocol ☐ SK 1.5 mU IVPB over 1 hour ☐ rPA 10U IV push now then repeat in 30 minutes ☐ TNk 0.5/kg, up to a maximum of 50 mg and no less than 30 mg by IV push over 50 seconds ☐ Repeat ECG in 30 minutes ☐ Planned PCI within 24 hours	STEMI or NSTEMI Reperfusion ☐ Criteria Not Met ☐ Stat Angioplasty within 90 minutes of arrival (Include GP IIb/IIIa Receptor antagonist if NSTEMI)	Lytic Contraindication ☐ GI Bleed　☐ Dissection ☐ Previous ICB　☐ Trauma ☐ Major Surgery last 3 wks ☐ Cerebral Aneurysm, AVN, Tumor Relative Contraindication ☐ Pregnancy ☐ CPR> 10 minutes ☐ SBP> 180 or DBP> 120 mmHg ☐ Hemorrhagic retinopathy ☐ Ischemic CV ☐ On Warfarin	Thrombolytics Time:
Anticoagulation ☐ Heparin not indicated ☐ Start Heparin 1000 U/hour 6 hours after streptokinase (SK) ☐ Heparin 60 U/Kg IV Bolus, then 12 U/Kg/hr infusion as adjunct to tPA, rPA, and TNK ☐ Enoxaparin 1 mg/kg Subcutaneously stat x 1 dose	Heparin and Enoxaparin Contraindications ☐ Active GI Bleed ☐ Recent ICH		Heparin or Enoxaparin
Glycoprotein IIB/IIIA Requires Cardiology Consultation Abciximab Eptifibatide Tirofiban	Glycoprotein IIB/IIIA Contraindication ☐ Refer to lytic contraindications		Antithrombotic Therapy Time:
Physician Signature Date:　Time:			Nursing Signature Date:　Time:

NC = nasal cannula, NS = normal saline, rPA = reteplase, tPA = tissue plasminogen activator, SK = streptokinase, TNK = tenecteplase, NTG = nitroglycerin, ASA = aspirin, COPD = Chronic Obstructive Lung Disease, CHF = Congestive Heart Failure, CPR = Cardiopulmonary Resuscitation, ICH = intracranial hemorrhage, GI = gastrointestinal.

Figure 16–12. Ischemic chest pain protocol.

A list of elements of management for the EP was made available when "chest pain" was selected as the chief complaint and impression of a cardiac cause was suspected.

ACHIEVING QUALITY THROUGH CDSS

This CDSS ischemic chest pain protocol, in addition to the emergency care staff, has facilitated better performance on various important quality indicators. As of April 3, 2008, according to the United States Department of Health and Human Services, the percent of heart attack patients given aspirin at arrival to the medical center was 95% (252 charts reviewed), which compared favorably to the United States average of 93%. The percent of heart attack patients given aspirin at discharge if appropriate is 95%, better than both the United States average and the average of hospitals within the vicinity at 90% and 93%, respectively. At Maimonides, the percent of heart attack patients given beta blockers upon arrival when appropriate is 93% (182 patients reviewed), which compared favorably to the United States average of 88% and similar to that of local area hospitals (93%).

HEPARIN WEIGHT-BASED NOMOGRAM: TRANSFORMATION TO AN AUTOMATED SYSTEM

Following recommendations from the Academic Emergency Medicine consensus conference on CPOE and CDSS, we designed instructional medication order sets during implementation of the electronic medical record system. The instructional order sets included several instructional elements that are commonly requested by nursing or physicians when prescribing. The instructional order sets included name of the medication, dosing regimen, dosing rate by weight, dosage concentration and diluents needed to prepare the medication, titration and monitoring parameters, and specific desired endpoint (see Fig. 16-11A, B).

TJC national patient safety goal 3E was announced in 2008 to reduce the likelihood of patient harm associated with anticoagulation therapy. Organizations should implement a defined anticoagulation management program to individualize the care provided to each patient receiving anticoagulation therapy. Prior to this announcement, we had already identified problems with anticoagulation management. Achieving therapeutic activated partial thromboplastin time (aPTT) with heparin was less than optimal and the customary dose that was used was not adjusted based on the patient's weight. For example, management with the standard heparin dosing (SHD) consisted of the administration of an intravenous heparin bolus of 5,000 units and a continuous infusion of 1,000 units/hour. As a result in 2003, we developed an ED-initiated CPOE factor-based, weight-adjusted dosing nomogram that reflected the anticoagulation, patient, and heparin factors that needed to be considered when rationalizing and responding to the aPTT in patients at risk for bleeding and that would permit for continuity of care, with the goal of rapidly achieving therapeutic aPTT and maintaining therapeutic aPTTs.[13] After appraising the current anticoagulation process, we were able to demonstrate improved time to therapeutic anticoagulation using this CPOE-based nomogram and improved maintenance of

achieving therapeutic aPTT.[13] CDSS facilitated the pharmacist activity of managing anticoagulation to improve upon quality indicators.

Based on this design, weight-adjusted doses could be easily selected. Instead of needing to build the order, to facilitate the ordering process, just a one-step selection of the dose-weight permitted the complete order (with instructions to pop-up), saving a significant amount of time.

An advantage of the instructional order support to nursing is that they can use the order to prepare and administer medication orders to achieve a target goal. This process facilitates rapid treatment during medical emergency of the critically ill.

PHARMACIST ROLE IN REVIEWING MEDICATION ORDERS DESPITE CDSS AND CPOE

The EDP is still called upon to execute and assure the appropriateness of these orders and to help in procurement because nursing is extremely busy in the ED. Because these instructional order sets were pre-formatted by a team including the EDP, the prospective review of these orders may be streamlined and facilitated. The EDP assigns students to ensure that target goals of the order are being met.

Despite the decision and instructional order sets, because there is frequent turnaround in physicians and nurses who work in the ED, we often experience orders that have been built, instead of selecting common orders that were available for use. The pharmacist should help assure that new EPs, residents, and nurses understand the common order sets available to them.

With prospective review, the use of built orders that are uncommon raises a red flag immediately, and the pharmacist cancels the order and re-orders the formulary product in the common medication section, with the instructional order for the nurse to carry out.

The development of these order sets is a dynamic process that requires constant surveillance and management. However, safeguards reduce the time to order verification and streamline the prospective review of the medication order.

Wears and Berg suggest the clinical workplace should be considered a "complex system in which technologies, people, and organizational routines dynamically interact."[4] Furthermore, there should be careful consideration for the workflow and cultural interactions of the organization in which the application is to be deployed to avoid risk of the technology failing to achieve its desired goals.

SUMMARY

The future is in customization of healthcare, and over the past decade, we have collaborated with emergency medicine in the design of optimal CPOE and CDSS systems that have facilitated emergency care and pharmaceutical care. The EDP must be involved in assuring that considerations for medication management are made and implemented.

The advantages of implementing CPOE and CDSS are that these systems can help ensure that the EPs, nurses, and the pharmacy team are alerted to potential clinically relevant contraindications or warnings. Permits for the translation of knowledge to practice of evidence-based medicine assures customization of dosing and instruction in administration of the high-risk medication.

References

1. Graham ID, Logan J, Harrison MB, et al. Lost in knowledge translation: Time for a map? *J Contin Edu Health Prof* 2006; 26:13–24.
2. Knowledge Management Specialist. KM technology: IT and knowledge management. Available at http://www.library.nhs.uk/knowledgemanagement/ViewResource.aspx?resID=94108&tabID=289. Accessed April 1, 2007.
3. Kawamoto K, Houlihan CA, Balas EA, Lobach DF. Improving clinical practice using clinical decision support systems: A systematic review of trials to identify features critical to success. *Br Med J* 2005;330:765.
4. Garg AX, Adhikari NKJ, McDonald H, et al. Effects of computerized clinical decision support systems on practitioner performance and patient outcomes. *JAMA* 2005;293: 1223–1238.
5. Wears RL, Berg M. Computer technology and clinical work. *JAMA* 2005;293:1261–63.
6. Bates DW, Kuperman GJ, Wang S, et al. Ten Commandments for effective clinical decision support making the practice of evidence based medicine a reality. *J Am Med Inform Assoc* 2003;10:523–530.
7. Saleem JJ, Patterson ES, Militello L, et al. Exploring barriers and facilitators to the use of computerized clinical reminders. *J Am Med Inform Assoc* 2005;12:438–447.
8. Koppel R, Metlay JP, Cohen A, et al. Role of computerized physician order entry systems in facilitating medication errors. *JAMA* 2005;293:1197–1203.
9. Handler JA, Feied CF, Coonan K, et al. Computerized physician order entry and online decision support. *Acad Emerg Med* 2004;11:1135–41.
10. Miller RA, Gardner RM, Johnson KB, Hripcsak G. Clinical decision support and electronic prescribing systems: A time for responsible thought and action. *J Am Med Inform Assoc* 2005;12:403–9.
11. Holroyd BR, Bullard MJ, Graham TAD, Rowe BH. Decision support Technology in Knowledge Translation. *Acad Emerg Med* 2007;14(11):942–947.
12. Dellinger R, Levy M, Carlet J, et al. Surviving Sepsis Campaign Management Guidelines Committee. Surviving Sepsis Campaign Guidelines for management of severe sepsis and septic shock. *Crit Care Med* 2008;36(1):296–327.
13. Cohen V, Murphy DG, Williams J. Review of the current ACS Practice Guideline to develop an ischemic chest pain protocol. *J Pharm Pract* 2002:(15)3:250–266.
14. Jellinek SP, Cohen V, Likourezos A, et al. Analyzing a health-system's use of unfractionated heparin to ensure optimal anti-coagulation. *J Pharm Technol* 2005;21:69–78.

17

Target Medication Reconciliation in the Emergency Department

Objectives

- Describe the process of medication reconciliation in the emergency department (ED)
- Discuss resistance to medication reconciliation and illustrate its need in the ED
- Review barriers to medication reconciliation in the ED
- Describe a multidisciplinary process for medication reconciliation in the ED

Currently of greatest angst in healthcare today is the process that has come to be known as "medication reconciliation." According to the Lunar III study group, conducted by the Emergency Nursing Association, medication reconciliation is considered one of the most difficult The Joint Commission (TJC) safety goals to accomplish.[1]

MEDICATION RECONCILIATION

Medication reconciliation is defined as the formal process of addressing discrepancies between a patient's current medications and the medications about to be prescribed. This includes a process for comparing the patient's current medications with those ordered for the patient while under the care of the organization, and a complete list of the patient's medications is communicated to the next provider of service when a patient is referred or transferred to another setting, service, practitioner, or level of care within or outside the organization. The complete list of medications is also provided to the patient on discharge from the facility.[2]

RESISTANCE TO MEDICATION RECONCILIATION

As part of the health-system, EDs are faced with meeting this national patient safety goal despite resistance from leading emergency medicine organizations that state that the net resources to comply with this standard are too much for the perceived benefit that will come from medication reconciliation.[3] Despite this resistance, medication reconciliation may reduce errors that can occur during the intake phase when a complete and accurate medication list would not otherwise be obtained. Examples of mistakes that have occurred include the transcription error of Desogen®, an oral contraceptive, for digoxin, and digoxin was prescribed on a daily basis; or the transcription error from a patient list of use of methotrexate prescribed daily when it was intended for weekly administration prescribed by the rheumatologist. The patient died due to the severe complications.[4–5] Errors in hand-off communications between providers may also occur. A patient who received a loading dose of digoxin in the ED without clear documentation received another loading dose on the inpatient unit, resulting in severe bradycardia.[1] A patient receiving Lovenox® in the ED was started on a heparin protocol on the inpatient unit and suffered an intracranial bleed.[5] Thus, although there is much discussion over the ability of the ED to fulfill this requirement, medication reconciliation, as one report stated, "did not come out of the blue." Medication errors due to incomplete collection of patient's medication lists and lack of reconciliation at the time of prescribing and during transitions has led to harm and death for decades; it is time to fix this problem.

As the Institute of Medicine described, pharmacists may be relied upon to lead the organization to the development of a safe medication use system, and they can be the catalyst to a consistent medication reconciliation process.

BARRIERS TO MEDICATION RECONCILIATION

Barriers to implementation of a medication reconciliation process are significant. For example, ED personnel are particularly burdened in the process of reconciliation due to the difficulty in gathering a current medication list under emergent situations, or the limited time frame that exists to reconcile medications. Also, ED patients are often distraught and unprepared when they arrive to the ED. Patients seldom carry a current list of their medications. Often, these lists are inaccurate and incomplete with only the drug name and possibly the associated dose; they lack the information of drug frequency, route, and last dose taken.[6] Patients are also rarely asked about over-the-counter drug use, vitamin, and herbal products. Patients are also likely to forget drug patches, respiratory inhalers, and other nontraditional sources of medications, i.e., "insulin pens."

Physician attitudes toward obtaining a complete medication list are also problematic. For example, because some patients are "treated and released" from the ED, there is a perception that reconciliation is not needed because there is minimal risk. Another emergency physician (EP) perception is that house staff is responsible for completing this step when admission orders are written.

It is our view that anything less than a reasonably complete and accurate list is useless information and a waste of valuable staff time. The EDP initiated a multidisciplinary committee to create a process and workflow to ensure compliance to this National Patient Safety Goal (NPSG).

MULTIDISCIPLINARY PROCESS FOR MEDICATION RECONCILIATION

Ideally, a pharmacist may be best suited to conduct medication histories to improve the medication reconciliation process within the ED and absolve the responsibility from other providers responsible for emergency care.[7,8,9] However, a safe medication use system is one in which all providers are involved to ensure layers of safety. Medication reconciliation may take the pharmacist away from more essential tasks within the department, i.e., assuring safety and quality during medical emergencies. Thus, our goal was to design a collaborative practitioner reconciliation process that was built upon existing infrastructure and involved all healthcare professionals.

Our experience of implementing a medication reconciliation process included several phases. First, we attempted to gain clarity of what is actually required and accepted from prime source documents from the Joint Commission (TJC). Second, we evaluated the current workflow and our current infrastructure including automation,[8] to identify what we could build upon to integrate the medication reconcilia-

tion process without exorbitant expenditure. Third, we evaluated the human resources that would be responsible for conducting the reconciliation.

MEDICATION RECONCILIATION AND AAEM, ACEP, AND ENA

Based on a consensus recommendation of the American Association of Emergency Medicine (AAEM), the American College of Emergency Physicians (ACEP) and the Emergency Nurses Association (ENA), there are three levels of intensity of the medication reconciliation process in the ED. *Screening reconciliation* includes routinely obtaining from *each* patient at each ED visit a list of the patient's current medications (usually done by the triage nurse).

Focused reconciliation, as directed by the emergency physician (EP), based on medical relevance, should include seeking additional information about the patient's medica-

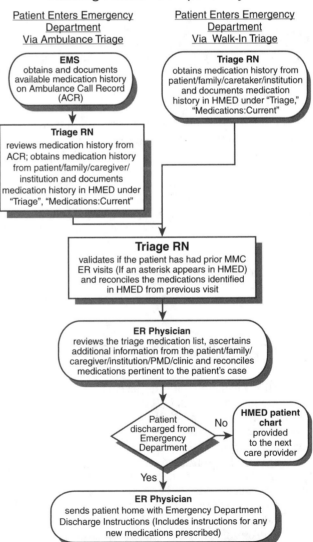

Figure 17–1. Flowchart of emergency department medication reconciliation process.

tions (exact drug list, dosage/route) from the patient's pharmacy, primary care physician, and family.

A *full reconciliation* for admitted patients should be completed by the receiving inpatient unit and pharmacist. This consensus recommendation from the AAEM, ACEP, and ENA is in full compliance with NPSG requirement 8A since each level includes obtaining a list of the patient's current medications to be used when ordering or prescribing medications in the ED. Therefore, this approach is acceptable to the Joint Commission in meeting requirement 8A.[10]

MAIMONIDES PROCESS

Our process is consistent with the consensus recommendation (Fig. 17-1).

The ED triage nurse records the screening reconciliation medication list on to the electronic medical record available for clinicians to use to reconcile with any medications given in the ED (Fig. 17-2).

Recent data published suggests that an electronic medication reconciliation does not result in longer triage times overall. In a prospective multicenter before and after trial at an urban academic ED with 60,000 visits per year, the median triage time was not significantly different between pre-reconciliation period (15 minutes:12 seconds with a range of 10 minutes:07 seconds to 23 minutes:57 seconds) and post-reconciliation period (15 minutes:09 seconds, with a range of 9 minutes:58 seconds to 23 minutes:49 seconds, $P > 0.05$). However, as the number of medications reconciled increased, the median triage time increased from 12:52 for 1 medication, 14:22 for 2 to 3 medications, and 17:16 for >4 medications, ($P < 0.05$). As part of the methods within this study, investigators required the nurse to obtain the complete medication regimen including dose and frequency, resulting perhaps in longer times than would otherwise be if only obtaining the name of the medication.[11]

Based on this study, it was agreed upon that obtaining the dose regimen at triage would be too difficult because of factors such as language problems, distraught patients, and incomplete information.

Instead the nurse would be responsible for producing the names of medications the patient is taking.

The EP would then evaluate, screen, and reconcile the list against medications to be give in the ED and upon discharge if released from the ED.

In the context of this safety goal, the EP compares the medications that the patient/client/resident has been taking prior to the time of admission or entry to a new setting with the medications that the organization is about to provide to avoid errors of transcription, omission, duplication of therapy, drug-drug, and drug-disease interactions.

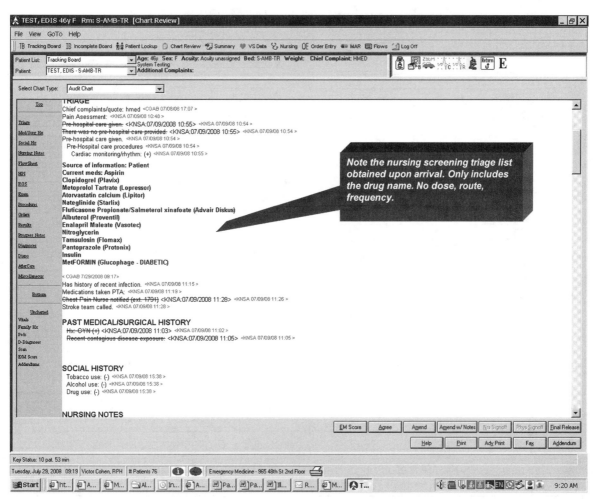

Figure 17–2. Screening reconciliation at triage.

A full medication reconciliation is completed using the inpatient hospital medication reconciliation form (Fig. 17-3) by the admitting physicians for patients admitted to the institution and is part of the initial history and physical.

The complete list includes dosage regimens reconciled by the admitting team. This process is implemented and audited by the inpatient medication management team and a medication reconciliation and safety officer.

Chan et al. conducted a study and noted that there were 1457 patients who had a new medication prescribed and 333 patients had a change in their current regimen as a result of reconciliation. Thus, coinciding with recommendations by the emergency societies, a focused reconciliation should be conducted by the EP when he or she is making changes in prescribed medications, i.e., changing the dose of warfarin or when a drug-induced disease visit is suspected. We use an automated system to reconcile medications at discharge for those patients who will be treated and then released from the ED (Fig. 17-4).[12]

The newly prescribed medications are screened and compared to home medications using the electronic medication record drug interaction database. The EP may add changes to the home medication list or prescribe to hold use of a medication until the patient has been seen by their primary care provider.

In certain circumstances, communication of the list of the patient's current medications is not completed because it is not deemed necessary according to TJC.[11]

These circumstances include those such as "minimal medication use," when no medications are used during the encounter, no new medications are prescribed or provided to the patient for use after discharge, there are no changes to "current medications," the next provider of care already has the patient's current medication information or only medications that act locally and have negligible systemic effects are used.

One note of caution, the ED pharmacist must ensure there is compliance with the process. Monthly audits must be completed to assure that the ED component is being achieved. Currently, we audit our inpatient setting and are devising a process to audit the treated and released patient population. This audit is essential to the sustainability of this process. A report of use of this embedded pathway can be conducted and quantified for the purpose of quality assurance.

Of note, during a medical emergency and as part of a screening process, the EDP initiates a medication history as needed and as it pertains to the clinical presentation to assist in assessing risk for a drug-induced disease or co-administration of potentially interacting medications.

MEDICATION RECONCILIATION FORM (MRF)

REMINDER - DO NOT Use The Following Abbreviations: U, QD, QOD, TIW, CC, μg. as directed, MS, MSO4, MgSO4. Use 0.1 not .1.

Source of Medication History: ☐ Patient ☐ Family ☐ Rx Bottle ☐ Medication List ☐ Other: ________

☐ Pharmacy ________ Phone #: ________

Allergies and Reaction Description: ________

Diagnosis: 1° ________ 2° ________

Prescribers Are To Use This Tool To Facilitate The Medication Reconciliation Process

CURRENT MEDICATION AT ADMISSION
(MD, RN, NP or PA **must** complete) (Include Rx, OTC, Herbal Products)

☐ Not on medication at home

DRUG	DOSE	ROUTE	FREQUENCY	INITIALS & TITLE

LIP RECONCILIATION OF ADMISSION MEDICATION ORDERS

Order Exactly?			ONLY Indicate Area of Modification				Reason for Modification
Yes (☒)	No (☒)	D/C (☒)	DRUG	DOSE	Route	FREQ.	Comments / Changes

1st REVISION 11/08/07

This Signature Verifies that I have Obtained And Reviewed The Patient's Current Medication List Upon Admission And That It Has Been Reconciled With The Patient's Admission Medication Orders.

LIP Signature: ________ Print ________ Date: __/__/__

5000-7

HP

Created and designed by the Medication Reconciliation Team, Maimonides Medical Center Including Pharmacy, Nursing and Performance Improvement Task Force.

Figure 17–3. Full medication reconciliation, which is completed upon admission.

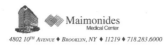

EMERGENCY DEPARTMENT
DISCHARGE INSTRUCTIONS

PATIENT NAME:	TEST, FINALFOUR	MR NUMBER:	71202739
		ACCOUNT NUMBER:	100400034619
ATTENDING PHYSICIAN:	Kenneth Sable, MD	DATE OF BIRTH:	5/5/1977
RESIDENT PHYSICIAN/PA:		DATE/TIME OF SERVICE:	07/27/06 15:39

MEDICATION RECONCILIATION

The medication list below represents the information provided to the Emergency Department staff at arrival, as well as throughout your visit today. Any changes made to your current medications by your Emergency Department physician are listed below next to the specific medications that were modified. You must bring this list to your primary physician or other healthcare provider/clinic as soon as possible to ensure safe continuation of your medical care. It is also important to speak to your pharmacist about any new medications prescribed and any other medications/supplements that you are currently taking.

Labetalol hcl - stop taking until you see your doctor
Lamictal
Lasix - take 80mg daily instead of 40mg × 3 days
Ambien
Amikin
Zyrtec
Zestril

PRESCRIPTIONS GIVEN:

Amoxicillin 500 MG Tablet, Take 1 Tablet, by mouth, 3 times a day, for 7 days. Take until all medication is finished., Disp: #21, -Refills: None
Diphenhydramine (Benadryl) 25 MG Capsule, Take 1 Capsule, by mouth, every 6 hours, as needed for itching., Disp: #20., -Refills: None.

Figure 17–4. Automated focused reconciliation for treated and released patients.

SUMMARY

In summary, a multidisciplinary emergency department team is needed to design a strategy to comply with current TJC standards for medication reconciliation.[6] The EDP must be aware of currently accepted standards of medication reconciliation and how they differ in the ED setting. The EDP must know the current workflow, technology, and resources available to design the most efficient medication reconciliation process. Medication reconciliation has a role in error prevention, and continuous quality improvement is needed to assure that this important safeguard is being completed. Auditing the ED specific medication reconciliation process will identify areas in need of improvement and should be a required task for the ED clinical pharmacy service to assure sustainability of this safeguard.[10]

References

1. Paparella S. Medication reconciliation: Doing what's right for safe patient care. *J Emerg Nurs* 2006;32(6):516–520.
2. The Joint Commission. http://www.jointcommission.org/PatientSafety/NationalPatientSafetyGoals/08_hap_npsgs.htm. Accessed 11/09/07.
3. No Authors Listed. Organizations join forces against Joint Commission medication rules. *ED Manage* 2006;18(8):85–87.
4. Institute for Safe Medication Practices. Building a case for medication reconciliation. *ISMP Medication Safety Alert* 2004;10:8.
5. Institute for Safe Medication Practices. Hazard Alert! Action needed to avert fatal error from concomitant use of heparin products. *ISMP Medication Safety Alert* 2001;6:4.
6. Selin Calgar, Henneman P, Blank F, Henneman EA. Emergency Department Medication Lists Are Not Accurate. SAEM Abstract, 2007 Annual Meeting 2006; 48(4):146.
7. Carter MK, Allin DM, Scott LA, Geauer D. Pharmacist-acquired medication histories in a university hospital emergency department. *Am J Health-Syst Pharm* 2006;63:2500– 2503.
8. Hayes BD, Donovon JL, Smith BS, Hartman CA. Pharmacist-conducted medication reconciliation in an emergency department. *Am J Health-Syst Pharm* 2007;64:1720–1723.
9. Young D. Maryland tackles emergency care crisis. *Am J Health-Syst Pharm* 2007;64:568–576.
10. The Joint Commission. http://www.jointcommission.org/NR/rdonlyres/9ECF1ED6-E04E-41DE-B7BC-174590CEDF33/0/07_NPSG_FAQs_8.pdf accessed 11.09.07.
11. Chan TC, Killeen JP, Castillo EM, et al. Impact of Electronic Medication Reconciliation on Triage Times for Patients Seen in the Emergency Department. SAEM Abstract, 2007 Annual Meeting. 2006;48(4):146.
12. Kramer JS, Hopkins PJ, Rosendale JC, et al. Implementation of an electronic system for medication reconciliation. *Am J Health-Syst Pharm* 2007;64:404–422.

18

Emergency Care Pharmacotherapy Considerations in Special Populations: Geriatric, Pediatric, and Obstetric

Objectives

- Illustrate increased use of emergency departments (EDs) by the elderly
- Highlight the greater complexity and severity of emergency care for the elderly
- Review indicators suggesting less-than-optimal quality for the elderly
- Propose geriatric emergency department interventions (GEDIs)
- Propose geriatric emergency care pharmacotherapeutic interventions (GEPIs)
- Review how to reduce medical errors in pediatric emergency care
- Describe EDP role in pediatric emergency care pharmacotherapy
- Review customized tools to expedite emergency care pharmacotherapy and ensure safety for pediatric emergencies
- Describe common obstetrical emergencies and their pharmacotherapy in the ED
- Review appropriate prescribing in pregnancy and lactation

INCREASED USE OF EMERGENCY DEPARTMENTS BY THE ELDERLY

Care for the elderly is increasingly being sought in emergency departments (EDs), where older patients typically present with complex medical conditions, stay longer for more extensive diagnostic testing and treatment regimens and require special needs during their visits.[1] In 2002 approximately 58% of 75-year-old patients had at least one visit to the ED compared with 39% of those of all other ages, and ED use increased with increasing age.[2]

COMPLEXITY AND SEVERITY OF EMERGENCY CARE FOR THE ELDERLY

Once in the ED, older persons are more likely to have an emergent or urgent condition, be hospitalized, and be admitted to a critical care unit.[3] Elderly patients are also more likely to receive a greater number of diagnostic tests, spend longer times in the ED, and have higher charges than younger patients.[4]

> *"Our patients never have one problem. They almost always have a heart attack compounded by a urinary tract infection compounded by muscle breakdown. . . . There's never one clear explanation for the pathological phenomenon we see in a lot of our patients. The reason? Maimonides patients tended to be exceptionally old or exceptionally foreign."*
>
> *John Marshall*
> *Emergency Medicine Residency Program Director*

INDICATORS OF LESS-THAN-OPTIMAL QUALITY FOR ELDERLY RECEIVING EMERGENCY CARE

The current model of ED care may not be meeting the needs of the older adult. Older adults are at greater risk for medical complications, functional decline, and poorer health-related quality of life than before their visits to the ED.[5] Furthermore, the special care needs of older adults are not aligned with the priorities of how the ED physical space is designed and how care is rendered. Space is planned with the intent of quick patient evaluation and turnover; traditional EDs are designed to maximize resources.

Hwang et al. described lack of customization of EDs for the geriatric patient at the expense of improving throughput. Privacy is lost as curtains, rather than walls, serve as barriers between beds in an open-space ED, allowing for greater staff maneuverability and placement of multiple patients in shared bays during periods of overcrowding. Older patients are at risk of pressure ulcers as they remain for hours to even days on narrow-thin mattresses or stretchers. Geriatric patients are at risk of falls because floors in the ED consist of slippery linoleum or hard vinyl components designed for easy cleanup. These floors are a hazard for those elderly patients with gait impairment. Elderly patients are at risk of confusion and disorientation due to lack of exposure to diurnal changes because many EDs are on the first floor but are windowless to preserve privacy; lighting is limited to glaring overhead fluorescent lamps. Delirium may be worsened in the elderly, especially those with hearing impairment and communication difficulties, because EDs are rarely quiet and noise can occur from multiple sources.[6]

Hwang et al. also described the mismatch of ED care rendered and how it could be optimally delivered to older adults. Rapid triage and diagnosis may be impossible in older patients with multiple comorbidities, polypharmacy, and functional and cognitive impairments who often present with subtle clinical symptoms and signs of acute illness. Time pressures to make a quick diagnosis can result in an incorrect diagnosis or missed diagnosis. Elders in the ED who are unaccompanied may not be able to advocate for themselves because of delirium, dementia or sensory impairments compete with younger more vocal adults for the attention of the busy clinical staff. Elderly patients may also be at risk of delirium and infection due to bladder catheterization as a means to reduce the risk of falls caused by patients ambulating to restrooms or because of limited time for staff to change diapers or provide bedpans. As a result Adams et al. called for a new model for emergency care for geriatric patients because the current system of ED care is not designed for the older person.[7]

PROPOSED GERIATRIC EMERGENCY DEPARTMENT INTERVENTIONS (GEDIS)

In response to the needs of the growing number of older adults seen in the ED, geriatric emergency department interventions (GEDIs) that would include better clinical staff education in geriatric emergency medicine and nursing care, evidence-based protocols for geriatric syndromes, and ideally appropriate structural modifications have been proposed. Several of the proposed GEDIs are in Table 18-1.

The need to customize emergency care for the elderly also includes optimizing safe and effective use of pharmacotherapy for the elderly.

Customization of emergency care pharmacotherapy for the elderly should begin with implementing full medication reconciliation upon arrival. This can be rationalized for several reasons. The geriatric patient has more complex medication regimens that increase the risk of drug-drug interactions, omissions, and incorrect commissions. The geriatric patient has multiple conditions that increase risk for drug–disease interaction. The geriatric patient has a lower threshold for morbidity if a medication error occurs. Furthermore it is not uncommon for the elderly to be boarded for longer periods in the ED. A full reconciliation can prevent these risks and assure quality of healthcare.

One barrier to implementation of full medication reconciliation in the ED is that the Joint Commission has accepted a 24-hour window upon admission in which medication reconciliation may be completed.

TABLE 18-1 Proposed Geriatric Emergency Department Interventions (GEDI)[6]

GEDI	Goal
Protocol Interventions: Cognitive impairment and delirium	Early identification of patients at risk for these conditions to assist in disposition, treatment, or discharge planning
Risk of adverse health outcomes, return visit, or hospitalization screening	Decrease risk of return visits or hospitalization
Abbreviated comprehensive geriatric assessments	
Minimal use of urethral catheters and other tethering devices	Reduce immobility
	Reduce risk of nosocomial infection and delirium
Discharge coordinator	Improve continuity of care
	Decrease return visits
	Increase patient satisfaction

Adapted with data from Hwang U, Morrison SR. The geriatric emergency department. *J Am Geriatr Soc* 2007;55(11):1873–1876.

This essentially bypasses the emergency care staff of conducting a full reconciliation in these special circumstances.

Because elderly patients present a unique circumstance to the ED by staying longer than other patients, having more diagnostics, receiving more treatments, and being more fragile to medication error or at greater risk of inattention to their continuity of care by healthcare staff, exceptions should be made for the elderly population to ensure safe and effective medication use while in the ED.

Continuity of care is also an issue amongst the elderly boarded in the ED. Even with a full medication reconciliation, admitting physicians may be unfamiliar with specialty medications, medication names, and dosing regimens often resulting in incorrect transcriptions or omissions.

Prescribing during a shift change amongst healthcare staff may result in medication error because of the speed and accuracy trade off. That is, the physicians are trying to leave by the end of their shift while they still have to complete their tasks for the care of the patient.

Thus, an elderly person may go with an incorrect medication for at least 24 hours, reducing the overall quality of care. Attention to continuity and transitions of care is of even greater relevance for the elderly to optimize quality of care.

The transition of nursing care within the ED to the boarding area may also result in errors or omissions in documentation and can have catastrophic consequences. For example, an enoxaparin order is entered and administered by the ED nurse at 4 AM, but may not be charted. The transition care team physician may enter an order for enoxaparin at 7 AM as a now dose plus the usual regimen. Because of no documentation of the dose given in the ED, the transition care nurse may re-administer the dose This gap in safeguards can be filled by the morning pharmacist who sees the unverified order, obtains the weight of the patient to assure appropriate dosing, and discusses with the patient if they received any dose while in the ED. This review should be mandated in this special population, but it requires a dedicated pharmacist in the ED.

The limited pre-formatted formulary drugs listed in the CPOE system increases the risk of transcription errors in this special population. Because the elderly population may be taking numerous specialty medications that are not listed in the CPOE system, the admitting physician must use a type-in format to enter the order into the system to prescribe the patient's home medications, including medication name, doses, route, and schedule. This is often a source for error and multiple discrepancies.

Medications used to treat psychiatric or behavioral disorders may not be continued appropriately or timed correctly, which can profoundly impact an older person's mental status. An EP may aggressively manage an older person's agitation with normal doses of Haldol (i.e., 5 mg) and Ativan (2 mg stat × 1 dose) without conducting an assessment of why the patient's mental status is impaired or what may be at the root of the elderly person's delirium. Furthermore, the management of the delirium may be too aggressive for the older person because his or her pharmacokinetic and dynamic variables are not optimal relative to younger patients. Because the EP is driven to enhance throughput, the admitting physicians manage care from a distance, and the hospitalist simply may not take into account these special pharmacotherapeutic considerations, quality of care for the elderly may not be optimal.

Quality of patient care is also an issue for the elderly in the ED because the elderly can stay boarded in the ED for 24–48 hours during peak seasons. The Assessing Care of Vulnerable Elders (ACOVE) investigators developed a comprehensive set of quality assessment tools for ill older persons. ACOVE is a standard designed to measure overall care delivered to vulnerable elders at the level of a health system or plan that targets four specific domains of care: prevention, diagnosis, treatment, and follow-up. This standard also covers the spectrum of care in 22 conditions that are important in the care of older persons. A sampling of the quality of pharmacologic care standards (Table 18-2) focuses on 1) prescribing of indicated medications, 2) avoidance of inappropriate medications, 3) education, continuity, and documentation, and 4) medication monitoring.[3,10]

However, due to the current model of emergency care, these indicators are not addressed until patients are admitted. Three of these quality pharmacologic care indicators are on the Hospital Quality Alliance's Hospital Quality Measures list, which uses quality measures to gauge how well an entity provides care to its patients and are used to improve the care provided by the nation's hospitals. Thus, a prolonged stay in the ED can have deleterious effects on the performance of these measures, and more importantly on the quality of care provided to elders.

PROPOSED GERIATRIC EMERGENCY CARE PHARMACOTHERAPEUTIC INTERVENTIONS (GEPIS)

We describe additional modifications to the current emergency medicine model to address the current mismatch in emergency care pharmacotherapy and enhanced provisions of care needed for the elderly within the ED, termed geriatric emergency care pharmacotherapeutic interventions (GEPIs) (Table 18-3).

In most emergency departments, the ED pharmacist provides the human resource to promote a customized geriatric approach. However, securing a pharmacist in the ED to provide enhanced quality of care services is often deterred by administration due to lack of funds.

PEDIATRIC EMERGENCY CARE AND MEDICAL ERROR

Twenty million children in the United States obtain care in EDs annually.[10] According to Chamberlain et al., pediatric EDs are particularly prone to increasing the risk of cognitive error due to issues that distract from cognitive tasks associated with managing the patient.[11] Overcrowding issues, workflow interruptions, fluctuating ED volumes that may be caused by media-released reports of potential outbreaks can cause cognitive errors. Resources are used by clinical staff to manage patient flow instead of attending to medical problems of the pediatric patients. Furthermore, errors are

TABLE 18-2 ACOVE Quality of Pharmacologic Indicators

Quality Indicator

Patients with symptomatic heart failure and LVEF ≤ 40% offered treatment with an ACE-I

Patients with heart failure, LVEF ≤ 40%, and NYHA class I-III disease offered a β-blocker unless the patient has a documented contraindication

Patients with an acute myocardial infarction receive aspirin therapy within 1 hour of presentation and a β-blocker within 12 hours; Patients with established coronary heart disease and an LDL cholesterol level > 130 mg/dL should be offered cholesterol-lowering medication

Patients admitted to the hospital with pneumonia should receive antibiotics within 8 hours of hospital arrival

Patients with chronic pain treated with opioids should be offered a bowel regimen

Physicians should review the medication lists of patients who present with symptoms of dementia to assess for initiation of medications that might correspond chronologically to the onset of dementia symptoms

Physicians treating patients with mild-moderate Alzheimer's disease should discuss treatment with a cholinesterase inhibitor with the patient and the primary caregiver; The physician should discuss or refer the patient and caregiver for discussion about patient safety; Patients prescribed a new medication should have a clearly defined indication for that medication documented in the medical record

Diabetic patients with proteinuria should be offered therapy with an ACE-I

Patients treated with warfarin or who have a history of peptic ulcer disease or gastrointestinal bleeding and who are being treated with a COX nonselective NSAID should be offered concomitant treatment with either misoprostol or a PPI

Patients started on antidepressant therapy should not receive tertiary amine tricyclics, MAOIs (unless atypical depression is present), benzodiazepines or stimulants (except methylphenidate) as first or second line therapy

Diabetic patients who are not on other anticoagulant therapy should be offered daily aspirin therapy

Atrial fibrillation patients with any "high-risk" conditions* should be offered oral anticoagulation therapy

Patients with risk factors for peptic stress ulcers should receive prophylaxis with a H_2-blocker, sucralfate, or a proton-pump inhibitor

Patients with osteoarthritis should be offered acetaminophen as a first-line agent unless there is a documented contraindication to its use

Patients with osteoporosis should be offered supplementation with calcium and vitamin D; Patients with osteoporosis should be offered treatment with HRT or bisphosphonates or calcitonin

*High-risk conditions include: impaired left ventricular function, female older than 75 years of age, hypertension or systolic blood pressure greater than 160 mmHg, prior ischemic stroke, transient ischemic attack, systemic embolism.

LVEF, left ventricular ejection fraction; ACE-I, angiotensin-converting enzyme inhibitor; NYHA, New York Heart Association; LDL, low density lipoprotein; COX, cyclooxygenase; NSAID, non-steroidal antiinflammatory drug; MAOI, monoamine oxidase inhibitor; HRT, hormone replacement therapy.

TABLE 18-3 Proposed Geriatric Emergency Care Pharmacotherapy Interventions (GEPI)

GEPI	Goal
Pharmacotherapeutic consultation and treatment plan for delirium during stay in the ED and other elderly specific ailments	Develop emergency care pharmacotherapy protocols for delirium and other disease states in the elderly
Medication reconciliation	Reduce polypharmacy and continuity of care related errors
Prospective review of medication order for the elderly	Reduce incorrectly transcribed orders, omissions, incorrectly timed orders, incorrect dosing regimens (based on pharmacokinetic and dynamic considerations), and risk for duplication in administration
Implementation of ACOVE quality of pharmacological standards	Address quality of pharmacological care in the ED for elderly patients boarded for > 12 hours
Medication Therapy Management Services (MTMS)	Reduce ED visits due to suspected drug-induced disease, such as noncompliance. Elderly who are treated and released but prescribed medications are enrolled in the MTMS program to improve quality of life after visiting the ED

more likely to occur from 4 PM until 8 AM and on weekends, suggesting that staffing issues can also be a cause of cognitive error.[12]

The nature of pediatrics and care in the pediatric emergency department (ED) is prone to error.[11] For example, pediatric patients may be pre-verbal so they cannot self report their symptoms, nor can they confirm their identity. Diverse family circumstances may result in multiple caregivers and a high risk for inaccurate medical history. According to Chamberlain et al., family apprehension and anxiety are distractions to ED staff because they must manage their anxiety. Handoffs, especially with the complex patient, increases risk for cognitive error. Lack of inpatient beds is not only an inconvenience to the patient, but increases the risk of cognitive error because the ED will have to assume responsibility for inpatient care.

Chamberlain et al. suggests that these forces cause clinicians to make medical decisions using limited information with limited time. Heuristics, as described earlier, are important, and efficient medical decision tools may lead to cognitive error or bias and result in medical error.[11]

Chamberlain described how errors were most commonly associated with non-peak times 4 PM to 8 AM. Triage systems may result in misadventures; diagnostics tests, such as radiographic readings, may be in error (pneumonia versus no pneumonia); and blood cultures may be collected and interpreted erroneously, resulting in additional charges and unwanted antibiotic use. The authors conclude that there is a body of evidence regarding medical errors, but the data needs to be improved.[11]

REDUCING ERRORS IN PEDIATRIC ED

Chamberlain et al. describes several approaches to reducing errors. Weight-based and length-based equipment and medication retrieval systems reduce the cognitive burden of dosage calculation. This is essential during resuscitative efforts because a delay in therapy constitutes an error. Kovac et al. concluded that training and practice are essential components of a safety-enhancing strategy; teamwork training similar to that of the military is also important.

Computerized physician order entry systems (CPOE), as described in earlier chapters, have been associated with reducing medication errors. These systems permit dosage calculation, just-in-time decision support in the form of warnings when dose exceeds limits, or warning of interactions or allergies and feedback systems of prescribing practices. Furthermore, the most elementary of errors, transcription errors can be averted using CPOE systems.

Chamberlain described the ED of the future and provided a fictitious case of a 3-week-old baby visiting the ED for fever at 4 AM. He described the ideal systems, which included the following scenario. The nurse at triage conducts a 1-minute quick assessment; a transporter takes the family to a room for a short registration procedure. A complete nursing assessment, which includes length and weight, is performed. The nurse prepares the intravenous line and obtains blood and urine cultures, which are linked by barcode to the patient's bracelet and based on the clinical pathway. Antibiotics are prepared by a pharmacist, in accordance with the pathway, and are checked with the physician for correct dose. A computer flashes with warnings of the risk of a resistant strain in 10% of patients who are prescribed

this antibiotic. The system then searches the in-house intranet antibiogram data for resistance patterns and trends and most current recommendations for this specific condition. Furthermore, the software warns the physician to consider changing the dosage interval from every 6 hours to every 8 hours because of patient's age. Two nurses subsequently crosscheck the concentration and volume and ask about medication allergies and begin administration after scanning the identification band and barcode to check the correct identity and weight.

ED PHARMACISTS IN THE PEDIATRIC EMERGENCY DEPARTMENT

In Chamberlain's future depiction of the pediatric ED, a procurement, distribution, and clinical role of the pharmacist emerge. Mialon et al. described a children's medical center that triages more than 120,000 patients annually. The authors reported the EDP's activities in a pediatric ED. The pharmacist's activities, described by the authors, were comprehensive (Table 18-4), and they provide information for establishing the clinical role.

Some distinguishing features of this service include participating on all trauma and code teams until the patient is deemed to be stable and aiding in management of poisons, including educating other personnel on toxins and their appropriate treatments.

The authors did not describe the specialty emergency care pharmacotherapy pediatric issues. The EDP must be involved in this area because in this highly specialized area, data are not well established and needs more attention.

Furthermore, there are no published tools to expedite pharmacist response during emergency care situations involving children. What should the pharmacist know? What should the pharmacist be ready to provide in this unique setting? What are common errors that the pharmacist should look for to avert a catastrophic event?

CUSTOMIZED TOOLS TO EXPEDITE EMERGENCY CARE PHARMACOTHERAPY FOR PEDIATRIC EMERGENCIES

Cardiopulmonary arrest has an extremely poor prognosis, with reported survival of 0–17%. An ill-prepared emergency care staff can worsen this rate. Cardiopulmonary resuscitation (CPR) events can be chaotic but also confusing if participants lack understanding of the roles of individual resuscitation team members and have inadequate training or education. This confusion can be aggravated by inadequate hospital policies on the content and location of the emergency drug cart and diverse range of ages and weights, thus requiring a wide array of medication dosages and fluid requirements.

Resuscitation medications come in a variety of concentrations and dosages, and pediatric- specific concentrations exist but are not mandated to be purchased by the pharmacy department. Because of the need to simplify labor and reduce time and cost associated with procurement, pharmacy departments may include concentrations of cardiac resuscitation medications that require very small quantities when given to a pediatric patient. This creates the potential for delays in drug administration owing to the reconstitution during resus-

TABLE 18-4	ED Pharmacist Responsibilities in a Pediatric Emergency Department

1. Seek out interventions by making rounds in the medical, trauma, and observation units. Clinical pharmacist offers suggestions and assists in preventing medication errors.
2. Suggest appropriate medication and/or dose recommendations when needed.
3. Assist with intravenous drip calculations, medication dosing, and compatibility in code and trauma situations.
4. Perform pharmacokinetic dose checks and make recommendations on dose adjustments for antiepileptic medications, phenytoin, theophylline, digoxin, aminoglycosides and therapeutic drug monitoring of other medications as needed.
5. Serve on medical and trauma code response teams. Attend all incoming transport patients until deemed stable or transferred to another area.
6. Manage the poison/toxicology patient, including review of toxin and its appropriate treatment. Recommends appropriate use of antidotes.
7. Inform on adverse medication events/reactions: document their occurrence. Collaborate with other ED team members to design strategies for minimizing errors.
8. Inform on medication side effects, interactions (drug-drug, drug-disease), and incompatibilities.
9. Respond to drug information questions from ED staff and patients.
10. Verify medication orders and facilitate rapid turnaround times from pharmacy.
11. Fill ED-issued outpatient prescriptions.
12. Document clinical and cost saving interventions and routine provision of drug information.
13. Educate medical staff on formulary considerations and cost effective selections.
14. Acquire medications for indigent patients from pharmaceutical companies
15. Supervise and manage all distributional functions within the ED. Serve as liaison to pharmacy and the ED to optimize and expedite drug delivery
16. Facilitate transfer of patients to floor, i.e., ICU pharmacist of medication needs after arrival.
17. Manage drug shortage by recommending alternatives.
18. Provide and attend physician, nursing, and pharmacy rounds and in-services on emergency-related topics.
19. Perform formal or informal consultations as requested by ED staff.
20. Identify unknown medications.
21. Recruit, maintain, and educate ED pharmacy staff.
22. Recommend alternate routes of administration.
23. Serve as preceptor of pharmacy students, interns, fellows, and residents.
24. Recommend judicious use of laboratory draws for therapeutic drugs (Phenytoin, vancomycin).
25. Conduct medication history, reconcile the medications, and document in the chart and notify the caregiver as needed.
26. Verify allergy history and reaction associated with it and document in the chart.
27. Serve as investigational drug study liaison.
28. Conduct CQI, quality assurance activities, MUE or DUEs.
29. Provide discharge counseling.
30. Provide a link to information for patients discharged home.
31. Use laboratory data to evaluate efficacy and achievement of therapeutic outcomes and provide follow up consultation on inpatient floor.
32. Discuss compliance and compliance issues.
33. Evaluate and study outcomes of pharmacist presence in the ED for continued justification of position.

Adapted from Mialon PJ, Williams P, Wiebe RA. Clinical pharmacy services in a pediatric emergency room. *Hospital Pharmacy* 2004;39(2):121–124.

citation and potential medication errors. During a resuscitation event, code team members need to validate the dose, affirm the concentration, and calculate the quantity needed to withdraw into a syringe for administration—all cognitive tasks that under severe stress and potential for distractions increases the risk for medication error.

We have developed operational tools for EDP so, when needed, we have a guide map and a dosing scheme to assist in facilitating the EDP involvement and avoid human error. As seen in Table 18-5, a pediatric-specific dosing guide is on hand for the pharmacist to recommend and use as a resource in the event of a pediatric emergency. Furthermore, Table 18-6 lists the sequence of events for facilitating the management of rapid sequence induction for intubation in children.

The dosing guide is weight adjusted and is based on the concentration that is expected to be in the code cart and provides the volume required to dispense. This guide reduces the number of tasks needed to calculate the volume to withdraw and reduces the risk of cognitive and technical error. The guide provides a balance check for the physician and nurse and expedites the care during these events. Furthermore, we created pre-formed orders within the decision support system to corresponds to drip rates to be initiated on the SMART pump infusion technology.

| TABLE 18-5 | Pediatric-Specific Resuscitation Dosing Guide |

Medication Usual Dose Dosage Conc	1 kg	5 kg	10 kg	15 kg	20 kg	25 kg	30 kg	35 kg	40 kg
Adenosine[1] 100 mcg/kg 1st dose (Rapid IVP)	0.04 mL (0.1 mg)	0.17 mL (0.5 mg)	0.34 mL (1 mg)	0.50 mL (1.5 mg)	0.70 mL (2.0 mg)	0.9 mL (2.5 mg)	1.0 mL (3 mg)	1.2 mL (3.5 mg)	1.4 mL (4 mg)
200 mcg/kg 2nd dose X 1 3 mg/mL	0.07 mL (0.2 mg)	0.34 mL (1 mg)	0.70 mL (2 mg)	1 mL (3 mg)	0.07 mL (0.2 mg)	1.7 mL (5 mg)	2 mL (6 mg)	2.4 mL (7 mg)	2.7 mL (8 mg)
Atropine[1] 0.02 mg/kg (min 0.1 mg; max: child 0.5 mg adolescent 1 mg) 0.1 mg/mL	1 mL (0.1 mg)	1 mL (0.1 mg)	2 mL (0.2 mg)	3 mL (0.3 mg)	4 mL (0.4 mg)	5 mL (0.5 mg)	6 mL (0.6 mg)	7 mL (0.7 mg)	8 mL (0.8 mg)
Ca Chloride[1] 20 mg/kg (q 10 min) 100 mg/mL (10%)	0.2 mL (20 mg)	1 mL (100 mg)	2 mL (200 mg)	3 mL (300 mg)	4 mL (400 mg)	5 mL (500 mg)	6 mL (600 mg)	7 mL (700 mg)	8 mL (800 mg)
Dextrose (infant 10%)[2] 0.5 g/kg 0.10 g/mL (10%)	5 mL (0.5 g)	25 mL (2.5 g)	50 mL (5 g)	—	—	—	—	—	—
Dextrose (peds 25%)[2] Patients < 8 YO 0.5 g/kg 0.25 g/mL (25%)	—	—	20 mL (5 g)	30 mL (7.5 g)	40 mL (10 mg)	50 mL (12.5 mg)	—	—	—
Dextrose 50%[2] 0.5 g/kg 0.5 g/mL (50%)	—	—	—	—	—	25 mL (12 5 g)	30 mL (15 g)	35 mL (17.5g)	40 mL (20 g)
Epinephrine[1] 0.01 mg/kg 1st dose 0.1 mg/mL (1:10,000)	0.1 mL (0.01 mg)	0.5 ml (0.05 mg)	1 mL (0.1 mg)	1.5 ml (0.15 mg)	2 mL (0.2 mg)	2.5 mL (0.25 mg)	3 mL (0.3 mg)	3.5 mL (0.3 mg)	4 mL (0.4 mg)
0.1 mg/kg 2nd and all subsequent doses (q3–5 min) or all ETT doses 1 mg/mL (1:1000)	0.1 mL (0.01 mg)	0.5 ml (0.05 mg)	1 mL (1 mg)	1 mL (1.5 mg)	2 mL (0.2 mg)	2.5 ml (2.5 mg)	3 mL (3 mg)	3.5 mL (3.5 mg)	4 mL (4 mg)
Etomidate[3] (For age 10 and above) 0.3 mg/kg 2 mg/mL	0.15 mL (0.3 mg)	0.75 mL (1.5 mg)	1.5 ml (3 mg)	2.25 mL (4.5 mg)	3 mL (6 mg)	3.75 mL (7.5 mg)	4.5 mL (9 mg)	5.25 mL (10.5 mg)	6.0 mL (12 mg)
Fentanyl[2a] 2 mcg/kg (over 3–5 min) 50 mcg/mL	0.04 mL (0.002 mg)	0.2 mL (0.01 mg)	0.4 mL (0.02 mg)	0.6 mL (0.03 mg)	0.8 mL (0.04 mg)	1 mL (0.05 mg)	1.2 mL (0.06 mg)	1.4 mL (0.07 mg)	1.6 mL (0.08 mg)
Furosemide[4] 0.5–2 mg/kg 10 mg/mL (max. 6 mg/kg/dose)	0.05 mL (0.5 mg)	0.25 mL (2.5 mg)	0.5 mL (5 mg)	0.75 mL (7.5 mg)	1 mL (10 mg)	1.25 mL (12.5 mg)	1.5 mL (15 mg)	1.75 mL (17.5 mg)	2 mL (20 mg)

(continued)

TABLE 18-5 Pediatric-Specific Resuscitation Dosing Guide *(continued)*

Medication Usual Dose Dosage Conc	1 kg	5 kg	10 kg	15 kg	20 kg	25 kg	30 kg	35 kg	40 kg
Ketamine[5] 1–2 mg/kg IVP 10 mg/mL	0.1 mL (1 mg)	0.5 mL (5 mg)	1 mL (10 mg)	1.5 mL (15 mg)	2 mL (20 mg)	2.5 mL (2.5 mg)	3 mL (30 mg)	3.5 mL (3.5 mg)	4.0 mL (40 mg)
Ketamine[5] 4–7 mg/kg IM 10 mg/mL	0.4 mL (4 mg)	2 mL (20 mg)	4 mL (40 mg)	6 mL (60 mg)	8 mL (80 mg)	10 mL (100 mg)	12 mL (120 mg)	14 mL (140 mg)	16 mL (160 mg)
Lidocaine[2b] 1 mg/kg (Q 10–15 min X 2) 20 mg/mL (2%)	0.05 mL (1 mg)	0.25 mL (5 mg)	0.5 mL (10 mg)	0.75 mL (15 mg)	1 mL (20 mg)	1.25 mL (25 mg)	1.5 mL (30 mg)	1.75 mL (35 mg)	2 mL (40 mg)
Midazolam[4a] 0.2 mg/kg 1 mg/mL	0.2 mL (0.2 mg)	1 mL (1 mg)	2 mL (2 mg)	3 mL (3 mg)	4 mL (4 mg)	5 mL (5 mg)	6 mL (6 mg)	7 mL (7 mg)	8 mL (8 mg)
Morphine[6] 0.1 mg/kg 5 mg/mL (max 15 mg)	0.02 mL (0.1 mg)	0.1 mL (0.5 mg)	0.2 mL (1 mg)	0.3 mL (1.5 mg)	0.4 mL (2 mg)	0.5 mL (2.5 mg)	0.6 mL (3 mg)	0.7 mL (3.5 mg)	0.8 mL (4 mg)
Naloxone (ped)[7] Known single injection 0.01 mg/kg 0.02 mg/mL	0.5 mL (0.01 mg)	2.5 mL (0.05 mg)	5 mL (0.1 mg)	7.5 mL (0.15 mg)	10 mL (0.2 mg)	——	——	——	——
Naloxone (reg)[7] 0.1 mg/kg (Q 2–3 min) 0.4 mg/mL	0.25 mL (0.1 mg)	1.25 mL (0.5 mg)	2.5 mL (1 mg)	3.75 mL (1.5 mg)	5 mL (2 mg)	6.25 mL (2.5 mg)	7.5 mL (3 mg)	8.75 mL (3.5 mg)	10 mL (4 mg)
Bicarbonate (ped)[1] Patients < 1 year old 1 mEq/kg 0.5 mEq/mL (4.2%)	2 mL (1 mEq)	10 mL (5 mEq)	20 mL (10 mEq)	——	——	——	——	——	——
Bicarbonate (reg)[1] 1 mEq/kg 1 mEq/mL (8.4%)	——	——	10 mL (10 mEq)	15 mL (15 mEq)	20 mL (20 mEq)	25 mL (25 mEq)	30 mL (30 mEq)	35 mL (35 mEq)	40 mL (40 mEq)
Propofol[5] Patients > 3YO 2.5 – 3.5 mg/kg IVP 10 mg/mL	0.25 mL (2.5 mg)	1.25 mL (12.5 mg)	2.5 mL (25 mg)	3.75 mL (37.5 mg)	5 mL (50 mg)	6.25 mL (62.5 mg)	7.5 mL (75 mg)	8.75 mL (87.5 mg)	10 mL (100 mg)
Rocuronium[5] 0.6 mg/kg 10 mg/mL	0.06 mL (0.6 mg)	0.3 mL (3 mg)	0.6 mL (6 mg)	0.9 mL (9 mg)	1.2 mL (12 mg)	1.5 mL (15 mg)	1.8 mL (18 mg)	2.1 mL (21 mg)	2.4 mL (24 mg)
Succinylcholine[5] Infants 2 mg/kg 20 mg/mL	0.1 mL (2 mg)	0.5 mL (10 mg)	1 mL (20 mg)	1.5 mL (30 mg)	2 mL (40 mg)	2.5 mL (50 mg)	3 mL (60 mg)	3.5 mL (70 mg)	4 mL (80 mg)
Succinylcholine[2c] Child 1.5 mg/kg 20 mg/mL	0.075 mL (1.5 mg)	0.375 mL (7.5 mg)	0.75 mL (15 mg)	1.125 mL (22.5 mg)	1.5 mL (30 mg)	1.875 mL (37.5 mg)	2.25 mL (45 mg)	2.625 mL (52.5 mg)	3 mL (60 mg)
Thiopental[4b] 5 mg/kg 20 mg/mL	0.25 mL (5 mg)	1.25 mL (25 mg)	2.5 mL (50 mg)	3.75 mL (75 mg)	5 mL (100 mg)	6.25 mL (125 mg)	7.5 mL (150 mg)	8.75 mL (175 mg)	10 mL (200 mg)
Vecuronium[4c] 0.1 mg/kg standard dose 1 mg/mL	0.1 mL (0.1 mg)	0.5 mL (0.5 mg)	1.0 mL (1 mg)	1.5 mL (1.5 mg)	2 mL (2 mg)	2.5 mL (2.5 mg)	3 mL (3 mg)	3.5 mL (3.5 mg)	4.0 mL (4 mg)

(continued)

TABLE 18-5 Pediatric-Specific Resuscitation Dosing Guide *(continued)*

Medication Usual Dose Dosage Conc	1 kg	5 kg	10 kg	15 kg	20 kg	25 kg	30 kg	35 kg	40 kg
Vecuronium 0.2–0.3 mg/kg RSI 1 mg/mL	0.2 mL (0.2 mg)	1 mL (1 mg)	2 mL (2 mg)	3 mL (3 mg)	4 mL (4 mg)	5 mL (5 mg)	6 mL (6 mg)	7 mL (7 mg)	8 mL (8 mg)
Vecuronium 0.01 mg/kg nonde-polarizing dose 1 mg/mL	0.1 mL (0.01 mg)	0.05 mL (0.05 mg)	0.1 mL (0.1 mg)	0.15 mL (0.15 mg)	0.20 mL (0.2 mg)	0.25 mL (0.25 mg)	0.3 mL (0.3 mg)	0.35 mL (0.35 mg)	0.04 mL (0.4 mg)

REFERENCES
1. American Heart Association. Pediatric Advanced Life Support. *Circulation* 2005;112:167–87.
2. Taketomo CK, Hodding JH, Kraus DM. *Pediatric Dosage Handbook. 10th Ed.* Hudson, OH: Lexicomp, 2003:366–69.
2a. Taketomo CK, Hodding JH, Kraus DM. *Pediatric Dosage Handbook. 10th Ed.* Hudson, OH: Lexicomp, 2003:479–83.
2b. Taketomo CK, Hodding JH, Kraus DM. *Pediatric Dosage Handbook. 10th Ed.* Hudson, OH: Lexicomp, 2003:671–74.
2c. Taketomo CK, Hodding JH, Kraus DM. *Pediatric Dosage Handbook, 10th Ed.* Hudson, OH: Lexicomp, 2003:1044–46.
3. Amidate package insert. Bedford, OH: Bedford Laboratories; 2004 Mar.
4. Phelps SJ, Hak EB. *Pediatric Injectable Drugs. 7th Ed.* Bethesda, MD: ASHP, 2004:180–81.
4a. Phelps SJ, Hak EB. *Pediatric Injectable Drugs. 7th Ed.* Bethesda, MD: ASHP, 2004:274–75.
4b. Phelps SJ, Hak EB. *Pediatric Injectable Drugs. 7th Ed.* Bethesda, MD: ASHP, 2004:374–75.
4c. Phelps SJ, Hak EB. *Pediatric Injectable Drugs. 7th Ed.* Bethesda, MD: ASHP, 2004:410–11.
5. Micromedex Healthcare Series (internet database). URL: http://www.thomsonhc.com. Available from internet. Accessed 2008 May 29.
6. Epocrates (internet database). URL: http://www.epocrates.com. Available from internet. Accessed 2008 May 30.
7. Narcan package insert. Chadds Ford, PA: Endo Pharmaceuticals, Inc; 2001 Oct.

EMERGENCY MEDICINE OBSTETRICAL PHARMACOTHERAPY

Emergency Medicine Obstetrical Pharmacotherapy

Antiemetics
Antibiotics
Anticonvulsants
Diazepam
Hydralazine
Antihypertensive agents (Methyldopa, labetalol)
Magnesium
Methotrexate
Morphine
Oxygen
Oxytocin
RhoGAM
Saline

Emergency physicians commonly encounter obstetric patients to whom they must prescribe medications.[14–15] Common obstetric emergencies in which the EDP may participate include ectopic pregnancy, vaginal bleeding in each trimester, preeclampsia and eclampsia. EDPs need to expedite delivery and/or review the appropriateness for use of a variety of medications (as seen in the medication box), and the EDP must anticipate this need and assure safe and effective use.

In contrast to the obvious sign of vaginal bleeding, the cause of an obstetric patient's problem may not be so obvious because the initial complaint may include only nausea, vom-iting, abdominal pain or tenderness. Yet, temporizing pharmacotherapy for symptom control needs to be initiated. In most cases, routine assessment of airway, breathing, circulation and interventions of intravenous saline fluids, oxygen are initially instituted while placing the patient on a cardiac monitor. The risk of shock must be anticipated with these diagnoses as fluids and blood products may be needed early on.

For symptom control, antiemetics or analgesics may be initiated. Antibiotics are indicated if the ectopic pregnancy is septic. The female may be at risk of sepsis once delivered. Intravenous magnesium sulfate is used for treatment of eclampsia, defined as a seizure associated with pregnancy. If refractory to magnesium, a benzodiazepine may need to be instituted. Magnesium sulfate may also be initiated as prophylaxis against seizures in pre-eclampsia patients. Pre-eclampsia is defined as hypertension during pregnancy that may progress to eclampsia if not controlled. Depending on the severity, intravenous hydralazine is the drug of choice, but methyldopa or labetalol, may be used in less severe cases.

Oral methotrexate may be indicated in an otherwise stable patient with an ectopic pregnancy as an alternative to surgery. However, this treatment has strict indications and requires referral and consultation by an OB/GYN specialist. Oxytocin is used primarily for producing rhythmic contractions, preventing postpartum bleeding, and for its vasopressive qualities. Its use is advantageous in cases of vaginal bleeding, which may be a symptom of a threatened abortion or an abortion. The oxytocin can help with the delivery and removal of the ectopic or the fetus.

RhoGAM is indicated to remove risk of antibody formation as it acts as an immunosuppressant. RhoGAM is prescribed in a pregnant patient presenting with a vaginal bleed because there is a risk to subsequent pregnancies. The fetuses' blood may mix with the maternal blood; if a specific antigen (Rh) is not the same, this mix may increase the risk

TABLE 18-6 Pediatric Rapid Sequence Induction for Intubation (RSII)*

GET READY

M	MONITORS: Pulse oximeter, cardiac, exhaled CO_2
S	SUCTION: Tonsil tip (Yankauer)
O	OXYGEN: Tubing, non-rebreather mask, (correct size) Ambu bag (without pop-off valve)
A	AIRWAY EQUIPMENT: Oral and nasopharyngeal tubes, ETT [(16 + age in years)/4] = mm, *also 1 size smaller and larger ETT, stylets, benzoin, precut tape, (working) laryngoscope with blades
P	PERSONNEL & PHARMACY: 1–2 nurses, respiratory therapist, another physician; RSII drugs, Working (free-flowing) IV line

GET SET

INDICATIONS	RESPIRATORY FAILURE	HEAD TRAUMA/ICP
PREMEDICATION	Oxygen 100% by mask without bagging (unless needed)	
	Atropine 0.01 mg/kg IV Push	
		Lidocaine 1 mg/kg IV Push
	(*Optional* defasciculation) Succinylcholine **0.1 mg/kg** IV Push (only for succinylcholine paralysis)	
SEDATION	Ketamine 2 mg/kg IV Push	Thiopental 5 mg/kg IV Push
PARALYSIS	Succinylcholine 1.5 mg/kg IV Push OR Rocuronium 0.6 mg/kg IV Push	

GO

WAIT!	30–60 seconds for full paralysis
SELLICK MANEUVER	Cricoid Pressure
INTUBATION	Limit attempt to 30 seconds or desaturation
CHECK & SECURE	Bilateral breath sounds, good saturation, chest rising; meticulous taping

POST-INTUBATION

	INITIAL DOSES	CONTINUOUS INFUSIONS
PARALYSIS	Vecuronium or Pancuronium 0.1 mg/kg IV Push	Vecuronium 1 mcg/kg/min: Add 6 mg to 100 cc IVF, run @ kg = cc/hr
ANALGESIA	Morphine 0.1 mg/kg IV Push **OR** Fentanyl 2 mcg/kg IV Push	Fentanyl 0.1 mcg/kg/min: Add 600 mcg to 100 cc IVF, run @ kg = cc/hr
SEDATION	Midazolam **OR** Diazepam 0.1 mg/kg IV Push	Midazolam 1 mcg/kg/min: Add 6 mg to 100 cc IVF, run @ kg = cc/hr

*****PHYSICIAN MUST KNOW INDICATIONS, CONTRAINDICATIONS, AND SIDE EFFECTS OF ALL DRUGS.** Refer to the following pages for volume needed for initial doses. Revised: May 29, 2008

---

of antibody formation to the fetuses' blood and an immune response to the subsequent fetus may result in hemolysis. An obstetric emergency pharmacotherapy tool is seen in Table 18-7 to assist in safe and effective use of these medications while in the ED.

ASSURING SAFE AND EFFECTIVE DRUG INFORMATION AND PRESCRIBING IN PREGNANCY AND LACTATION

The emergency physician often needs to prescribe drugs for various problems encountered in pregnancy or is faced with a woman already taking a medication who coincidentally learns she is pregnant or is lactating.[16] In a survey we recently conducted, 60% (N=45) of emergency physicians consult pharmacy for safety information, another role for the EDP.[17]

From a safety perspective, we have observed emergency physicians using pocket handbooks (i.e., Tarascon's Pharmacopoeia), which may be outdated, for information regarding the pregnancy risk to prescribe or inform a lactating patient. In this same survey, most physicians were unaware of pregnancy-related informational resources available to them during prescribing. Surprisingly, when asked to rate the willingness to prescribe by FDA category (A, B, C, D, X) of pregnancy, 98% were willing to

| TABLE 18-7 | Obstetrical Emergency Pharmacotherapy |

Drug	Dosing Regimen	Clinical Pearls
Hydralazine	5–10 mg IV every 15–20 minutes and titrate as needed; switch to PO as soon as possible	• Anticipate need when pregnant female has abdominal tenderness and BP > 140/90 • Preserves uterine blood flow • Resolution is delivery • Treatment goal is 130–150/90–105 • Hypotension may cause fetal compromise also
Labetalol	20 mg IV over 2 minutes; follow with 40 mg in 10 minutes, then 80 mg every 10 minutes until max dose of 220 mg ; start a maintenance infusion at 2 mg/minute	• Use when hydralazine is not tolerated
Magnesium	Seizure (Eclampsia) prophylaxis and treatment 6 grams over 15 minutes; then 2 grams/hour IV; Repeat 2 grams bolus IV over 15 minutes if seizure re-occurs	• Goal Mg level of 4–7 mEq/L • Check maternal deep tendon reflex (may be lost at high magnesium levels) • Respiratory rate every 5 minutes • Urine output • Cardiac arrest at 13 mEq/L use 1 gram of calcium gluconate 10 mL of a 10% solution IV over 2 minutes
Methotrexate	50 mg/m^2 IM day 1	• Review Indications for use • OBGYN should be consulted • Repeat if hCG decline is < 15% in 4–7 days • Instruct patient on complications
Nicardipine	Infuse at 5 mg/hour and titrate at 2.5 mg/hour up to 15 mg/hour	• Use when hydralazine is not tolerated
Oxytocin	**Labor induction**: 0.5–1 milliunit/minute IV; titrate to 1–2 milliunits/minute to desired contraction pattern **Post partum bleeding**: 10 units after delivery IM Or 10–40 units by IV infusion in 100 mL of IV fluids at a rate to control uterine atony **Adjunct to abortion**: 10–20 milliunits/minute	• Considered a high risk drug by ISMP • Available as 10 units/ml • Use an infusion pump to administer • Compatible with NS or D5W, and mixtures
RhoGAM (Immunosuppression)	300 mcg IM only (contains polysorbate 80)	• 300 mcg sufficient to prevent Rh sensitization if volume entering circulation is < 15 mL • >If > 15 mL conduct fetal red cell count to determine dose • Give dose as soon after delivery • Some products are administered IM or IV (Contains polysorbate 80) be sure to check which is stocked by the blood bank • Observe for 20 minutes for signs of hemolysis, anemia, renal insufficiency.

Adapted from *Pearlman's Obstetric and Gynecologic Emergencies.*

TABLE 18-8	Drugs to Avoid in Pregnancy During Emergency Care

ACE inhibitors
Antiepileptic drugs
Ergotamines
Nitroprusside sodium
Quinolones
Tetracyclines
NSAIDS
Warfarin

Adapted from *Pearlman's Obstetric and Gynecologic Emergencies.*

prescribe category A drugs; 93% were willing to prescribe category B drugs. However, only 21% were willing to prescribe category C, and none were willing to prescribe category D and X. There is a disconnect with respect to FDA pregnancy categories, what they mean, and what information should be used to determine relative safety as 66% of the medications stored in our ED are in category C.

The FDA is in the process of revising the current letter category system because it oversimplifies risks and does not facilitate updating of labeling as new information becomes available. Furthermore, the Teratology Society for Public Affairs Committee recommended that the FDA pregnancy ratings be deleted from drug labels and be replaced by narrative statements. This process is in its infancy and is not yet in place.[16–17] This new system, however, appears to be even more complex. The EDP may play a greater role in assisting prescribers with the interpretation and application of this information to provide the best outcomes for the pregnant patient.

Several excellent pregnancy resources are available and accessible to clinicians in the ED. Briggs' *Drugs in Pregnancy and Lactation*, REPROTOX and TERIS in MicroMedex® are just a few. However, using these resources takes time, more than is available in the ED, and may not be fully conclusive as to whether a drug should be used.

W. Hansen in *Pearlman's Obstetric and Pregnancy Emergencies* provides a practical tool to expedite the acquisition of accurate information on what drugs can be used in concurrent illnesses associated with pregnancy and drugs that should be avoided. These lists are included in the emergency medicine pharmacotherapist obstetric tool box (see Tables 18-7, 18-8, and 18-9). We suggest, however, if there is ever a concern of risk, use the resources described and inform the patient on the risk versus benefit.

TABLE 18-9	Drugs That Are Safe to Use in Concurrent Illnesses of Pregnancy

	Drugs of Choice		**Drugs of Choice**
Pain	Morphine, Hydromorphone	Antihypertensives	Methyldopa, Labetalol and most Beta Blockers
	Acetaminophen with or without Codeine		Hydralazine
	Acetaminophen with Hydrocodone or propoxyphene	Antivirals	Acyclovir
Asthma Meds	Albuterol, Metaproterenol		Valacyclovir
	Beclomethasone dipropionate, Flunisolide	Antifungals	Nystatin
	Prednisone		Pyrethrins with piperonyl butoxide, Permethrin
	Aminophylline or Theophylline	Antipsychotics	Haloperidol
Antibiotics	Cefazolin	Anxiolytics	Diazepam
	Cefuroxime		Chlordiazepoxide
	Cephalexin		Alprazolam
	Ceftriaxone		Hydroxyzine
	Clindamycin	Antireflux	Famotidine, Ranitidine
	All macrolides		Metoclopramide
	Nitrofurantoin	Vaginal anti-infectives	Clotrimazole, Nystatin, terconazole
	Ampicillin all Beta lactams	Cardiac agents	Adenosine
	Piperacillin with or without tazobactam		Digoxin
Anticoagulants	Enoxaparin	Antimigraine	Acetaminophen, butalbital, caffeine
	Heparin	Vaccines	Tetanus vaccine and immune globulin
Antiemetics	Pyridoxine B$_6$		Rabies vaccine and Immunoglobulin
	Diphenhydramine		Influenza
	Promethazine		Pneumococcal
	Prochlorperazine		Diphtheria-tetanus
	Metoclopramide		
Anticonvulsants	Diazepam	OTC Colds/ allergies	Chlorpheniramine
	Magnesium sulfate		Pseudoephedrine

Adapted from reference 16: Pearlman's Obstetric and Gynecologic Emergencies

SUMMARY

Use of the ED by special populations continues to increase. Quality of care in the ED for special populations must be optimized. New safeguards for geriatric emergency care pharmacotherapy have been proposed. Pediatric EDs also constitute a natural risk for medication error that pharmacists may have a role in preventing. Dosing tools and protocols, in addition to automation, are several strategies to reduce this risk. Furthermore, a list of responsibilities for a pharmacist attempting to establish pediatric ED services has been provided. Few reports describe the role of the EDP in obstetric emergencies or in advising on drug use in pregnancy. Thus, based on our experience and published data on common obstetric emergencies, we provided some practical tools to assist pharmacists who may be asked about these issues or who may be responding during an obstetric emergency.

References

1. Wilber ST, Gerson LW, Terrell KT, et al. Geriatric emergency medicine and the 2006 IOM reports on the future of emergency care. *Acad Emerg Med* 2006;13:1345–1351.
2. Older Americans Health Factsheet. National Center for Health Statistics 2005 [online]. Available at http://www.cdc.gov/nchs/data/factsheet/olderadulthtlt.pdf Accessed September 25, 2006.
3. Baum SA, Rubenstein LZ. Old people in the emergency room. Age related differences in emergency department use and care. *J Am Geriatr Soc* 1987;35:398–404.
4. Singal BM, Hedges JR, Rousseau EW, et al. Geriatric patient emergency visits. Part I: Comparison of visits by geriatric and younger patients. *Ann Emerg Med* 1992;21:802–807.
5. Magid DJ, Masoudi FA, Vinson DR, et al. Older emergency department patients with acute myocardial infarction receive lower quality of care than younger patients. *Ann Emerg Med* 2005;46:14–21.
6. Hwang U, Morrison SR. The geriatric emergency department. *J Am Geriatr Soc* 2007;55(11):1873–1876.
7. Adams JG, Gerson LW. A new model for emergency care of geriatrics patients. *Acad Emerg Med* 2003;10:271–274.
8. Wegner NS, Shekelle P, Davidoff F, et al. Quality indicators for assessing care of vulnerable elders. *Ann Intern Med* 2001;135:641–758.
9. Beck A, Scott J, Williams P, et al. A randomized trial of group outpatient visits for chronically ill older HMO members: The Cooperative Health Care Clinic. *J Am Geriatric Soc* 1997;45:543–49.
10. Wenger NS, Shekelle PG, Solomon DH, et al. The quality of pharmacologic care for vulnerable older patients. *Ann Intern Med* 2001;135:642–646.
11. Chamberlain JM, Patel KM, Pollack MM. Association of emergency department care factors with admission and discharge decisions for pediatric patients. *J Pediatr* 2006;149(5):644–649.
12. Kozer E, Berkovitch M, Koren G. Medication errors in children *Pediatr Clin North Am* 2006;53(60:1155–68.
13. Mialon PJ, Williams P, Wiebe RA. Clinical pharmacy services in a pediatric emergency room. *Hosp Pharm* 2004;39(2):121–124.
14. Giustina-Della K, Chow G. Medications in pregnancy and lactation. *Emerg Med Clin North Am* 2003;21585–613.
15. Mick NW, Peters JR, Egan D, Nadel ES, Walls R, Silvers S. Part Six Obstetric/Gynecologic and Urogenital Emergencies. In: *Blueprints Emergency Medicine, Second Edition.*
16. Hansen W. Drug Use in Pregnancy. In: *Pearlman's Obstetrics and Gynecologic Emergencies: Diagnosis and Management.* http://www.accessemergencymedicine.com.
17. Cohen V, Stanfield L, Jellinek S, Likourezos A. A Survey on Drug Information References Used by Emergency Medicine Clinicians for Prescribing Decisions in Pregnant Patients. Abstract Presented at the 2008 ASHP Midyear Clinical Meeting, Orlando, Florida.

Part IV

Fostering Interest in Emergency Medicine Pharmacotherapy

In Part IV, we discuss the apex of the pyramid that, if in place, will help navigate the safe medication use system and fill daily gaps in safety and quality. We describe how to foster the role of the pharmacist in emergency medicine. We establish the structure for which processes may be created and performance can be evaluated to assess its value—a missing link in current clinical pharmacy services provided in the emergency department (ED).

The clinical pharmacy service is composed of clinical managers who lead the service, post-graduate year one (PGY1) and two (PGY2) residents who are responsible for day-to-day operations, pharmacy interns, and board-certified technicians who facilitate the clinician's role in the provision of optimal pharmacotherapy and assuring safety. In chapter 19, we describe the PGY1 and PGY2 pharmacy practice residents role in ensuring that gaps in each stage of the drug order and delivery process are filled. Their roles and activities are described, and the academic-based clinical pharmacy services role in fostering this involvement will be reviewed. A discussion of whether an ED residency should be considered a PGY1 or PGY2 or both is provided. In chapter 20, we describe an emergency medicine pharmacy intern model to foster postgraduate training in emergency medicine pharmacotherapy. In chapter 21, we describe the use of board-certified pharmacy technicians to facilitate clinical pharmacy services in the ED. If achieved, the PharmER pyramid model will assure the provision of a sustainable service that perpetually adjusts itself to assure safety and quality of emergency medicine pharmacotherapy.

19

Education for Emergency Medicine Pharmacotherapy: A Blueprint for PGY2 Specialty Training

Objectives

- Describe the post-graduate year one (PGY1) resident's role, activities, and structure in the emergency department (ED)
- Describe the post-graduate year two (PGY2) resident's role, activities, and structure in the ED
- Develop PGY2 learning experiences, outcomes, goals, and objectives
- Review current standards of the emergency medicine pharmacy practice specialty residency
- Describe the 2007 Emergency Medicine (EM) Model of Practice
- Discuss integration of the 2007 EM model into American Society of Health-System Pharmacists (ASHP) Goals and Objectives for PGY2

PGY1 RESIDENT ROLE AND ACTIVITIES IN THE ED

In 2003, with more than 5 years of providing an internal medicine rotation for undergraduate pharmacy students within the ED, we realized that the ED can also serve as a location for a post graduate pharmacy resident. The advantages of the ED include providing a general medicine experience equivalent to that seen in other traditional internal medicine units, with the advantage of the hands-on experience of witnessing cases evolve in front of their eyes.

With this in mind in 2003, we designed a post-graduate year one residency (PGY1) using the ED as a source for

rotations in Internal Medicine. The PGY1 resident was required to conduct medication histories, interventions, conduct profile reviews for all boarded patients, assure timely delivery of all medications to boarded patients through the unit dose distribution services, provide discharge counseling of patients who requested their medications from the outpatient pharmacy, and report any adverse drug events or medication errors that may have occurred out of hospital or in the ED. The PGY1 resident would also conduct a medication use evaluation and provide in-services to the nursing and medical staff. We observed that the pharmacy interns and PGY1 were extremely successful at providing this service to the ED, and it was well accepted by nursing and medical staffs. It was also clear that the PGY1 resident was not comfortable with responding to resuscitation or an emergency care or critical care situation, and that only in the presence of the clinical manager would the PGY1 or intern be willing to act. The PGY1 residency was subsequently accredited by the American Society of Health-System Pharmacists Commission on Credentialing in 2003. From our observations, the ED can serve as an alternative practice site for PGY1 residency requirements.

Currently, the Maimonides PGY1 residents are required to do two rotations in the ED. The first is an internal medicine rotation that includes managing the boarded patient medications, and the second rotation is a critical care/resuscitation rotation. The PGY1 resident is also required to work short call to the ED from 3 PM –11 PM, one day a week, and one weekend a month from 8 AM –8 PM. During these times, the PGY1 resident is autonomous and conducts drug consults to the ED and acts as a liaison for any drug-related issues. A portion of this time is used for academics.

To further increase coverage to the ED, we expanded the PGY1 residency and created a second position. The funding for the PGY1 residency supported the subsequent requests for funding of a PGY2 specialty residency in emergency medicine. In 2007, we officially opened two PGY2 specialty residency positions in emergency medicine and recruited and filled one of the two positions.

PGY2 RESIDENT ROLE AND ACTIVITIES IN THE ED

The PGY2 specialist role expedites safe and effective medication use during emergency and critical care in the ED and manages and supervises the needs of the boarded patients and lower acuity issues. Daily activities include responding to all emergency care notifications and verifying emergency care medication orders. The resident is responsible for assisting central pharmacy with verification of all medication orders for boarded patients and assisting in supervising the drug order and delivery process.

Each rotation has its own dynamics. A weekly schedule may appear as follows: Two days a week, the PGY2 resident is autonomous yet under the guidance of the clinical pharmacy manager specialist and is responsible for prospective verification of boarded patient medication orders written in the ED. Two days a week, the PGY2 resident is provided academic time to engage in emergency care of patients, without the restraint of verifying the boarded patients medication orders. On Wednesdays, the resident attends the emergency medicine core seminar that includes morbidity and mortality reports, didactic presentations, and a research meeting. In addition, the resident is provided administration time in the afternoon to document their activities or prepare for their lectures or other scholarly activities.

During the academic days, ideally the resident is responsible for following up with five patients per day, as they pertain to the corresponding disorders to fulfill direct patient care goals (Outcomes R2-R4, P1–P2F and P5 as described in the ASHP PGY2 standards) for that rotation.[1] However, because we can never be assured of the disease states and acuities that will be observed on any given day, the resident documents any case requiring emergent care and records the experience for that case in a log book or via the use of FARM (findings, assessment, recommendations, monitoring) notes.

CERTIFYING MASTERY OF GOALS AND OBJECTIVES

The preceptor assures the acquisition of knowledge by the PGY2 resident through providing hands-on instruction on how to manage the case in real-time when it is occurring or through didactic instruction or through provision of reading material. To achieve mastery of emergency medicine pharmacotherapy conditions, the resident is required to observe a total of five patients with varying acuities of the disease state to pass through the continuum of "knowledge-application-do-and able to teach." Once this continuum is achieved, the resident has achieved the objective for that complaint and will no longer be evaluated. However, the expectation is that the PGY2 resident now understands the myriad of acuities that can occur with a given complaint

and is proficient in the pharmacotherapy management of them with minimal facilitation from the preceptor. Of note, the PGY1 and PGY2 residency experience in the ED can be neatly demarcated by the responsibility as it pertains to emergency care. Not all PGY1 residents would shy away from a resuscitation or emergency care situation, but the difference between PGY1 and PGY2 is that the PGY2 resident is held accountable for managing emergency care and resuscitation as part of their achievement of the residency goals and objectives. The PGY1 resident is not held to that level of mastery.

Daily from 3 PM to 4 PM, the resident is provided with a pharmacotherapy lecture on a rotational topic to supplement the practical experiences. This partition model provides a good mix of academic time with practical experience and permits the PGY2 to develop some autonomy as well. The PGY2 learns the generalist pharmacist role while given time to master the specialist role of the emergency medicine pharmacotherapy.

The PGY2 resident rotates with the three other residents to service the ED one weekend a month and will be on call in the ED 1 to 2 days a week from 3 PM to 11 PM, similar to the PGY1 resident. The four residents are able to provide weekend coverage for 12 hours a day and daily coverage of the ED 18 hours a day to promote safe and effective medication use.

Of note, the more time a pharmacist spends in the ED the more opportunity he or she has to identify areas that need improvement as it pertains to medication use.

DOCUMENTATION OF ACTIVITIES

The resident is required to submit evidence of his or her performance. The PGY2 resident must conduct a number of interventions, document interventions on a personal digital assistant, and document two FARM notes per short-call. Furthermore, the PGY2 must document medication histories, report adverse drug events, and/or medication errors that are encountered, and conduct a medication use evaluation as it pertains to the emergency department. The resident is responsible for two journal clubs, an oral in-service and a major presentation associated with the conditions assigned during the designated rotation. It is the expectation that advanced practice residents should be able to review and master a topic on a weekly basis, and thus, it is reasonable to expect that five emergency medicine topics are mastered by the resident during each rotation. Completion of topics for each rotation depends on what is encountered in the ED.

A credentialing book is provided to each PGY2 resident, and they must demonstrate levels of proficiency with each condition as it pertains to the pharmacotherapy and management of each disease state experienced. A pharmacotherapist is responsible to attest to the resident's competency for the list of topics. A log book is used to verify and document the residents' pharmacotherapy knowledge and competence in the performance and mastery of the drug indication, contraindications, selection of appropriateness, dosing, anticipation of adverse events and drug interactions, as well as the prescribing, procurement, monitoring and assuring optimal administration. Completion of a log book is required for certification.

Four stages are documented as it pertains to mastery of each disease state. First, cognitive skills are demonstrated after the resident has experienced one patient and demonstrates knowledge of emergency medicine pharmacotherapy. Second, technical skill must be displayed; the resident applies that knowledge by managing a case with some facilitation. The third level is demonstrated when the resident can act, as part of their practice, at all times with little facilitation; and the fourth level is demonstrated when the resident is able to teach the disease state, its emergency medicine pharmacotherapy management, and can identify inadequacies in care. We require a total of five patients to pass through each stage to verify that the resident is proficient in the emergency medicine pharmacotherapy of each complaint and their associated conditions.

DEVELOPMENT OF NATIONAL OUTCOMES, GOALS AND OBJECTIVES: STANDARDS FOR PGY2 RESIDENCY IN EMERGENCY MEDICINE PHARMACOTHERAPY

As of 2007, there are three American Society of Health-System Pharmacist's accredited emergency medicine residency programs in the country and one pending accreditation[2]. In addition, there are numerous non-accredited PGY2 emergency medicine specialty residencies.

Graduate medical education pass-through funding for emergency medicine pharmacotherapy is not available. Few hospitals who do offer emergency medicine specialties will lack the incentive to seek accreditation for these programs. This may delay the development of a national standard of practice. Irrespective there is probably, no one standard that can represent the variation of ED activities across the country. However, creating a standard may help in developing common performance goals that can demonstrate the value of this service. We contend that the current emergency care crisis needs pharmacy input; thus, incentives in the form of funding is needed to assure implementation and growth. Furthermore, to accelerate implementation, ASHP standards are needed to provide a blueprint for health-systems to implement this service. We reviewed the literature for standards in practice and have designed a potential blueprint for a PGY2 emergency medicine pharmacotherapy residency (Appendix C).

With only a few PGY2 emergency medicine residencies there are no published reports describing specific ED outcomes, goals, objectives, and instructional objectives. Furthermore, the current ASHP PGY2 standards for advanced practices of pharmacy are appropriate but are non-specific for the required body of knowledge and skills needed in emergency medicine pharmacotherapy.

We conducted an evidence-based review of knowledge and skills needed in emergency medicine pharmacotherapy, fused them with the observations made in practice, and developed a set of outcomes, goals, and objectives that we have used that may, in addition to other EM ASHP-accredited institutions' goals and objectives, become a blueprint for nationally accepted outcomes.

The design of this set of goals and objectives are based on a review of the 2007 Emergency Medicine model[3] for medical residency training. We have identified elements of the 2007 emergency medicine (EM) model of practice that relate to pharmacy practice, and have integrated our activities associated with improving safety and quality of emergency care. In the subsequent section, we describe the activities, tasks, and components of the 2007 EM model for which the pharmacists can have a role.

DESCRIPTION OF THE 2007 EMERGENCY MEDICINE MODEL OF PRACTICE

In 1975, the American College of Emergency Physicians and the University Association for Emergency Medicine (now the Society for Academic Emergency Medicine, SAEM) conducted a practice analysis of the emerging field of Emergency Medicine. This work resulted in the development of the **Core Content of Emergency Medicine**, which included a listing of common conditions, symptoms, and diseases seen and evaluated in EDs; this work has evolved into the 2007 EM model[3], a three-dimensional description of emergency medicine clinical practice and is available at the following link (http://www.acgme.org/acWebsite/ RRC_110/110_clinModel.pdf).[3]

THREE-DIMENSIONAL MODEL OF EMERGENCY MEDICINE PRACTICE

There are three components to the EM Model: 1) physician-conducted assessment of patient acuity; 2) a list of the tasks that must be performed to provide appropriate emergency medical care; and 3) a listing of common conditions, symptom and disease presentations. Together, these three components describe the clinical practice of EM and differentiate it from the clinical practice of other specialties.[3] All of these dimensions are employed concurrently by a physician when providing patient care. For example, the EP's initial approach is determined by the acuity of the patients' presentation. While assessing the patient, the physician completes a series of tasks to collect information. Through this process, the physician is able to select the most likely etiology of the patients' problem from the listing of conditions. Through continued application of all three components, the physician makes the most probable diagnosis and subsequently implements a treatment plan for the patient.

INTERGRATION OF THE 2007 EM MODEL INTO ASHP GOALS AND OBJECTIVES FOR PGY2

Using the EM Model and applying it to the ASHP educational goals and learning objectives for PGY2, we designed the goals, objectives, and criteria for the emergency medicine pharmacotherapy residency.

PATIENT ACUITY

The first goal for the PGY2 must be to master the ability to differentiate varying acuities, such as critical, emergent, and lower. For example, the *critical patient* is defined as a patient who is presenting with symptoms of a life-threatening illness or injury with a high probability of mortality if immediate intervention is not begun to prevent further airway, respiratory, hemodynamic, or neurologic instability. *Emergent* illness is defined as patients with presenting symptoms of an illness or injury that may progress in severity or result in complications with a high probability for morbidity if treatment is not begun quickly. *Lower acuity* is defined as a patient who presents with symptoms of an illness or injury but has a low probability of progression to more serious disease or development of complications.[8]

An example of differentiation in acuity is seen with the patient complaining of chest pain. The patient, who is a 50-year-old hypertensive, diabetic man with crushing chest pain and is diaphoretic, has a blood pressure of 60 systolic and is clutching his chest. This patient would be placed in a critical acuity frame, and physician tasks include immediate intervention needed to manage and stabilize the vital signs where a high probability exists of mortality without immediate intervention.[3]

This frame of acuity differs from that of a 74-year-old woman who has a history of angina and presents with 3 to 5 minutes of dull chest pain typical of her angina. She has stable vitals signs, and her pain is relieved by nitroglycerin. She will be placed in an emergent acuity frame, and physician tasks include monitoring, vascular access, evaluation, and treatment performed quickly because progression in severity, complications, or morbidity may occur without immediate treatment.[3]

This again differs from the 12-year-old female with non-traumatic sharp chest pain that lasts several days and intensifies with movement of the torso. She will be placed in a lower acuity frame; symptoms will be addressed promptly. However, progression to major complications is unlikely.[3] Pharmacists must be able to differentiate the acuity and anticipate the complications with a tiered and appropriate pharmacotherapeutic response. This knowledge is gained only through experience while in the ED.

PHYSICIAN TASKS

The second goal for the PGY2 to take into consideration is the 2007 EM model list of physician tasks for which pharmacists must be prepared to participate. This list includes emergency stabilization, therapeutic interventions, pharmacotherapy, observation and reassessment, consultation and disposition, prevention and education, documentation, and multi-tasking as part of team management.[3]

PROCEDURAL PHARMACOTHERAPY

A third goal for the PGY2 is to be aware of the procedures and skills of an EP that may be facilitated by pharmacotherapy, for example, airway techniques including airway adjuncts, intubation (naso, orotracheal and rapid sequence), and mechanical ventilation. Other procedures requiring the use of pharmacotherapy are anesthesia including local and regional, sedation, analgesia for sedation, blood, fluid, and component therapy. Diagnostic procedures, their significance, and complications when conducted by emergency physicians, include procedures such as anoscopy, arthrocentesis, bedside ultrasonography, cystourethrogram, lumbar puncture, nasogastric tube, paracentesis, pericardiocentesis, peritoneal lavage, slit lamp examination, thoracentesis, and tonometry. Organ-specific procedures, conducted by EPs, include bladder catheterization and testicular detorsion, head and neck control of epistaxis with anterior packing, cautery, posterior packing and balloon placement, use of laryngoscope, needle aspiration of peritonsillar abscess, removal of rust ring, and tooth replacement.

The EDP needs to understand varying hemodynamic access techniques to appropriately titrate and monitor vasopressors and vasodilators, such as arterial catheter insertion, central venous access from various locations, and intraosseous infusion devices. Pharmacists may be asked to assist with pharmacotherapy in obstetric procedures such as in abnormal and normal deliveries. Other techniques for which pharmacists should be familiar and that may have pharmacotherapeutic implications include foreign body removal, gastric lavage, gastrostomy tube placement, pain management, physician restraints, sexual assault examination, trephination of nails, wound closure techniques, and wound management.

Most likely, pharmacists will be involved in procedures associated with resuscitation, such as cardiopulmonary resuscitation and neonatal resuscitation. Pharmacists must have a familiarity with skeletal procedures such as assisting physicians with fracture/dislocation immobilization techniques, fracture/dislocation reduction techniques, and spine immobilization techniques. Pharmacists may also be involved in assisting with cutaneous and transvenous cardiac pacing, defibrillation or cardioversion, and other invasive thoracic techniques. Lastly, pharmacists must ensure the use of universal precautions when in the ED.

EMERGENCY MEDICINE ADMINISTRATIVE COMPONENTS

A fourth goal for the PGY2 resident is to be aware of how a pharmacist may play a role in administrative components of the 2007 EM model,[3] such as financial (cost containment, reimbursement with capture of medications), facility design including design of a satellite or medication room, information management, patient throughput and crowding and policies and procedures. Pharmacists are frequently needed to assist with performance improvement such as in patient safety and error reduction and translation of practice guidelines. Pharmacists play a role in pre-hospital care as it relates to multi-casualty incidents and protocol development. The pharmacist will also be involved in institutional and community-wide emergency preparedness and end-of-life issues. Pharmacists may collaborate with EPs in research, including evidence-based interpretation of the medical literature and performance of research. Pharmacists are also involved in risk management and regulatory issues.

With these four goals, obtained from the 2007 EM model, the PGY2 ASHP goals and objectives, and more than a decade of observations, we developed a list of outcomes, goals, objectives, and instructional objectives (see Appendix: Educational Outcomes, Goals, and Objectives for Postgraduate Year Two (PGY2) Pharmacy Residencies in Emergency Medicine). Furthermore, we structured this textbook to be a lead in to emergency medicine pharmacotherapy residency and to accelerate the PGY2 acclimation and growth to the field of emergency medicine. The order of goals and objectives correspond to the chapters in this text.

SUMMARY

A continuum of education for emergency medicine pharmacotherapy has been suggested. A set of goals and objectives have been developed to foster an emergency medicine pharmacotherapy postgraduate residency year two training program. This set of goals and objectives was composed from an integration of the 2007 EM model and the ASHP PGY2 standards. This blueprint may assist fellow EDPs and organizations to initiate an emergency medicine residency and help grow this important practice. Furthermore, the use of this blueprint may assist in achieving the future 2020 vision in which all pharmacists practicing in the healthcare setting are residency trained.[4] This may also contribute to the needed pharmacy resources that are estimated from the pharmacy manpower project.[5]

References

1. ASHP PGY2 Practice Foundation skills http://www.ashp.org/ s_ashp/cat1c.asp?CID=3549&DID=5577 Accessed July 30, 2008.
2. National Matching Services Inc. ASHP resident matching positions beginning in 2009 available at http://www.natmatch.com/ ashprmp/index.htm. Accessed in December 2008
3. The EM Model of medical residency training. http://www. acgme.org/acWebsite/RRC_110/110_clinModel.pdf. Accessed December 10, 2007.
4. American College of Clinical Pharmacy. A vision of pharmacy's future roles, responsibilities, and manpower needs in the United States. *Pharmacotherapy* 2000;20:991–1022.
5. Johnson TJ. Pharmacist work force in 2020: Implications of requiring residency training for practice. *Am J Health-Syst Pharm* 2008:65:166–170.

20

Designing an Undergraduate PharmD Intern Practice Model in the Emergency Department

Objectives

- List course objectives for an Emergency Medicine undergraduate clerkship
- Describe instructional methods and content for an Emergency Medicine Undergraduate Clerkship
- Describe course session for an Emergency Medicine Undergraduate Clerkship
- Describe assessment criteria for an Emergency Medicine Undergraduate clerkship
- Describe course references for an Emergency Medicine Undergraduate clerkship
- Discuss daily activities, personal attributes, and advantages and challenges of an Emergency Medicine Undergraduate clerkship

With preventable medication errors as one of the main contributors to morbidity and mortality in the ED, it is essential to stimulate interest in emergency medicine pharmacotherapy at an early juncture among doctor of pharmacy students. However, there are no published examples on the conduct of an elective rotation in emergency medicine pharmacy practice. Over the past decade, students from the Arnold & Marie Schwartz College of Pharmacy and Health Sciences have been assigned to the ED as part of an advanced atypical internal medicine.

In this chapter, we outline course objectives, instructional methods and content, and grading criteria for the purpose of assisting pharmacy faculty in developing a similar course at their respective institutions. Outcomes and experiences learned in offering this course over the last 10 years at the Arnold & Marie Schwartz College of Pharmacy and Health Sciences are also discussed.

EMERGENCY MEDICINE UNDERGRADUATE CLERKSHIP

COURSE OBJECTIVES

The objectives of this course are seen in Table 20-1:

These course objectives align well with current American Association of Colleges of Pharmacy Center for Advancement of Pharmaceutical Education (CAPE)[3] educational outcomes and curricular endpoints for pharmacy education (Fig. 20-1), course-specific endpoints (Fig. 20-2), and course-specific goals and learning or behavioral objectives (Fig. 20-3).[3]

INSTRUCTIONAL METHODS AND CONTENT

This four-credit elective rotation requires students to meet daily for a routine 8-hour day, including lunch.

COURSE SESSION DESCRIPTION

The methods used for conveying information within this course included a variety of techniques. While modeling, facilitation, and coaching were the foundation upon which the course was built, the faculty (that may have included other preceptors and colleagues who cover the ED) provide didactic presentations in issues concerning the emergency medicine provision of safety and quality of pharmacotherapy because there is little concentration on emergency care pharmacotherapy during the pharmacy school curriculum.

text continues on page 198

TABLE 20-1 Objectives for an Emergency Medicine Elective

- Outline the workflow and pharmacy operations in the ED
- Demonstrate the use of automation in the ED
- Illustrate procedures for pharmacist review of medication orders for boarded and emergency patients
- List procedures with procuring and dispensing medications for boarded and emergency patients
- Demonstrate how to conduct medication interviews
- Demonstrate the information needed to be generated by the pharmacist and how to record that data into the ED CPOE systems
- Demonstrate how to conduct and streamline drug therapy assessments
- Demonstrate how to identify drug-related problems and intervene as needed as it pertains to boarded and emergency care situations
- Illustrate various methods to record interventions in and ED setting
- Illustrate how to record adverse drug events and medication error incidents
- Demonstrate how to provide target in-services to ED nursing as it pertains to medication safety and quality
- Demonstrate how to design and present lectures to ED medical residents
- Demonstrate how to review and present journal articles in emergency care pharmacotherapy in an active learning strategy
- Demonstrate how to assure quality through patient safety
- Demonstrate how to survey for medication discrepancies with high risk medications or high risk patients
- Illustrate how to respond quickly to drug information questions
- Demonstrate how to expedite and facilitate acquisition of non-floor stock medications
- Illustrate how to conduct a project to evaluate performance on ED specific quality indicators
- Describe how to provide medication therapy management services through the ED

This Course will assist the student in meeting the following curricular endpoints:

- Gather and organize accurate and comprehensive patient information to identify ongoing or potential drug therapy problems.(A1a)
- Interpret and evaluate patient and drug-related data needed to identify actual or potential drug therapy problems.(A1b)
- Design, implement, and defend a course of treatment based on evidence that best addresses the patient's health needs.(A1c)
- Prepare, dispense, and/or administer a pharmaceutical product for patient use based on professional practice guidelines.(A1d)
- Counsel patients to ensure appropriate pharmaceutical care outcomes, and institute programs to maximize compliance to drug regimens. (A1e)
- Educate patients about behaviors that promote health (including drug adherence), maintain wellness, prevent, and control disease.(A1f)
- Monitor patients to optimize therapeutic efficacy and minimize side effects. Develop strategies to manage and minimize potential adverse events.(A1g)
- Display respect and sensitivity for patient and family attitudes, behaviors and lifestyles, paying particular attention to cultural, ethnic and socioeconomic influences while incorporating cultural preferences, spiritual, and health beliefs and behaviors into the patient care plan.(A1h)
- Provide clinical preventive services (based on pharmacists practice activity domains) to improve outcomes and quality of life.(C1b)
- Communicate and collaborate with patients, care givers, physicians, nurses, other health care providers, policy makers, members of the community and administrative and support personnel to engender a team approach to patient care.(D1)
- Retrieve, analyze, and interpret the professional, lay, and scientific literature to provide drug information and counseling to patients, their families or care givers, as well as other health care providers.(D2)
- Demonstrate expertise in informatics (D3)
- Carry out duties in accordance with legal, ethical, social, economic, and professional guidelines (D4)
- Evaluate and resolve ethical dilemmas that arise in practice and find a solution that is acceptable to all parties involved.(D4a)
- Maintain professional competence by identifying and analyzing emerging issues, products, and services.(D5)

Figure 20–1. Emergency medicine clerkship and curricular endpoints.

This Course will assist the student in meeting the following course-specific endpoints:

- Obtain necessary information from the patient, caregiver, and/or other members of the healthcare team.(A1a)
- Identify relevant information in the patient profile or medical record. (A1a)
- Interview the patient and caregiver employing effective communication strategies. (A1a)
- Identify the patient's primary complaint(s) and reason(s) for seeking medical care.
- Perform selected aspects of physical assessment, as appropriate.(A1a)
- Protect the confidentiality of patient information. (D4)
- Evaluate information obtained from the patient's history and physical assessment. (A1b)
- Assess any patient history of allergies and intolerances. (A1b)
- Evaluate laboratory tests results and pharmacokinetic data. (A1b)
- Perform any additional patient calculations needed (e.g. creatinine clearance, ideal body weight, body surface area, body mass index).(A1b)
- Identify the cause and significance of adverse drug effects. (A1b)
- Evaluate the significance of actual or potential drug interactions. (A1b)
- Assure that there is no excessive medication use or unnecessary drug duplication. (A1b)
- Determine the extent to which medical conditions or diseases are treated and controlled. (A1b)
- Identify signs or potential indicators of drug misuse or abuse. (A1b)
- Develop a complete medical and drug therapy problem list. (A1a, A1b)

   - Use relative priority to direct the pharmacotherapeutic plan
   - Differentiate active from inactive problems.
   - Rank patient problems based on urgency and severity.
   - Identify any preventative and health maintenance issues
   - Explain to patients or caregivers the drug, dosage, indication, and storage requirements for a given drug.
   - Educate patients or caregivers on the symptomatology, significance, frequency, and treatment of adverse drug reactions.
   - Explain any action that should be taken in the event of a missed dose.
   - Demonstrate proper administration technique for a given drug delivery system.
   - Facilitate patients assuming an active role in their self-care and overall health.
   - Choose communication methods that are sensitive to the social and cultural background of the target audience.
   - Confirm patient understanding of counseling provided and clarify if needed.

- Educate patients or caregivers about the proper use of medical goods and devices. (A1e, A1f)

   - Identify print, audiovisual, and/or computerized sources of patient education information on medical devices and goods that meet the patient's needs.
   - Demonstrate and verify the proper use of medical goods and devices to ensure effective use.
   - Communicate storage, calibration, and maintenance information for medical goods and devices.

- Identify and analyze emerging issues, products, and services that may impact patient-specific and population-based pharmaceutical care.(D5)
- Assess one's own knowledge and abilities independently. (D5)
- Set personal knowledge and ability goals and take responsibility for attaining them.
- Recognize self-limitations and seek appropriate assistance/clarification.(D5)
- Review topics relevant to patient care activities to enhance knowledge base and preparedness. (D5)
- Accept feedback and implement suggestions for improvement. (D5)
- Manage time appropriately and efficiently. (D5)
- Exhibit intellectual curiosity to ensure ongoing professional competency.(D5)

Figure 20–2. Course-specific endpoints.

Course-specific goals and learning/behavioral objectives using Bloom's Taxonomy:

The student will learn the following objectives as it applies to the management of emergency department patients with low, emergent and critical acuity, and those who are boarded in the ED:

Acquisition of Knowledge:

- Identify types of medication discrepancies that occur in the ED.
- Identify concerns with continuity of care as the patient transitions from the ED to admission or discharge.
- Identify possible drug-induced disease.
- Conduct a patient's ED case presentation, including the hospital course.
- Rank potential for drug-related problems based on risk and need for resolution.
- Chart ED compliance with quality indicators.
- Describe use of emergency care medications such as vasopressors, vasodilators, thrombolytics, and anticoagulants.
- Prepare a presentation to the ED staff.

Psychomotor Skills:

- Perform a medication interview upon arrival to the ED.
- Detect the indication, any contraindications, drug-drug, drug-disease interactions with medications administered in the ED with those taken prior.
- Check if medication dosing is optimized, weight-based and adjusted as deemed necessary.
- Conduct screening and brief interventions for public health concerns, i.e. smoke cessation, vaccination.
- Demonstrate empathy for patients in the ED.
- Produce medical information necessary to assist the ED pharmacist prospective review of medication orders.

Enhanced Thinking Skills:

- Evaluate if correct administration of medication occurred, and if not, document the associated event.
- Evaluate if medications administered in the ED achieved desired endpoint, and if not, recommend necessary management.
- Explain how to manage drug-related events presenting to the ED or associated with ED care.
- Compare medications prescribed by admitting physician with those the patient claims is taking for omissions or commissions (medication reconciliation).
- Reflect on the ED pharmacist role in basic life support measures.
- Reflect on the ED pharmacist role in advance cardiac life support.

Changes in Attitude, Values, and/or Feelings:

- Judge the clinical significance of drug interactions and contraindications.
- Justify and defend the use of alternative pharmacotherapy from what has been prescribed.
- Persuade clinicians to conform to hospital policies for medication management.
- Question the pharmacotherapy selections.
- Resolve drug therapy-related problems.
- Select the optimal pharmacotherapy for the condition.
- Advocate for pharmacist role in public health and the ED.

Figure 20–3. Course-specific goals and learning/behavioral objectives using Bloom's Taxonomy.

Every effort was made to provide students with a real-life experience of the emergency department and the ED clinical pharmacy service as part of the team. Pharmacy students attend medical emergencies with the preceptor, such as responding to cardiac arrest, toxicologic emergencies, rapid sequence intubations, emergent infectious diseases, vascular emergencies, neurologic emergencies, and drug-induced diseases, and may experience a variety of other general medicine conditions.

This rotation is conducted as a 4-week rotation. During this time, the student experiences clinical presentations of conditions listed in the EM 2005 model, and this is a point for discussion during the daily morning report conducted at 11 AM to review with the student the important emergency care pharmacotherapeutic considerations and fill gaps in student knowledge. Students attend the Wednesday emergency medicine core seminar that includes morbidity and mortality rounds.

Often during the first week of patient care, the student is first learning how to comprehensively present the clinical case from the emergency medicine perspective and is focusing on learning medical terminology and reviewing clinical presentations. Salient features important to safe and effective medication use in the ED and how they counter from traditional pharmacotherapy principles are discussed daily. Components of the PharmER pyramid are discussed during the afternoon sessions for 1 hour.

Week 1: Course Overview, Introduction to the ED, and the Role of the Pharmacist in ED Workflow, Operations, and Automation

During the first week, emergency medicine is introduced to the student. The current problems with patient safety and quality in emergency medicine and the role the pharmacist plays in helping to solve those problems and the structure of the clinical pharmacy service in the ED are discussed and reviewed. The first several sessions include modeling the workflow of the pharmacist in the ED, describing automation of the CPOE systems, and reviewing enhancements that facilitate pharmaceutical care modes of delivery. These sessions are provided to the student for 1 hour during the end-of-the-day report.

Week 2: Patient Safety and Quality in the ED

During the second week session, we focus on patient safety, which includes topics such as those described by Cosby et al. for teaching patient safety in emergency medicine and the five goals as listed in Table 20-2.

Concepts, content, teaching methodology and recommended reading have been suggested and are incorporated into a patient safety rotation in emergency medicine for the pharmacy interns.[2]

Week 3: Describe the PharmER Pyramid

During week three and while the student has already experienced the ED physically, we introduce the student to the PharmER pyramid model and the cognitive structure of ED clinical pharmacy services. We describe how the PharmER pyramid model establishes structure within the ED, how this structure's performance can be assessed through evaluation of processes that can show positive outcomes, and how if not established, any safeguard process initiated in silo will not have the far-reaching effects of a safe medication use system. A description of the processes undertaken to establish the clinical pharmacy services structure is described and the building blocks of the PharmER pyramid are reviewed Tools to expedite pharmacist response to medical emergencies and various high-risk medications are discussed.

Week 4: Medical Emergencies and Important Personal Attributes for Success in the ED

A session on team play is conducted with the student, as traditionally throughout college, and in community settings, pharmacists are autonomous workers with little team expe-

rience. In the ED, team play is an essential part of assuring quality. Often, it appears that the ED code team members are not communicating with each other, in actuality, the team members are completing their designated tasks to assist in the resuscitation and stabilization of the patient. This is a skill that the pharmacy student needs to attain.

Besides usual discussion of traditional pharmacotherapy, a concentrated week on emphasis in emergency care pharmacotherapy is conducted. We also conduct special sessions on how to design pharmacy operations and what resources to have when responding to medical emergency to assure preparedness and added quality. Also unique to the emergency department, during the medical emergencies, students may be asked by the preceptor to quickly obtain a non-floor stock medication or unique antidote from the pharmacy, they may be asked to scan through the literature for important drug information to ascertain significance of drug interactions, and to immediately review treatment alternatives due to patient modifiers that preclude the use of classic drug therapy during the emergency. Pharmacy students may assist in physician procedures, such as assisting with CPR or assisting with ventilating the patient until the respiratory therapist arrives, all under direct supervision of the preceptor.

ASSESSMENT CRITERIA

Successful completion of the elective rotation requires the student to participate in several educational and clinical activities. Specific evaluative activities and their respective weight toward the final grade course were as follows:

- Identify medication discrepancies and intervene and write a FARM note (10%)
- Daily patient care activities (medication interviews and reconciliation, ADR reporting, expedite medication acquisition, team play, and patient-specific care plans) (40%)
- Conduct ED performance improvement activity participation (10%)
- Behavioral assessment and reliability (10%)
- Prepare two journal clubs specific to emergency medicine (10%)
- Prepare two case-based emergency care pharmacotherapy presentations (20%)

COURSE REFERENCES

Although there are no emergency care pharmacotherapy-specific texts available as of yet, there are course references that are essential to the pharmacy student's success and are listed:

- Cohen V. Safe and Effective Medication Use in the Emergency Department. Bethesda, MD: American Society of Health-System Pharmacists, 2009.
- Tintinalli JE, Kelen GD, Stapczynski JS. Emergency Medicine: A Comprehensive Study Guide, 6th Edition. New York: McGraw-Hill, 2003.

TABLE 20-2 Patient Safety Curriculum

- Increase awareness of medical error: Bringing a safety culture to medicine
- Definition and models of error
- Cognitive error and medical decision making
- Learning from experience of others
- Complications from invasive procedures
- Medical error from a system perspective
- Living with the reality of medical error

- Slaven EM, Stone SC, Lopez FA. Infectious Diseases: Emergency Department Diagnosis and Management. New York: McGraw-Hill, 2006.
- Davis MA, Votey SR, Signs and Symptoms in Emergency Medicine, 2nd Edition. Philadelphia PA: Mosby-Elsevier, 2006.
- Wolfson AB, Hendey GW, Hendry PL, Linden CH, Rosen CL. Harwood-Nuss' Clinical Practice of Emergency Medicine, Third Edition. Philadelphia: Lippincott Williams & Wilkins, 2005.
- Flomenbaum N, Goldfrank L, Hoffman R, Howland M. Goldfrank's Toxicologic Emergencies, Eighth Edition. New York: McGraw-Hill, 2006.
- Lacy CF, Armstrong LL, Goldman MP, Lance LL. Lexi-Comp's Drug Information Handbook. Lexi-Comp, 2008.
- Bosker G, Talan DA, Goldman HB, The Manual of Emergency Medicine Therapeutics. St. Louis: Mosby, 1995.
- Dipiro JT, Talbert R, Yee G, Matzke G. Pharmacotherapy: A Pathophysiologic Approach, Seventh Edition. New York: McGraw Hill, 2008.
- Koda-Kimble MA, et al. Applied Therapeutics; The Clinical Use of Drugs. Philadelphia: Lippincott Williams & Wilkins, 2008.
- Majerus TC, Dasta JF. Practice of Critical Care Pharmacy. Maryland: Aspen, 1985.
- Zipperer L, Cushman S. Lessons in Patient Safety. National Patient Safety Foundation. Chicago, IL. 2001
- Salyer SW. Essential Emergency Medicine for the Healthcare Practitioner. St. Louis, Elsevier, 2007.
- Mahadevan SV, Garmel GM. An Introduction to Clinical Emergency Medicine: Guide for Practitioners in the Emergency Department. New York: Cambridge University Press, 2005.
- Hamedani AG, Lai MW, Noble VE, Shah KH. Pocket Emergency Medicine. Philadelphia: Lippincott Williams & Wilkins.

Through the intranet, we have a plethora of electronic resources available to students, such as the following:

- Micromedex, Thomson.
- McGraw Hill's Access to Emergency Medicine www.accessemergencymedicine.com
- Pubmed, National Library of Medicine.
- e-medicine, WebMD.
- UpToDate, Inc., www.uptodate.com

HANDS-ON LEARNING

The emergency department offers many valuable opportunities to pharmacy interns to do meaningful work that allows them to contribute to the pharmacy, learn something new, and grow and develop as a pharmacist. The emergency department provides a great venue for facilitating observation of the practical application of pharmacotherapy for various emergency care topics (Fig. 20-5). This list of emergency care topics is used to validate the pharmacy intern's experience during the emergency care pharmacotherapy rotation.

Perhaps the most important for faculty involvement in pharmacy student education is at the patient's bedside. For medical students, the emergency department is frequently the first place where students feel autonomy for patient care, which requires decision making, synthesis of information and a sense of responsibility and accountability [2]; similar experience can be gained by pharmacy students. The skilled educator can support these feelings in the pharmacy student while assuring patient safety and targeting the degree of supervision to the student's particular needs. Throughout the course of the rotation, it is likely that a student will progress in his or her ability to assist with managing the pharmacotherapy of routine patients, and the educator's role can adapt to accommodate the advancement of the student's capability. [1]

PHARMACY INTERN ACTIVITIES

We have created an intern practice model with designated duties and responsibilities that interns will be held accountable for completing. To align with practices and principles of emergency care, which requires safe but expedient care, we use a blend of duties and responsibilities that include distributional and clinical pharmacy services. All duties and responsibilities are under direct supervision of an ED pharmacist.

In contrast to other settings (internal medicine, critical care), the intern's greatest challenge is to adapt to the frenetic pace of the ED, multiple patient acuities, and the broad mix of patients. Undergraduate pharmacy students at all times should shadow a pharmacy practitioner. The student can prove extremely useful.

Pharmacy interns are tasked with obtaining medication lists, heights, and weights, calculating creatinine clearance, reviewing the electronic medical record, and collecting pertinent data to support the verification of medication orders by the pharmacist.

Patient profiles are provided to the pharmacy interns to facilitate their medication regimen review for boarded patients. Prospective review of emergency medications must be done through the emergency medicine electronic medical record.

Encounter forms unique to the emergency department are provided to the student to facilitate data acquisition (Fig. 20-4).

The encounter forms include important elements needed to expedite the pharmacy intern's ability to identify medication-related discrepancies within the ED. We provide the intern with the prospective review form and general monitoring form for data collection and drug therapy assessment. A "FARM note" (Findings, Assessment, Recommendations, and Monitoring) must be written after each intervention. Pharmacy interns are provided a palm pilot to document their clinical interventions.

PERSONAL ATTRIBUTES

Personal attributes that are beneficial to a pharmacy intern while on rotation in the ED include the ability to multitask. Kinesthetic learners find this setting most conducive

Patient Decal

EMERGENCY MEDICINE

PHARMACOTHERAPY ASSESSMENT

PHARMACIST-PATIENT ENCOUNTER

Chief Complaint/HPI _____

_____

_____

_____

_____

_____

_____

_____

_____

_____

_____

_____

Temp _____	Height _____	VD _____
Pulse _____	Weight _____	Ke _____
RR _____	ABW _____	T1/2 _____
BP _____	IBW _____	Peak _____
Pulse Ox _____	Scr _____	

Positive signs on exam:

Laboratory values/ Diagnosis:

Risk Score:

Medical Impression/Plan:

PHARMACOTHERAPY ASSESSMENT FARM NOTE

EMERGENCY MEDICINE PHARMACOTHERAPY MONITORING

Hr/Day 0	Hr/Day 1	Hr/Day 2	Hr/Day 3	Hr/Day 4	Outcome Achieved: Yes No

Figure 20–4. Emergency medicine pharmacotherapy assessment.

STUDENT TOPIC CHECKLIST

Maimonides Medical Center

Emergency Care Pharmacotherapy Clerkship

Please check the boxes below.

Student (Name) _____ has monitored and delivered patient-specific care on the following disease states:

☐ Cardiopulmonary Resuscitation
☐ Rapid Sequence Intubation
☐ Monitored Anesthesia Care
☐ Trauma
☐ Respiratory Emergencies
  • Status Asthmatics, Pulmonary Edema, Foreign Body Obstruction
☐ Gastrointestinal Emergencies
  • Upper and Lower GI Bleed, Variceal Bleed, Acute Abdomen, Ruptured Appendicitis, Drug Induced GI Disturbance
☐ Genitourinary Emergencies
  • Hematuria, PID, STD, Renal Colic
☐ Infectious Emergencies
  • Sepsis, Septic Shock, Pneumonia, Urosepsis, Orbital Cellulitis
☐ Neurologic Emergencies
  • Stroke, Intracranial hemorrhage, Headache
☐ Oncologic Emergencies
  • Tumor Lysis Syndrome, Neutropenia, Fever, Cardiomyopathy
☐ Toxicologic Emergencies
  • Acetaminophen, Sedative Hypnotics, Digoxin, Coumadin, etc.
☐ Arrhythmias
  • Atrial Fibrillation/Flutter, Stable Ventricular Tachycardia
☐ Renal disorders and/or electrolyte /fluid disorders
  • Acute Renal failure, Rhabdomyolysis
☐ Psychiatric disorders
  • Delirium, Agitation, Aggression,
☐ Venous thromboembolism
  • DVT, PE
☐ Thyroid disorders
  • Thyroid Storm

Figure 20–5. Student topic checklist.

because movement helps them think. Being a team player is also an essential skill for success.

ADVANTAGES AND CHALLENGES OF AN EMERGENCY MEDICINE UNDERGRADUATE CLERKSHIP

ADVANTAGES

Advantages to an intern of an advanced practice experience in the emergency care setting include gaining experience in providing direct patient care, gaining experience in clinical manifestations of diseases and drug-induced diseases, distinguishing clinically important drug interactions and contraindications, gaining experience in multi-tasking, team work, interpersonal, and time management skills, developing experience on important emergency medicine references and scanning techniques for rapid drug information, using and navigating through healthcare technologies, witnessing and participating in emergency care for emergently ill patients, and implementing safe practices, continuity of care, and public health (Table 20-3).

The emergency care staff is also involved in training the pharmacy intern. The pharmacy interns will perform rounds with the ED medical residents at 7AM until 8AM, and at 3PM. Medical residents and attending physicians may demonstrate physical assessment and procedure skills; nursing may provide training in the use of infusion pumps, and respiratory technicians train in the use of a nebulizer therapy.

CHALLENGES

There are many challenges associated with an emergency medicine clerkship. Pharmacy interns will be faced with comprehending the variations in acuity (low, emergency, and critical) as defined (Table 20-4). These distinctions are essential in emergency medicine to manage the surge of patients that may occur.

TABLE 20-3	Advantages of Advance Practice Experience in Emergency Care

- Experience the initial clinical manifestations of the condition
- Distinguish from clinical significant contraindications and drug interactions
- Experience drug-induced diseases as they initially manifest
- Experience working on a team
- Experience multitasking
- Use interpersonal skills such as justification and persuasion
- Contribute to direct patient care
- Triage medication-related problems and prioritize
- Improve time management skills
- Provide rapid drug information through scanning techniques
- Identify reliable sources of drug information that can be incorporated into practice
- Review and apply evidence-based medical literature in practice
- Experience the use of an electronic medical record and tracking board
- Observe procedures for stabilization and medications used during these procedures
- Gain a sense of satisfaction for providing patient care
- Receive hands-on training
- Practice patient safety

However, the emergency medicine physician's tasks as described by the 2007 model of clinical practice of emergency medicine includes principles of pharmaceutical care; thus, pharmacy interns will be quickly absorbed on the emergency care team. Success of this course is highly dependent on students who are willing to experience new settings and are flexible enough to enjoy experiences that vary daily, in contrast to the more structured inpatient environments.

ASSESSMENT TOOLS AND OUTCOMES

Sample assessment forms are seen in Figures 20-6 and 20-7 for the patient-specific care plan and FARM note.

A total of 30 students have successfully completed the atypical Internal Medicine and Emergency Medicine specialty elective since 1998. Overall, student acceptance has been very good as evidenced by the students' verbal and written comments in reflective essays.

The emergency medicine clerkship has fostered interest as students have committed to doing a pharmacy practice residency experience at the hospital and have gone on to specialty training in emergency medicine. Furthermore, the elective rotation allows students to quickly identify their interest, or lack there of, as it pertains to emergency medicine

pharmacotherapy. Some students may be interested in more established areas, such as internal medicine or infectious disease, as opposed to leading the way in a new specialty area, which is only now becoming fully recognized.

A major challenge for colleges of pharmacy interested in developing an emergency medicine pharmacotherapy course similar to the one described here is identifying a cohort of faculty members with expertise in emergency medicine and who would be dedicated to being present and onsite within the ED, not at an alternative location.

SUMMARY

There are no published reports of undergraduate pharmacy students and their role in an emergency department. Colleges of pharmacy have reported offering the emergency department as elective rotations[2]; however, there are no standard published reports of a syllabus, goals, objectives, tasks, or activities. Educators argue that the emergency department is no place for pharmacy students due to its frenetic, chaotic, and high-risk nature. We contend that the emergency department is an ideal learning environment for the undergraduate

TABLE 20-4	Patient Acuity Definitions	
Critical	**Emergency**	**Lower Acuity**
Patient presents with symptoms of a life-threatening illness or injury with a high probability of mortality if immediate intervention is not begun to prevent further airway, respiratory, hemodynamic, and/or neurologic instability.	Patient presents with symptoms of an illness or injury that may progress in severity or result in complications with a high probability for morbidity if treatment is not begun quickly.	Patient presents with symptoms of an illness or injury that have a low probability of progression to more serious disease or development of complications.

Sample PH 633– Emergency Care Pharmacotherapy Clerkship

Patient Specific Care Plan Scoring Assessment

Student: _____ Student ID #: _____

Site: _____ Preceptor: _____ Date: _____

Please assess the pharmacy student using the key below, by writing the number that best describes his/her performance for each activity, since the inception of this rotation.

Poor / Unsatisfactory	Needs Improvement	Average	Above Average	Excellent
0–59.4	59.5–69.4	69.5–79.4	79.5–89.4	89.5–100

I. Collection of Patient Data Base and Other Pertinent Information and Assessment of Patient-Specific Disease States	Score
1. Collect accurate and complete patient information from appropriate sources (e.g., medical records, health care professionals, and patient/caregiver)	
2. Identify problem-specific patient information (subjective and objective) signs/symptoms (i.e., chief complaint, review of systems, etiology of problem, risk factors, vitals, physical exam, lab data, etc.)	
3. Identify complete problem list, in order of priority, by integrating above data as it pertains to emergency medicine specific considerations	
Subtotal: Average of Score × 0.10	

II. Evaluate Current Therapy, Select, Recommend and Justify Appropriate Therapy	Score
1. Determine the appropriate choice of medication(s) for the patient based upon individual patient need, characteristics (e.g., co-morbidities, cost, age, weight, absorption, renal/hepatic function, compliance) and current standard of care	
2. Identify non-pharmacologic therapy (e.g., pneumonic boots, diet, exercise)	
3. Describe the pharmacology of current therapy for the patient	
4. Identify correct alternative drug, dose, route, frequency based on drug-specific factors, patient-specific factors (e.g., indications, mechanism of action, side effects/tolerability) and current standard of care for the patient	
5. Identify desired clinical endpoints of therapy	
Subtotal: Average of Score × 0.45	

III. Monitoring/Counseling of Therapy	Score
1. Assess subjective and objective data in assessing efficacy of regimen and patient progress (e.g., improvement in SOB, heart rate) including frequency of monitoring	
2. Asses subjective and objective data to monitor in anticipation for adverse effects (e.g., diarrhea, hyperkalemia) including frequency of monitoring	
3. Assess for subjective and objective data to monitor in anticipation for drug-drug, drug-food, drug-supplement interactions if applicable	
4. Provide counseling to patients and/or caregivers relative to proper therapeutic self-management, risk reduction strategies and proper use of medical goods and devices	
Subtotal: Average of Score × 0.15	

IV. Ability to answer Questions	Score
1. Student is able to justify answers based on standard of practice	
Subtotal: Average of Score × 0.30	
Total I + II + III + IV = _____	

Final Score: _____

Preceptor's Signature: _____

Figure 20–6. Emergency care pharmacotherapy clerkship: Patient-specific care plan scoring assessment. Courtesy of Arnold & Marie Schwartz College of Pharmacy and Health Sciences, Long Island University.

Sample PH 633– Emergency Care Pharmacotherapy Clerkship

F.A.R.M. Note Documentation Scoring Sheet

Student: _____   Student ID Number: _____

Site: _____   Preceptor: _____   Date: _____

Poor / Unsatisfactory	Needs Improvement	Average		Above Average		Excellent		
0–59.4	59.5–69.4	69.5–79.4		79.5–89.4		89.5–100		
Findings are accurately and concisely summarized as it pertains to the evaluation and management of the emergency care issues								
Assessment is systematic, complete and appropriately documented as it pertains to the emergency care issue								
Recommendations are accurate, specific, complete, with no ambiguity as it pertains to the emergency care issues								
Monitoring parameters and frequency of monitoring are clearly written as it pertains to emergency care issues								
Documentation is accurate, with no spelling or grammatical errors as it pertains to emergency care issues								
Average of the scores will provide the total							Total	

Preceptor's Signature: _____   Date: _____

Figure 20–7.   Sample PH 633– Emergency care pharmacotherapy clerkship. Courtesy of Arnold & Marie Schwartz College of Pharmacy and Health Sciences, Long Island University.

pharmacy student to observe the array of clinical presentations that may occur and solidify what has been taught in pharmacotherapeutics. It is the precise environment for pharmacy students to begin building a foundation of clinical experiences that are not provided in any other setting. Furthermore, pharmacy students will determine immediately their interest by experiencing the emergency department.

References

1. Coates WC. An educator's guide to teaching emergency medicine to medical students. *Acad Emerg Med* 2004;11(3): 300–306.
2. Cosby KS, Croskerry P. Patient safety: A curriculum for teaching patient safety in emergency medicine. *Acad Emerg Med* 2003;10(1):69–78.
3. American Association of Colleges of Pharmacy Center for Advancement of Pharmaceutical Education, Educational Outcomes 2004. http://www.aacp.org/Docs/Main Navigation/Resources/6075_CAPE2004.pdf. Accessed March 17, 2008
4. Cue'llar LM, Ginsburg DB. *Preceptor's Handbook for Pharmacists.* Bethesda, MD: American Society of Health-System Pharmacists, 2005.
5. Kuo GM, Pinon M. Advanced (specialty) experiential education. In Cue'llar LM, Ginsburg DB. *Preceptor's Handbook for Pharmacists.* Bethesda, MD: American Society of Health-System Pharmacists.
6. Purcell K. How to develop, implement, coordinate and monitor introductory or advanced internship program. In Cue'llar LM, Ginsburg DB. *Preceptor's Handbook for Pharmacists.* Bethesda, MD American Society of Health-System Pharmacists, 170–179.
7. Nemire R. Differentiating between cognitive and affective learning. In Cue'llar LM, Ginsburg DB. *Preceptor's Handbook for Pharmacists.* Bethesda, MD: American Society of Health-System Pharmacists.
8. Eckel FM. Developing lifelong learning habits. In Cue'llar LM, Ginsburg DB. *Preceptor's Handbook for Pharmacists.* Bethesda, MD: American Society of Health-System Pharmacists.
9. Metting TL. Developing workplace skills. In Cue'llar LM, Ginsburg DB. *Preceptor's Handbook for Pharmacists.* Bethesda, MD: American Society of Health-System Pharmacists.
10. Huls CE. Effective methods, styles, and strategies of teaching and learning. In Cue'llar LM, Ginsburg DB. *Preceptor's Handbook for Pharmacists.* Bethesda, MD: American Society of Health-System Pharmacists.

21

Role of the Pharmacy Technician: Use of Board-Certified Support Personnel to Facilitate Clinical Pharmacy Services in the Emergency Department

Objectives

- Review the role of the pharmacy technician in the emergency department (ED)
- Describe and illustrate a nursing station review

ROLE OF THE PHARMACY TECHNICIAN IN THE ED

Pharmacists pursuing clinical pharmacy services need to make intelligent use of support personnel, such as pharmacy technicians, to the extent that the law permits.

Several reports of the role of the pharmacy technician in the ED have been published. In one report, the pharmacy technician took a role as the medication management technician (MMT) in the ED.[1]

In an initial survey of need, the MMT identified that the ED frequently was running out of stock items, and this was time consuming for everyone involved. Thus, initially the MMT assumed responsibility for the ordering and the storage of drugs and intravenous fluids. The MMT also reviewed stock lists, removed obsolete stock, added new items, and increased stock levels. Furthermore, the MMT reorganized and relabeled the shelving in all areas in the ED. As a result, the stock available for the code carts and labeling of the items improved.

The MMT also played a role in assisting with drug expenditure capture, identified high-cost medications, and provided lists of cheaper alternative medications. The results showed a reduction in spending despite an increase in ED visits.

The MMT reduced the number of calls to the on-call pharmacist from the ED for stock items, and there were been fewer shortages within the resuscitation room. The MMT also assisted in transfer of medications left behind and played a role in emergency preparedness and response.[1]

In another report, technicians conduct medication histories and successfully reconcile medications in the ED.[2]

Our pharmacy technicians are board certified and take on important medication management roles for the ED that facilitate the clinical pharmacists' ability to prospectively review medication orders and implement pharmaceutical care principles.

NURSING STATION REVIEW

Developed by the pharmacy supervisors, the technicians are responsible for conducting monthly nursing station reviews per location within the ED, using designated forms (Fig. 21-1).

ED

Resuscitation Room

Maimonides
Medical Center
Department of Pharmacy
Monthly Nursing Station Review

Date:_____Time:_____
Pharmacist:_____
Charge Nurse:_____

Circle the Appropriate responses

A.

1. **COUNTER TOPS**

Y N Counter Tops Clean & Free of Debris
Y N Absence of items under sink
Y N Absence of unauthorized drugs (recall/non-Formulary)
Y N Absence of exposed needles and syringes
Y N Medication cabinet locked if applicable
Y N Poison/ Antidote Chart properly displayed
Y N Conversion chart properly displayed
Y N Formulary with revisions available on MACS
Y N Up-to-Date pharmaceutical reference available (Micromedex)

2. **STOCK CABINETS**

Y N Stock Cabinets clean, orderly, & locked
Y N Contains only drug items
Y N Absence of unauthorized /non-Formulary items or samples
Y N Internal and External medications separated
Y N Medication labels clean, legible, & in date
Y N Absence of drug requiring refrigeration
Y N Floor stock content sheet posted from hospital Warehouse

3. **MEDICATION CASSETTES/CARTS**

Y N Stock Cabinets clean, orderly, & locked
Y N Contains only drug items
Y N Absence of unauthorized /non-Formulary items or samples
Y N Internal and External medications separated
Y N Medication labels clean, legible, & in date
Y N Absence of drug requiring refrigeration

4. **RAPID SEQUENCE INTUBATION CASSETTE**

Y N Contains only drug items
Y N Absence of unauthorized /non-Formulary items or samples
Y N Internal and External medications separated
Y N Medication labels clean, legible, & in date
Y N Absence of drug requiring refrigeration

5. **MEDICATION INFUSIONS CABINET**

Y N Labels clean legible and in date

B. **EMERGENCY CODE CART OR CARDIAC (2 CARTS) RESUSCITATION CART (CRC) - ADULT**

Y N CODE CART located within designated area
Y N CODE CART within date, locked, & signed Exp Date: _____
Y N CODE CART content sheet properly displayed
Y N Absence of exposed needles and syringes
Y N Nurse's Emergency Checklist Log Maintained

C. **EMERGENCY CODE CART - PEDIATRIC**

Y N CODE CART located within designated area
Y N CODE CART within date, locked, & signed Exp Date: _____
Y N CODE CART content sheet properly displayed
Y N Absence of exposed needles and syringes
Y N Nurse's Emergency Checklist Log Maintained

D. **REFRIGERATOR**

Y N Clean and free of ice accumulation

Y N Thermometer present

Y N Temperature range acceptable 36-46 F (2-8 C)

Y N Temperature _____

Y N Contains only drugs requiring refrigeration

Y N Absence of medications no longer needed by patient

Y N Medications in Date & Labels legible

Y N Is the refrigerator temperature recorded on Sign-in sheet of the Controlled Substance Log-Book

Y N If temperature out of range, was action noted? If not record each Missing date on the reverse of this sheet

Y N All paralytic agents stored and clearly labeled in red bins

PHARMACY MUST BRING ALL NOTED DEFICIENCES TO THE ATTENTION OF THE NURSE AT THE COMPLETION OF THIS INSPECTION. A COPY OF THIS REPORT WILL BE SENT TO THE NURSING UNIT AS WELL AS THE NURSING SUPERVISOR IN CHARGE.
COMMENTS: ALL "No" ANSWERS MUST BE EXPLAINED. (REFER TO LETTER SUBHEADING) Check { } IF ADDITIONAL SHEET ATTACHED.

Figure 21–1. Example of form used to conduct an ED nursing station review.

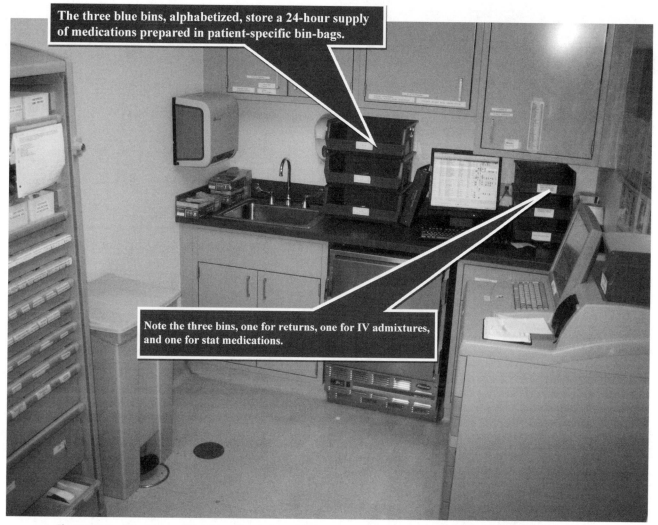

The three blue bins, alphabetized, store a 24-hour supply of medications prepared in patient-specific bin-bags.

Note the three bins, one for returns, one for IV admixtures, and one for stat medications.

Figure 21–2   Blue bins, within the restricted medication room, where technicians deliver medications.

Wherever mediations are stored in the ED, the technician must review that area for compliance to standards for appropriate storage, cleanliness, and inventory. The pharmacy technician is responsible for restocking floor stock on a daily basis and conducting hourly deliveries for specialty items that are not able to be sent down via the tube system.

Pharmacy technicians in the main pharmacy also continuously fill pharmacist-verified boarded patients' medications. These medications are then checked by a pharmacist and sent down to the emergency department by the technician during hourly runs to the ED from 8 AM until 12 midnight, and via the pneumatic tube system from 12 midnight to 8 AM the next morning. The technician places all intravenous admixtures into a designated bin, any stats into the stat bins, and any patient-specific medications into the patient-specific blue bin (Fig. 21-2). The technician also removes all medications placed in the discharge bin and returns them to the pharmacy for re-use.

The pharmacy technician is responsible for sending stat medications to the ED immediately as labels are generated to prevent time delays of urgent or emergent medications.

SUMMARY

This role of the pharmacy technician of managing the distributional, storage, inventory, and cleanliness of the medications in the ED is an essential component to facilitating direct patient care activities by the EDP. Without the pharmacy technician, EDPs would be inundated with managing these indirect patient care issues and would have little time for attending to pharmacotherapy during medical emergencies and managing emergency care pharmacotherapy.

References

1. Buglass A. Emergency Department – A role for pharmacy technicians. *Hosp Pharm* 2006;13:139.
2. Michels RD, Meisel SB. Program using pharmacy technicians to obtain medication histories. *Am J Health-Syst Pharm* 2003; 60:1982–1986.
3. Plaza C, Draugalis JR. Implications of advanced pharmacy practice experience placements: A 5-year update. *Am J Pharm Educ* 2005;69(3):296–303.

22

Future of Clinical Pharmacy Services in the Emergency Department

Objectives

- Review ASHP 2015 Health-System Pharmacy Initiatives
- Establish ED-based medication therapy management services
  - Emergency care pharmacotherapy research agenda
  - Screening and brief interventions
  - Vaccinations and wellness screening
  - Medication therapy management services in the ED

With regulatory requirements now leaning on EDs across the country to assure quality and improve safety, the time for clinical pharmacy services in the ED to make its mark is now.[1] Despite the barriers that will be placed in front of the pharmacy world to integrate,[2] these challenges will help create new services and new ideas on how to deliver emergency care; new collaborations and interfaces will force the healthcare world to further recognize the impact of a pharmacist and the evolution of this role's skill set. To achieve safe and effective medication use in all EDs, a national strategic plan is needed. Thus, in forecasting the future of emergency medicine pharmacy practice, we used the ASHP 2015 Health-System Pharmacy Initiatives (Fig. 22-1) to derive a set of goals and objectives to achieve.

GOAL 1: HELP INDIVIDUAL ED PATIENTS ACHIEVE THE BEST USE OF MEDICATIONS

Pharmacists will be involved in acquiring medication histories upon admission for a majority of hospital inpatients with complex and high-risk medication regimens in 50% of emergency departments. Pharmacists will manage therapy of the majority of emergency department patients with complex high-risk medication regimens, and high-risk regimens will be monitored by a pharmacist in 50% of emergency departments. The pharmacist will have organizational authority to manage medication therapy in collaboration with other members of the emergency care team in 50% of emergency departments. The pharmacist will provide discharge medication counseling to patients who receive treatment and are released from the emergency department and schedule medication therapy management follow up to ensure continuity of care in 50% of hospitals. Fifty percent of patients treated in the emergency department will recall speaking with a pharmacist in the ED. Percentages have been selected arbitrarily. However the number of phamacists currently participating in emergency care is not fully known.

ESTABLISH ED-BASED MEDICATION THERAPY MANAGEMENT SERVICES

The ongoing shift in the healthcare delivery system continues to occur. The number of elderly patients in the ED is increasing and reimbursement is shrinking, leading to earlier discharge of patients with higher levels of acuity. Consequently, EDs are faced with the responsibility of providing discharge planning for a growing number of sick or injured elderly patients. Inadequate discharge planning or intervention has resulted in costly revisits to the ED due to complications and recurrence of illness and injury.[4] These unacceptable outcomes have led to development of instruments to identify high-risk discharges. Yeaw et al. describes the high-risk discharge assessment instrument (HRDAI) as a tool used to detect high-risk indicators so that appropriate intervention and referral can be initiated. Primarily used by the nurse, the HRDAI requires that patients age 65 and older be assessed prior to discharge and repeated by the home care nurse to assess for risks.

The HRDAI contains eight categories of risk, each with its own set of specific indicators. Points are assigned to each indicator based on evidence-based findings. Several of these categories are drug related, such as identifying substance abuse and the potential for noncompliance and referring to pharmacists as medication managers to intervene and bridge components of healthcare delivery services.

Medication Therapy Management is a distinct group of services that optimize therapeutic outcomes for individual patients. Medication Therapy Management Services are independent of, but can occur in conjunction with, the provision of a medication or medication product. These services can be initiated through an ED where patients will be screened for the need of these services. The target market is extremely diverse but includes patients with various chronic disorders such as diabetes, asthma, thromboembolic disorders that require anticoagulation; hyperlipidemic patients; patients with pain syndromes; and those with substance abuse problems with alcohol, cigarettes, and illicit drugs. The predominant group of patients may include the elderly; however, patients with poor healthcare support, those with poor compliance with their medications, and patients taking multiple medications will also need services

*(Revised March 2008, new and revised objectives in **bold**)*

	Goal/Objective
Goal 1	**Increase the extent to which pharmacists help individual hospital inpatients achieve the best use of medications.**
Objective 1.1	Pharmacists will be involved in managing the acquisition, upon admission of medication histories for a majority of hospital inpatients with complex and high-risk medication regimens* in 75% of hospitals.
Objective 1.2	The medication therapy of a majority of hospital inpatients with complex and high-risk medication regimens will be monitored* by a pharmacist in 100% of hospitals.
Objective 1.3	**In 90% of hospitals, pharmacist will manage medication therapy for inpatients with complex and high-risk medication regimens*, in collaboration with other members of the health-care team.**
Objective 1.4	Hospital inpatients discharged with complex and high-risk medication regimens* will receive discharge medication counseling managed by a pharmacist in 75% of hospitals.
Objective 1.5	50% of recently hospitalized patients (or their caregivers*) will recall speaking with a pharmacist while in the hospital.
Objective 1.6	**In 90% of hospitals, pharmacist will ensure that effective medication reconciliation* occurs during transitions across the continuum of care.**

	Goal/Objective
Goal 2	**Increase the extent to which health-system pharmacists help individual non-hospitalized patients achieve the best use of medications.**
Objective 2.1	In 70% of health systems providing clinic care, pharmacist will manage medication therapy for clinic patients with complex and high-risk medication regimens*, in collaboration with other members of the health-care team.
Objective 2.2	In 95% of health systems providing clinic care, pharmacist routinely councel clinic patients with complex and high-risk medication regimens.
Objective 2.3	**In 90% of home care services, pharmacist will manage medication therapy for patients with complex and high-risk medication regimens*, in collaboration with other members of the health-care team.**
Objective 2.4	**In 90% of long term care facilities, pharmacists will manage medication therapy for patients with complex and high-risk medication regimens*, in collaboration with other members of the health-care team.**

	Goal/Objective
Goal 3	**Increase the extent to which health-system pharmacists actively apply evidence-based methods to the improvement of medication therapy.**
Objective 3.1	**In 90% of hospitals, pharmacist will be actively involved in providing care to individual patients that is based on evidence, such as the use of quality drug information resources, published clinical studies or guidelines, and expert consensus advice.**
Objective 3.2	**In 90% of hospitals, pharmacists will be actively involved in the development and implementation of evidences-based drug therapy protocols and/or order sets.**
Objective 3.3	**In 90% of hospitals, pharmacy departments will actively participate in hospital-wide efforts to ensure that patients receive evidence-based medication therapies required by the CMS hospital quality initiative, Joint Commission Core Measures, and/or state-based quality improvement and public reporting efforts.**
Objective 3.4	**In 70% of hospitals, pharmacists will actively be involved in medication- and vaccination-related infection control programs.**

A

Figure 22–1. ASHP Health-System Pharmacy Initiative. Reprinted with permission from the American Society of Health-System Pharmacy.

	Current Goal/Objective
Goal 4	**Increase the extent to which pharmacy departments in health systems have a significant role in improving the safety of medication use.**
Objective 4.1	90% of health systems will have an organizational program, with appropriate pharmacy involvement, to achieve significant annual, documented improvement in the safety of all steps in medication use.
Objective 4.2	80% of pharmacies in health systems will conduct an annual assessment of the processes used throughout the health system for compounding sterile medications, consistent with established standards and best practices.
Objective 4.3	80% of hospitals have at least 95% of routine medication orders reviewed for appropriateness by a pharmacist before administration of the first dose. (*Not including doses required in the context of emergencies or immediate procedures such as surgeries, labor and delivery, cardiac catheterization, etc.)*
Objective 4.4	90% of hospital pharmacies will participate in ensuring that patients receiving antibiotics as prophylaxis for surgical infections will have their prophylactic antibiotic therapy discontinued within 24 hours after the surgery end time.
Objective 4.5	85% of pharmacy technicians in health systems will be certified by the Pharmacy Technician Certification Board.
Objective 4.6	**50% of new pharmacy technicians entering hospital and health system practice will have completed an ASHP-accredited pharmacy technician training program*.**
Objective 4.7	**90% of new pharmacists entering hospital and health-system practice will have completed an ASHP-accredited residency.**

	Goal/Objective
Goal 5	**Increase the extent to which health systems apply technology effectively to improve the safety of medication use.**
Objective 5.1	75% of hospitals will use machine-readable coding to verify medications before dispensing.
Objective 5.2	75% of hospitals will use machine-readable coding to verify all medications before administration to a patient.
Objective 5.3	For routine medication prescribing for inpatients, 70% of hospitals will use computerized prescriber order entry systems that include clinical decision support.
Objective 5.4	In 65% of health systems, pharmacists will use medication-relevant portions of patients' electronic medical records for managing patients' medication therapy.
Objective 5.5	In 70% of health systems, pharmacists will be able to access pertinent patient information and communicate across settings of care to ensure continuity of pharmaceutical care for patients with complex and high-risk medication regimens.

	Goal/Objective
Goal 6	**Increase the extent to which pharmacy departments in health systems engage in public health initiatives on behalf of their communities.**
Objective 6.1	60% of pharmacies in health systems will have specific ongoing initiatives that target community health.
Objective 6.2	50% of pharmacies departments in health systems will be directly involved in ongoing immunization initiatives in their communities.
Objective 6.3	85% of hospital pharmacies will participate in ensuring that eligible patients in health systems receive vaccinations for influenza and pneumococcus.
Objective 6.4	80% of hospital pharmacies will participate in ensuring that hospitalized patients who smoke receive smoking-cessation counseling.
Objective 6.5	90% of pharmacy departments in health systems will have formal, up-to-date emergency preparedness programs integrated will their health systems' and their communities' preparedness and response programs.

B

Figure 22–1.   (continued)

and management support. The services that are provided vary according to the needs of the patient and include but are not limited to the following (Table 22-1).

Using HRDAI can lead to specific medication therapy management issues and may require follow up, not just for social services, but from a medication therapy manager after the ED visit.[4]

Furthermore, according to the Drug Abuse Warning Network (DAWN), described in Chapter 13, that monitors a sampling of ED charts for drug-related hospital ED visits and drug-related deaths to track the impact of drug use, misuse, and abuse in the U.S., more than 1,500 patients (2.5%) of patients who visit the ED at Maimonides are identified as DAWN cases (Table 22-2).

TABLE 22-1	Medication Therapy Management Services

- Performing or obtaining necessary assessments of the patient's health status; formulating a medication treatment plan
- Selecting, initiating, modifying, or administering medication therapy
- Monitoring and evaluating the patient's response to therapy, including safety and effectiveness
- Performing a comprehensive medication review to identify, resolve, and prevent medication related problems, including adverse drug events
- Documenting the care delivered and communicating essential information to the patient's other primary care providers
- Providing verbal education and training designed to enhance patient understanding and appropriate use of his/her medications
- Providing information, support services and resources designed to enhance patient adherence with his/her therapeutic regimens
- Coordinating and integrating medication therapy management services within the broader health care-management services being provided to the patient.

Adapted from *Medication Therapy Management Services: A Critical Review: Executive Summary.* http://www.lewin.com/content/publications/3179.pdf. Accessed July 30, 2008.

DAWN cases include suicide attempts, alcohol use in persons less than 21 years of age, adverse drug reactions, overmedication, malicious poisonings, accidental ingestions, and other drug-induced ED visits. Many of these visits and re-visits exponentially increase costs associated with healthcare and can be prevented or significantly reduced by implementing ED-based medication therapy management services.

The future will bring services such as those recently published by Zed et al., who established an ED-based deep venous thrombosis outpatient management program that has been shown to be safe, effective, and has a high level of patient satisfaction.

GOAL 2: APPLY EVIDENCE-BASED METHODS TO IMPROVE MEDICATION THERAPY

To apply evidence-based methods to improve medication therapy, 100% of ED pharmacists will be actively involved in ensuring that patients receive evidence-based pharmacotherapy. For example, therapies deemed a part of strategies that are known or proven to be associated with positive outcomes when part of early management that are

TABLE 22-2	Summary of 2006 Dawn Data Collection (Data Received Through 2-19-07)

Month	ED Visits	Charts Reviewed	DAWN Cases Identified
January	7536	7291	165
February	6385	6382	168
March	7168	7166	149
April	7147	7141	161
May	7303	4929	133
June	7075	4671	153
July	7078	4777	122
August	6759	4380	83
September	6984	4632	113
October	7262	4908	137
November	7058	2840	70
December	7985	0	0
Total	**85740**	**59117**	**1454**

The above terms are defined as follows:
ED Visits: any ED visit, including visits that result in admission, but **excluding any chart for patients that leave without being seen by a physician**.
Charts Reviewed: DAWN protocol requires 90–100% of all ED visits to be reviewed.
DAWN Case: any of the following types of visits; suicide attempts, drug detox, under-21 alcohol abuse, adverse reactions to medication (both OTC and RX), overmedication, malicious poisoning, accidental ingestion, or abuse of illegal drugs.
Please be aware that significant differences between charts reviewed and ED visits may be due to staffing changes or chart access.

designated as quality indicators will be assured and complied with to expedite treatment for pay for performance initiatives.

GOAL 3: INCREASE ED PHARMACISTS ROLE IN HEALTH-SYSTEMS TO IMPROVE SAFETY OF MEDICATION USE

To achieve this goal, all EDs will have organizational programs, with appropriate pharmacy involvement to achieve significant annual documented improvement in the safety of all steps in medication use. EDPs will conduct annual assessments of the processes used for compounding sterile medications, consistent with standards of best practices; 50% of EDs will have at least routine medication orders reviewed for appropriateness by a pharmacist before administration of the first dose. For doses required in emergencies or immediate procedures, EDPs attend and expedite the delivery 100% of the time while simultaneously assuring appropriateness.

GOAL 4: APPLY TECHNOLOGY EFFECTIVELY TO IMPROVE SAFETY OF MEDICATION USE

In the future, EDs will use machine-readable coding to verify medications before dispensing and administration; EDs will use computerized prescriber order entry systems that include some form of decision support and assure two-way interface amongst inpatient computer systems. The EDP will use medication-relevant portions of patient's electronic medical records for managing patient medication therapy, and EDs will have access across health-systems so EDPs will be able to access pertinent patient information and communicate across settings of care to ensure continuity of pharmaceutical care for patients with complex and high-risk medication regimens.

GOAL 5: INCREASE PARTICIPATION IN PUBLIC HEALTH INITIATIVES

The responsibility of managing pharmaceuticals during a disaster and assuring formal up-to-date emergency preparedness programs will be integrated with their health-systems and their communities' preparedness and response programs; EDPs should be involved in targeting community health. All EDPs will assist the ED in ongoing immunization initiatives in their communities. This initiative is in concert with principles of pharmaceutical care as first described by Hepler and Strand. Hepler and Strand described pharmaceutical care as the provision of drug therapy to achieve outcomes that im-

prove a patient's quality of life—these outcomes are: 1) cure of a disease, 2) elimination or reduction of symptoms, 3) arresting or slowing of a disease process, and 4) prevention of a disease or symptoms.[7] Thus, EDPs will participate in ensuring vaccination screening of patients visiting the ED, and assure administration of their vaccinations for influenza and pneumococcal and other appropriate vaccines.

EDPs will ensure that hospitalized patients who smoke receive smoke-cessation counseling, are screened, and are provided a brief intervention during their ED stay. The knowledge translation activities needed to enhance the delivery of clinical preventive and screening services in the ED is a current primary focus of emergency care personnel interested in public health initiatives. Current evidence-based medicine that supports ED-based clinical preventive service delivery is new and still evolving. Yet evidence supporting effective ED-based screening and preventive services has been published.[8–12] Emergency care personnel who have been interested in public health initiatives for years are in the process of identifying unique contextual elements that are likely to bring proven preventive and other public health initiatives into the emergency department.[11] Emergency care personnel have identified barriers to knowledge translation, and a group of emergency care personnel have provided recommendations focused on overcoming these barriers to provision of effective ED-based screening and preventive services.

First, the consensus group recommended including integrating principles of prevention, health behaviors, and health behavior interventions into the core curriculum of emergency medicine. Second, this group recommended that ED clinical information systems be re-configured to facilitate screening, intervention, and referral for patients who need prevention screening and health behavior change. Third, the delivery of clinical prevention services and health behavior interventions should be enhanced to ED patients by deploying other personnel and resources, including public health professionals to the ED. According to D'Onofrio and colleagues, unhealthy alcohol, tobacco, and other drug use is prevalent in ED populations. Evidence suggests that screening, intervention, and referral can change patterns of use and reduce negative consequences. ED practitioners can learn these skills. System changes, however, are needed to incorporate best practices.[11]

There are significant barriers to screening for alcohol, tobacco, and other drug use and providing intervention and referral in the ED. The chaotic environment, lack of sufficient staff and resources, and practitioner characteristics, such as low levels of confidence in skills and negative attitudes toward patients with drinking problems, are all barriers to screening.[4] In a survey conducted on screening and brief interventions among emergency clinicians, both supporters and non-supporters thought that lack of time was a major obstacle to screening and interventions. Brief interventions for alcohol abuse can take up to 30–60 minutes and were initially developed and performed by non-ED staff.

D'Onofrio et al. recommends three strategies to change practitioner behavior regarding screening and interventions, including the use of educational techniques that involve skill-based learning; eliciting opinion leaders in all practitioner groups, instituting system changes, such as prompts or screening questions on triage forms and computer-generated screening, and providing incentives to the staff [11]

As automation creates less distributional responsibilities for the pharmacist and as pharmacists become better accepted as providers of healthcare, independent of product, innovative clinical roles within the ED will emerge, and screening and brief intervention, initially an extension of conducting a medication interview, may be one of those roles. Pharmacist involvement in smoking cessation has been published; however, there are no studies to date of a pharmacist in the ED providing screening and brief interventions. Thus, a great opportunity awaits.[12]

With this expanding role of the EDP, a network of EDPs throughout the country will permit sharing of information in real time, and multicenter research studies, which encompass multiple centers or health systems to increase the magnitude of evidence-based pharmacotherapy medicine within the emergency department, will emerge.

This network will lead to consensus and evidence-based pharmacotherapy guidelines that align emergency medicine and pharmacotherapy principles and create a best practice standard associated with medication policies within the ED.

SUMMARY

In summary, these initiatives, such as medication therapy management services, preventive care through vaccinations, wellness services such as screening and brief interventions for smoking cessation or drug and alcohol abuse, medication noncompliance, and obesity can be implemented in the ED to further justify and rationalize pharmacists' involvement in the future of emergency care.

References

1. Institute of Medicine. To Err is Human: Building a Safer Health-System. Washington, DC: National Academy Press, 2001.
2. SoRelle R. EM Groups persuade Joint Commission to temper Pharmacy Review Policy. *Emerg Med News* 2007;29(9): 42–45
3. ASHP 2015 Health-System Pharmacist Initiatives. http://www.ashp.org/s_ashp/docs/files/2015_Goals_Objectives_0508.pdf. Accessed July 30, 2008.
4. Yeaw EM, Burlingame PA. Identifying high-risk patients from the emergency department to the home. *Home Healthcare Nurse* 2003;21(7): 473–480.
5. The Lewin Group. *Medication Therapy Management Services a Critical Review: Executive Summary.* http://www.lewin.com/ content/publications/3179.pdf. Accessed July 30, 2008.
6. Internal data delivered to Maimonides from the Drug Abuse Warning Network. http://dawninfo.samhsa.gov/ Accessed July 30, 2008.
6. Zed P, Filiatrault L, Busser JR. Outpatient treatment of venous thromboembolic diseases based in an emergency department. *Am J Health-System Pharm* 2005;62(6): 616–619.
7. Hepler CD, Strand LM. Opportunities and responsibilities in pharmaceutical care. *Am J Hosp Pharm* 1990;47:533–43.
8. Bernstein S, Cohen V. Public health considerations in knowledge translation in the emergency department. *Acad Emerg Med* 2007;11:1036–1041.
9. Lowenstein SR, Weissberg M, Terry D. Alcohol intoxication, injuries, and dangerous behaviors and the revolving emergency department door. *J Trauma* 1990;30:1252–7.
10. Graham DM, Maio RF, Blow FC, et al. Emergency physician attitudes concerning intervention for alcohol abuse/dependence delivered in the emergency department: A brief report. *J Addict Dis* 2000;19:45–53.
11. D'Onofrio G, Becker B, Woolard RH. The impact of alcohol, tobacco, and other drug use and abuse in the emergency department. *Emerg Med Clin North Am* 2006; 24:925–967.
12. Leschisin RK, Martin BA. Pharmacist-facilitated tobacco-cessation services in an inpatient setting. *Am J Health-System Pharm* 2007;64(22):2386–9.

Appendices

APPENDIX A: **Policies and Procedures** **213**

Policy and Procedure for Monitoring Medications and Supplies
for Emergency Response 213

Policy and Procedure for Code Team and PharmD Role 214

Policy and Procedure for Acute Stroke 216

Policy and Procedure for the Treatment of Thrombolytic for .... .218
Acute Myocardial Infarction (AMI)

APPENDIX B: **Dosing Guides and Tables** **221**

Adult ED Acute Area Medication Floor Stock Par Level List .... .222

Acute Care Area Medication Floor Stock List for Refrigerated Medications .... .223

Acute Care Area Controlled Drug Floor Stock List .... .224

Resuscitation Care Area Medication Floor Stock List .... .224

Resuscitation Care Area Controlled Drug Floor Stock List .... .226

Pediatric ED Controlled Drug Floor Stock List .... .227

Clinical Steps for Safe Antidote Ordering and Delivery Process in the ED 228

Bioterrorism Monthly Inventory List: Antidotes for Biological Agents 233

Antidotes for Chemical Agents 234

Radiologic and Nuclear Antidotes Monthly Inventory List 235

Pandemic Influenza Preparedness 237

Chronic Care Medications for Natural Disasters 239

Emergency Medicine Pharmacotherapist General Principles and
Guide for Managing Critical Care Infusions 242

APPENDIX C: **Educational Outcomes, Goals, and Objectives** **246**
for Emergency Medicine

Educational Outcomes, Goals, and Objectives for Postgraduate Year Two (PGY2)
Pharmacy Residencies in Emergency Medicine 246

Appendix A
Policies and Procedures

1.0 MEDICATIONS AND SUPPLIES

1.01 Inventory control

(1) The pharmacy department updates its inventory as it pertains to essential pharmaceutical supplies monthly using a monthly pharmaceutical inventory list as seen in the Appendix A (PERT manual). The monthly pharmaceutical inventory list includes the quantity of each drug expected to be needed during a public health emergency for various types of emergencies i.e. (chemical, biological, radiological, pandemic and natural disaster), the location, and the date of most recent expiration.

1.02 Mobilizing

1.02.1 Response

(1) Upon receiving notification of HIECS alert the supervisor of the pharmacy department will conduct a department specific disaster needs analysis specific to the hazards involved.

(2) The disaster needs analysis form as seen in *Appendix B* identifies that hazard, the estimated number of victims, and the amount of pharmaceutical assets on hand that are *quickly transferable*.

(3) The supervisor will estimate the amount needed to purchase for response, recovery, and replenishment and will assign a pharmacy staff member to execute standing orders and make contact with prime vendors (Amerisource Bergen)

1.02.1 Recovery

(1) The supervising pharmacist will immediately anticipate needs of pharmaceutical assets for recovery, and will plan with institutional leaders, account purchasing and the distributors designated recovery team a course of action.

(2) The account purchaser will be in contact via phone or by way of face to face meeting (pertinent contact numbers are seen in Appendix C (PERT manual) with Amerisource Bergen's designated recovery team representatives to assist with determining methods of delivery based on type of disaster (Earthquake, Facility or Hospital Fire, Flood, Tornado, other Internal or external disasters), and the conditions of transportation corridors.

(3) Amerisource Bergen will use pre-determined medication and quantity lists that are updated and maintained at both facilities (Appendix D, PERT manual)

1.03 Distributing

1.03.1 Response

(1) The supervising pharmacists will release a pharmacist to the location of the emergency for immediate response.(Job action sheet seen in Appendix E, PERT manual)

(2) Depending on the hazard the pharmacist along with a pharmacy technician will prepare the disaster cart with likely medications needed for response, i.e. Atropine for nerve agent.

(3) A response matrix for each hazard is available and alphabetically indexed in the PERT manual in the pharmacy department

1.03.2 Recovery

(1)   The supervising pharmacist will take direction from the pharmacy unit leader as to the plan of action to meet pharmaceutical resources needed during recovery as determined by the EOC and mutual aid partners of the Southern New York Emergency Partnership (SNYEP).

(2)   If needed the supervising pharmacist will delegate to a pharmacist the responsibility of auxiliary site pharmacy coordinator

(3)   Auxiliary site pharmacy coordinator will be responsible for mobilization, distribution, tracking, recording and replenishing pharmaceutical resources to the alternate site as deemed necessary by the pharmacy unit leader. A job action sheet is seen in Appendix F PERT manual.

(4)   In the event a point of distribution site is needed the supervising pharmacists will delegate an event specific pharmacist to assist in the operations, logistics, and resources needed and will communicate up the chain of command. A job action sheet is seen in Appendix G for POD preparation (PERT manual).

1.04   Tracking

(1)   The supervising Pharmacist will use a pharmaceutical asset tracking form to keep account of all assets dispensed as seen in Appendix H (PERT manual) during response.

(2)   The form will record the time and date of requisition, what location the item distributed, received or returned, to what location within the facility, or to what organization, the items that were distributed, the model #, quantity, estimated cost, the person receiving, and plan for replenishment.

(3)   During response the pharmacy technician will monitor inventory continuously to replenish stock in the location of the emergency.

(4)   The pharmacy technician will record all pharmaceutical assets distributed, returned, or received from distributors

1.05   Replenishment/Inventory rationing

(1)   The supervising pharmacists will review the policies for replenishing pharmaceutical assets early on during the disaster with the use of standing orders. Using the standing orders distributors will replenish inventory as requested by designated pharmacy personnel.

(2)   Mutual aid partners from the Southern New York Emergency Management region will be a channel for additional pharmaceutical assets during response and recovery.

(3)   In the event that no additional assets will be available from other sources i.e. federal, local, and state resources the department of pharmacy has set a policy for rationing medication use. The supervising pharmacist will implement this policy as seen in Appendix I in PERT manual.

1.06   Recording

(1)   Net expenditures of all assets dispensed during the response and recovery phase will be recorded and submitted to finance for reimbursements.

POLICY AND PROCEDURE FOR CODE TEAM AND PHARMD ROLE

MAIMONIDES MEDICAL CENTER DEPARTMENT OF EMERGENCY MEDICINE POLICY & PROCEDURE MANUAL

PURPOSE

To provide an immediate and organized response to patients in unstable condition in the Maimonides Medical Center Department of Emergency Medicine.

To improve the outcomes of those patients who need urgent resuscitation and stabilization.

To ensure the safety and humane treatment of patients with acute behavioral disturbances.

To enhance a culture of interdisciplinary teamwork among ED personnel.

To improve clinical job satisfaction among ED personnel.

POLICY

A 6-person Code Team comprised of physicians, nurses, and patient care technicians will be designated at all times, with pre-assigned roles. A clerk registrar will also report if the patient is unregistered. Security personnel will immediately report for all "Code White" alerts for patients with behavioral abnormalities.

Code Team assignments must be endorsed to replacement team members during breaks, lunches and at change-of-shift.

Any employee in the Department of Emergency Medicine may activate the Code Team Procedure.

Members of the Code Team must immediately interrupt any other activities when the Code Team Procedure is activated and report to the specified location within 30 seconds.

Code Team performance will be rehearsed regularly with drills.

PROCEDURE

A.   **Assignments:** Code Team assignments will be posted at all times and revised at 7:30 AM, 3:30 PM, 7:30 PM and 11:30 PM to reflect changes in assignment at change of shift. The ED Charge Nurse is responsible for updating the posted assignments.

Members of the Code Team will be given no other clinical or clerical responsibilities or assignments while the Code Team is activated or being drilled.

Members of the Code Team may assume primary clinical and documentation responsibilities for the patient being resuscitated, but are not obligated to do so or formally assigned the case. These responsibilities remain with the doctors, nurses and PCTs assigned through previous extant Policy and Procedure.

B. Roles:

1. Team Captain – Physician annotated on schedule
2. Head of Bed – Physician annotated on schedule
3. Patient's Right Arm – PCT
4. Patient's Left Arm –2nd Nurse Team 2
5. Foot of Bed – PCT
6. Med Cart –PharmD or 2nd Nurse Team 1
7. Security – for Code White

The Team Captain is responsible for organizing the resuscitation, including team assignments and positions as the situation dictates.

If the assigned Team Captain is for any reason delayed in reporting to the resuscitation, the first ED physician who arrives will assume the role until the assigned physician arrives.

All PCTs on duty must report to the code. The Team Captain will assign PCT roles and will dismiss any others.

If an attending physician, nurse or PCT who are not assigned to the Code Team are already involved with the care of a patient who deteriorates and requires Code Team activation, the attending physician may assume the Team Captain role and may assign the nurse and PCT to Code Team positions.

C. Activation: Any employee of the Department of Emergency Medicine or MMC employee regularly schedule to work in the ED may activate the Code Team procedure if they feel it is necessary.

1. The activation procedure can be done verbally or over the intercom (x3285–00).
2. The request must specify "Code Team" or "Code White" and the patient's location and can be repeated loudly and continuously until the team responds.
3. The Code Team is responsible for patients located within the department, including the CT suite, ED hallways, radiology suites, waiting rooms and restrooms, and the ambulance bay. The Code team may respond to patients directly outside the department on sidewalks contiguous to the ambulance bay and entrance as long as the site is known to be secure.
4. The Code Team will be activated only for patients who are real or impending cardiac or respiratory arrest or who demonstrate a state of hemodynamic shock or for a "Code White". The Emergency Severity Index (ESI) of the patient should be "1". This includes those patients with real or impending respiratory failure, hemodynamic instability, multiple blunt or penetrating trauma, active myocardial ischemia/acute injury, cardiopulmonary arrest and threatening behavior. These are patients who need multiple members of the ED to initially stabilize them in an organized and effective fashion.
5. A "notification" does not necessarily require Code Team activation and can await triage. If it is known that pre-hospital personnel are bringing a patient in arrest or hemodynamic shock, the Code team should be activated and should wait for the patient's arrival at the bedside.
6. If an ED employee notes an unconscious, seizing, traumatized, non-breathing or cyanotic person in a non-clinical area (e.g., waiting room, restroom, etc), they should activate the Code Team.

D. Responsibilities: Once summoned, the responsibility of the team is to immediately report to the patient's bedside, assume predefined resuscitation team roles and execute a stabilization procedure that meets or exceeds the standard of care and provides the patient the best opportunity to survive.

Team Leader   (Physician)

Announce leadership role and roles of rest of team, if necessary.

Establish and maintain control of entire team.

Verify pulse status if in doubt.

Assign person to obtain code cart, if needed.

Excuse, recruit, switch or replace team members, as needed.

Fill in for team members without losing control and oversight.

Order medications and procedures.

Keep team verbally appraised of patient's status.

De-Activation: The Team Captain can dismiss or replace members of the Code Team, depending on the clinical circumstance.

Pronounce death, if applicable.

Inform the charge nurse of any death pronouncements, if applicable, and complete required paperwork and .

HEAD of BED   (Physician)

Secure airway, if necessary.

Quick look with defibrillator paddles, if necessary or supervise nurse.

Electrical defibrillation or cardioversion, if necessary or supervise nurse.

Order medications for rapid sequence induction and paralysis, if necessary.

Secure advanced airway or intravenous access, if necessary.

Order STAT portable images if needed.

PATIENT'S RIGHT SIDE (PCT)

Help to expose patient adequately.

CPR at 100–120 compressions per minute, if necessary.

Assist with setting up suction and/or Ambu bag, if necessary.

Secure monitor leads.

12 lead EKG if needed.

Switch roles with Runner, as needed

PATIENT'S LEFT SIDE (Nurse)

Help to expose patient adequately.

Establish pulse status.

Quick look with defibrillator paddles, if necessary, under supervision of physician.

Electrical defibrillation or cardioversion, if necessary, under supervision of physician.

Immediately establish left antecubital access with at least 18g angiocatheter or inform the Team Leader of difficulties in doing so.

Push medications provided by Med Provider and verbally announce the administration of every medication. Await verbal response from Team Leader and Record Keeper.

Prompt Team Leader with repeat medication suggestions if necessary.

MED CART & RECORDER (PharmD or Nurse)

Help to obtain code cart, if necessary.

Open, prepare and carefully hand all ordered medications to Medication Pusher.

Prompt Team Leader with repeat medication suggestions if necessary.

Record the administration of all medications and changes in clinical status.

Insure that the monitor has paper and that rhythm strips are recorded.

Initiate complete of cardiac arrest form, if necessary.

Make sure Team Leader informs Charge Nurse of a death, if applicable.

FOOT of BED (PCT)

Obtain Code Cart if needed.

Get all equipment or unsecured medications that are not at the bedside as requested.

Do CPR relief as needed.

REGISTRAR/COMMUNICATIONS CLERK

Facilitate STAT registration as per protocol.

Make calls and pages at the request of the Team Leader.

SECURITY: Security Personnel

Report immediately to the patient's location when a "Code White" for abnormal or threatening patient behavior.

Clear the ED of all visitors without exception if the Code Team is activated for a patient any location other than resuscitation rooms 1–4.

Clear the resuscitation rooms 1–4 of all visitors without exception if the Code Team is activated for a patient in resuscitation rooms 1–4.

POLICY AND PROCEDURE FOR ACUTE STROKE

DEPARTMENT OF EMERGENCY MEDICINE POLICY & PROCEDURE MANUAL

CATEGORY	SUBJECT	MANUAL CODES
Thrombolytic Therapy in Acute Stroke		T 9.5
EFFECTIVE DATE	**REVIEWED**	**REVISED DATE**
May 2003	December 19, 2006	December 19, 2006
ISSUED BY	**APPROVED BY**	**CROSS REFERENCE** S 18

Protocol for Care of the Patient Receiving Thrombolytic Therapy

PURPOSE

To outline the physician and nursing responsibilities for assuring appropriate use of thrombolytic therapy for acute ischemic stroke within the Emergency Department.

RATIONALE FOR INFUSION

Administration of early thrombolytic therapy in ischemic stoke is based on the concept that early restoration of circulation in the affected territory by recanalization of an occluded intracranial artery preserves reversible damaged neuronal tissue in the penumbra. The recovery of this neuronal function reduces clinical neurological disability. Thrombolytic therapy is used to restore perfusion or improve perfusion within the intracranial arteries occluded within the ischemic zone, in order to salvage any adjacent dysfunctional tissue; restoration or perfusion to the ischemic area is a key therapeutic strategy and is fundamental to the current treatment of stroke.

GOAL OF THERAPY

The goal of this care is (1) to assure the use of thrombolytic therapy is indicated, and no contraindications exist (see scoring sheet, figure 1), (2) to monitor the patient for the effectiveness of therapy, as well as development of untoward effects.

A. CRITERIA FOR PATIENT SELECTION (PHYSICIAN RESPONSIBILITY)

1. Diagnosis of ischemic stroke causing measurable neurological deficit. Neurological signs should not be clearing spontaneously, nor should they be minor and isolated. Patients with major deficits should also be treated with **caution** because of the minimal benefit gained, and the noted risk.
2. Symptoms of stroke should not be suggestive of a subarachnoid hemorrhage
3. Onset of symptoms $<$ 3 hours before beginning treatment
4. No head trauma or prior stroke in previous 3 months
5. No myocardial infarction in the previous 3 months
6. No gastrointestinal/ urinary tract hemorrhage in previous 21 days
7. No major surgery in previous 14 days
8. No arterial puncture at a non-compressible site in the previous 7 days
9. No history of previous intracranial hemorrhage
10. Blood pressure not elevated (Systolic $<$185 mm Hg and Diastolic $<$ 110 mm Hg)
11. No evidence of active bleeding or acute trauma (fracture) on exam
12. Not taking oral anticoagulants or if anticoagulant being taken, INR $\leq$ 1.5
13. If receiving heparin in previous 48 hours, a PTT must be in normal range
14. Platelet count $\geq$ 100,000 mm³
15. Blood Glucose concentration $\geq$ 50 mg/dL
16. No seizure with postictal residual neuro-impairment
17. CT does not show a multilobar infarct
18. The patient or family understands the potential risks and benefits from treatment

B. GENERAL PREPARATION

1. Establish 2 peripheral IV lines or hep locks, one must be minimum 18 gauge.
2. Obtain a good quality 12 lead EKG

C. Alteplase (ACTIVASE) PREPARATION ADMINISTRATION

1. Reconstitute the 100 mg of Activase with 100 mL of sterile water for injection (SWFI), which is supplied in the kit
2. Utilize the transfer device and insert the piercing pin vertically into the center of the stopper of the vial of SWFI
3. Holding the vial of Activase upside-down, position it so that the center of the stopper is directly over the exposed piercing pin of the transfer device. Push the vial of Activase down so that the piercing pin is inserted through the center of the Activase vial stopper
4. Invert the 2 vials so that the Activase is on the bottom (upright). Approximately 2 minutes are required for the transfer device
5. Swirl gently to dissolve the Activase powder. DO NOT SHAKE

6. No other medications should be added to infusion solutions containing Activase
7. Slight foaming is not unusual and should be dissipate upon standing for several minutes
8. The solution should be observed for particulate matter and discoloration. A colorless pale yellow solution should be present
9. Infuse 0.9 mg/kg (maximum of 90 mg) over 60 minutes with 10 % of the dose given as a bolus over 1 minute. Refer to dosing chart below for weight adjusted dosing:

Dosing Chart

Weight	Total Dose	Bolus Over 1 minute	Maintenance dose over 60 minutes	Rate of infusion
40 kg	36 mg	3.6 mg	32.4 mg	32.4 mL/hour
50 kg	45 mg	4.5 mg	40.5 mg	40.5mL/hour
60 kg	54 mg	5.4 mg	48.6 mg	48.6 mL/hour
70 kg	63 mg	6.3 mg	56.7 mg	56.7 mL/hour
80 kg	72 mg	7.2 mg	64.8mg	64.8 mL/hour
90 kg	81 mg	8.1 mg	72.9 mg	72.9 mL/hour
100 kg*	90 mg	9.0 mg	81 mg	81 mL/hour
110 kg*	90 mg	9.0 mg	81 mg	81 mL/hour
120 kg*	90 mg	9.0 mg	81 mg	81 mL/hour

* Maximum dose 90 mg according to NINDS Trial

D. PATIENT MONITORING: (NURSING RESPONSIBILITY: INFORM MD OF ANY ABNORMAL FINDINGS)

I. Neurological Status:
   a. Neurological assessment every 15 minutes during the infusion, and every 30 minutes for the next 6 hours and then every hour until 24 hours from treatment
   b. Monitor for severe headache, acute hypertension, nausea, or vomiting, discontinue the infusion (If agent is still being administered) and obtain a CT of the brain on an emergent basis.

II. Vital Signs
   a. Monitor V/S every 15 minutes for the first 2 hours, every 30 minutes for the next 6 hours, and then every hour for the next 24 hours from treatment.
   b. Increase frequency of blood pressure measurements if systolic blood pressure is $\geq$ 180 mm Hg, or diastolic $\geq$ 105 mm Hg is recorded. Administer antihypertensive medications to maintain blood pressure below these levels

II. Monitor for Bleeding
   a. Monitor mouth, gums, and IV sites
   b. Check all body fluids for blood, including:
      1. urine
      2. sputum
      3. stool
      4. gastric fluid

c. Assesses and document neuro status every hour, including:
   1. LOC
   2. orientation
   3. motor responses
d. Monitor for symptoms of retroperitoneal bleeding:
   1. low back pain
   2. leg pain
   3. ecchymosis over flank area

IV. Ongoing Lab Monitoring/Orders
   1. Strict bed rest × 18 hours
   2. Automated noninvasive BP monitoring should not be used more than every thirty (30) minutes
   3. CBC, PT/PTT 4–6 hours post infusion

V. Specific Drug Administration
   1. Labetalol 10 mg: administer intravenously over 1–2 minutes for SBP 180–230 mm Hg or DBP 105–120 mm Hg.
   2. May repeat or double the dosage of labetalol every 10–20 minutes to a maximum of 300 mg
      i. Alternatively start with a bolus and then start a continuous infusion given at a rate of 2–8 mg/minute

VI. Tube Placements
   1. Delay placement of NGT, indwelling bladder catheters, or intra-arterial pressure catheters.

POLICY AND PROCEDURE FOR THE TREATMENT OF THROMBOLYTIC FOR ACUTE MYOCARDIAL INFARCTION (AMI)

DEPARTMENT OF EMERGENCY MEDICINE
POLICY & PROCEDURE MANUAL

CATEGORY	SUBJECT	MANUAL CODES
Thrombolytic Therapy		T 9.0
EFFECTIVE DATE	**REVIEWED**	**REVISED DATE**
August 31, 1992	March 1, 2005	February 4, 2005
ISSUED BY	**APPROVED BY**	**CROSS REFERENCE**

PROTOCOL FOR CARE OF THE PATIENT RECEIVING THROMBOLYTIC THERAPY

PURPOSE

To outline the Management of a patient receiving thrombolytic therapy for Acute Myocardial Infarction (AMI) in the Emergency Department.

RATIONALE FOR INFUSION

Thrombolytic Therapy is used to achieve thrombolysis within the coronary arteries, thus limiting the size of, or preventing infarction of myocardial tissue.

GOAL OF THERAPY

The goal of this care is to monitor the patient for the effectiveness of therapy, as well as development of untoward effects.

A. CRITERIA FOR PATIENT SELECTION (PHYSICIAN RESPONSIBILITY)

1. Assessment of Chest Pain (PQRST)
2. Assessment of 12 lead EKG
3. Assessment of signs and symptoms of AMI
4. Assessment of time from onset of chest pain
5. Absolute/Relative Contraindications
   a. Active bleeding
   b. Recent hemorrhage, Cerebrovascular Accident
   c. Bleeding diathesis
   d. Severe, uncontrolled hypertension, despite intravenous vasodilator therapy
   e. Recent surgery within 6 months
   f. Recent significant trauma
6. An allergy to streptokinase or a thrombolysis for MI with streptokinase within the last six months.

B. GENERAL PREPARATION

2. Establish 3–4 peripheral IV lines or hep locks and secure firmly
3. Obtain a good quality 12 lead EKG

C. TNKASE RECONSTITUTION INSTRUCTIONS

1. Withdraw 10 mL of sterile water for injection.
2. Inject entire contents into the TNKase vial, directing the diluent at the powder slight foaming upon reconstitution is not common. Let stand undisturbed for several minutes to allow bubbles to dissipate.
3. Gently swirl until contents are completely dissolved. DO NOT SHAKE solution. Solution should be colorless or pale yellow and transparent. Use upon reconstitution. If not used immediately refrigerate solution at 2–8 degrees Celsius (34–46 degrees) and use within 8 hours. DO NOT FREEZE.
4. Withdraw the appropriate volume of solution based on patient's weight (see dosing information). The recommended total dose should not exceed 50mg. Discard solution remaining in the vial.
5. Flush a dextrose containing line with saline containing solution prior to and following administration (precipitation may occur when TNKase is administered in an IV line containing dextrose).
6. Administer as an IV Bolus over 5 seconds.

Simple, weight-based dosing in 5 easy increments:

DOSING INFORMATION

PATIENT WEIGHT (kg)	PATIENT WEIGHT (lb)	TNKASE (mg)	RECONSTITUTED TNKASE (mL)
<60	<132	30	6
>60–70	>132 to <154	35	7
>70 to <80	>154–176	40	8
>80–<90	>176–198	45	9
>90	>198	50	10

D. RETEPLASE (RETAVASE)

Use aseptic technique throughout.

1. Remove the protective flip=cap from one vial of sterile water for injection. Open the package containing the 10 mL syringe with attached needle. Remove the protective cap from the needle and withdraw 10 mL of sterile water from the vial.
2. Open the package containing the dispensing pin. Remove the needle from the syringe, discard the needle. Remove the protective cap from the Luer lock port of the dispensing pin and connect the syringe to the dispensing pin. Remove the protective flip-cap from one vial of Reteplase.
3. Remove the protective cap from the spike end of the dispensing pin, and insert the spike into the Reteplase. Transfer the 10 mL of sterile water through the dispensing pin into the Reteplase.
4. With the dispensing pin and syringe still attached to the vial, swirl the vial gently to dissolve the Reteplase. DO NOT SHAKE.
5. Withdraw 10 mL of Reteplase reconstituted solution back in to the syringe. A small amount of solution (0.7 mL) will remain in the vial due to overfill.
6. Detach the syringe from dispensing pin, and attach the sterile 20-gauge needle provided.
7. The 10 mL bolus dose is now ready for administration.
8. Safely discard all used reconstitution components and the empty Reteplase vial according to hospital procedures.

E. STREPTOKINASE PREPARATION ADMINISTRATION

1. Reconstitute the 1,500,000 units vial of Streptokinase with 10 mL of D5w (withdraw 10 mL of D5W from the accompanying 100 mL D5W bag and inject into streptokinase vial)
2. Gently swirl the vial *Avoid Shaking
3. Observe for a colorless to slightly yellow color
4. Solutions containing large amounts of flocculations should be returned to pharmacy
5. Streptokinase should not be mixed with any other IV fluids or medications
6. Set up the bag of streptokinase solution for infusion via IV pump

7. Set the pump to deliver 100 mL over 1 hour (60 minutes)
8. Administer other medications as ordered, which are consistent with protocol
   a. Aspirin 160–325 mg orally chewed
   b. Nitroglycerin (Tridil®) or Morphine Sulfate for pain management
   c. Metoprolol (contraindicated bradycardia, hypotension and CHF)
   d. Heparin, initiated 8 hours after streptokinase completed
   e. IV antiarrhythmic as needed

F. ACTIVASE PREPARATION ADMINISTRATION

1. Reconstitute the 100 mg of Activase with 100 mL of sterile water for injection (SWFI), which is supplied in the kit
2. Utilize the transfer device and insert the piercing pin vertically into the center of the stopper of the vial of SWFI
3. Holding the vial of Activase upside-down, position it so that the center of the stopper is directly over the exposed piercing pin of the transfer device. Push the vial of Activase down so that the piercing pin is inserted through the center of the Activase vial stopper
4. Invert the 2 vials so that the Activase is on the bottom (upright). Approximately 2 minutes are required for the transfer device
5. Swirl gently to dissolve the Activase powder. DO NOT SHAKE
6. No other medications should be added to infusion solutions containing Activase
7. Slight foaming is not unusual and should be dissipate upon standing for several minutes
8. The solution should be observed for particulate matter and discoloration. A colorless pale yellow solution should be present
9. Loading Dose: 15 mg (15 mL) IV Push over 1–2 minutes. This may be obtained by withdrawing 15 mL from the above solution
10. Remainder of Dose: 85 mg via infusion over 90 minutes to begin by vented administration set and controller as follows:
    a. 50 mg (50 mL) over 30 minutes (set pump for 100 mL/hr)
    b. 35 mg (35 mL) over 60 minutes (set pump for 35 mL/hr)
11. Administer other medications as ordered, which are consistent with protocol.
    a. Aspirin 160–325 mg orally chewed
    b. Nitroglycerin (Tridil®) or morphine Sulfate for pain management
    c. Metoprolol (contraindicated bradycardia, hypotension and CHF)
    d. Heparin: (60 u/kg by intravenous bolus, (max 4,000 units bolus, given immediately after – Activase, followed by a continuous infusion of 1,000 Units/hr controlled by an infusion pump).
    e. IV antiarrhythmic as needed

G. PATIENT MONITORING: (NURSING RESPONSIBILITY: INFORM MD OF ANY ABNORMAL FINDINGS)

I. Vital Signs
Monitor V/S every 30 minutes, or more frequently where indicated, until chest pain subsides or thrombolytic therapy is completed. Thereafter, every 2 hours, or more frequently as needed.

II. Monitor for Bleeding
  a. Monitor mouth, gums, and IV sites
  b. Check all body fluids for blood, including:
    1. urine
    2. sputum
    3. stool
    4. gastric fluid
  c. Assesses and document neuro status every hour, including:
    1. LOC
    2. orientation
    3. motor responses
  d. Monitor for symptoms of retroperitoneal bleeding:
    1. low back pain
    2. leg pain
    3. ecchymosis over flank area

III. Monitor Patient for Effectiveness of Therapy:
Assess patient for:
  1. resolution of chest pain
  2. resolution of EKG changes
  3. appearance of reperfusion arrhythmias

IV. Ongoing Lab Monitoring/Orders
  1. Repeat 12 lead EKG 30 minutes - 1 hour after thrombolytic completed
  2. Strict bed rest × 18 hours
  3. Automated noninvasive BP monitoring should not be used more than every thirty (30) minutes
  4. Serial Cardiac enzymes every 8 hours
  5. CBC, PT/PTT 4–6 hours post infusion

V. Specific Drug Administration
  1. Metoprolol (Lopressor): 5 mg/5mL IV push over 1–2 minutes slowly every 5 minutes × 3, followed by Metoprolol 50 mg orally every 8 hours × 3 doses, then 100 mg PO every 12 hours
  2. Heparin Drip: 8 hours after streptokinase
    a. 5,000 unit IV Bolus followed by 25,000 units/250cc D5W, at 1000 Units/hour = 10 mL/hour or MD's order
  3. Nitroglycerin (Tridil®)
    50 mg/250cc D5w (Glass) titrate according to pain and vital signs
    60 mL/hr = 200 mcg/minute
    30 mL/hr = 100 mcg/minute
    15 mL/hr = 50 mcg/minute
    7–8 mL/hr = 25 mcg/minute
    3–4 mL/hr = 12.5 mcg/minute
    1–2 cmL/hr = 6.25 mcg/minute

Appendix B
Dosing Guides and Tables

ADULT ED ACUTE AREA MEDICATION FLOOR STOCK PAR LEVEL LIST

Generic Name	Dose Strength	Dose Form	Pharmacovigilance Code	Quantity
acetaminophen	650 mg	Suppository	GREEN	25
activated charcoal	50 g	Solution	RED	5
adenosine	6 mg/2 mL	vial	RED	5
albuterol	0.083% 3 mL	Inhalation solution	GREEN	30
ampicillin	1 g	vial	YELLOW	10
aspirin	81 mg	Chewable tablet	YELLOW	30
aspirin	325 mg	Enteric coated tablet	YELLOW	30
aspirin	325 mg	tablet	YELLOW	30
atropine	1 mg/10 mL	Brist.	YELLOW	16
belladonna/phenobarbital		elixir	GREEN	3
bupivacaine/HCl	0.5%	30 mL vial	GREEN	10
calcium chloride	10%	10 mL vial	RED	5
calcium gluconate	10%	10 mL vial	RED	5
cefazolin	1 g	vial	YELLOW	10
cefuroxime	750 mg	vial	YELLOW	10
clindamycin	600 mg/4 mL	vial	YELLOW	10
clonidine	0.1 mg	tablet	YELLOW	10
clonidine	0.2 mg	tablet	YELLOW	10
clopidogrel	75 mg	tablet	YELLOW	25
dexamethasone	4 mg/mL	5 mL vial	YELLOW	5
dextrose	50% 50 mL	Brist.	YELLOW	12
digoxin	0.5 mg/2 mL	vial	YELLOW	10
diltiazem	30 mg	tablet	RED	10
diltiazem	5 mg/mL	5 mL vial	RED	10
diltiazem	5 mg/mL	10 mL vial	RED	10
diphenhydramine	25 mg	tablet	YELLOW	10
dopamine	400 mg/250 mL D5W	premixed	RED	10
epinephrine	1:10,000	brist	RED	16
famotidine	20 mg	tablet	GREEN	20
famotidine	20 mg/2 mL	2 mL vial	GREEN	25
furosemide	10 mg/mL	4 mL vial	YELLOW	15
gentamicin	80 mg in 50 mL NaCl	premixed	RED	15
haloperidol	5 mg/mL	vial	YELLOW	10
heparin	1,000 units/mL	10 mL vial	RED	5
heparin	5,000 units/mL	10 mL vial	RED	5
heparin	25,000 units/250 mL D5W	premixed	RED	30
hydrocortisone	100 mg/2 mL	vial	YELLOW	10
ibuprofen	400 mg	tablet	YELLOW	30
insulin NPH (Lantus)	10 units/mL	10 mL vial	YELLOW	5
insulin regular (insulin aspart)	10 units/mL	10 mL vial	YELLOW	5
ipratropium	0.02%	Inhalation solution	YELLOW	30
ketorolac	30 mg/mL	vial	YELLOW	25
klor-con m 20	20 mEq	ER tablet	YELLOW	20
lidocaine HCl	1% 50 mL	vial	GREEN	10
lidocaine viscous	2%	solution	GREEN	10
magnesium sulfate	1 g/100 mL D5W	premixed	YELLOW	10
meclizine	25 mg	tablet	GREEN	20
metaproterenol	0.6%	Inhalation solution	GREEN	10
methocarbamol	500 mg	tablet	YELLOW	24
methylprednisolone	125 mg/2 mL	vial	GREEN	10
metoclopramide	10 mg/2 mL	vial	YELLOW	25
metoprolol	5 mg/5 mL	vial	YELLOW	10
metoprolol XL (take out)	50 mg	tablet	YELLOW	20
metoprolol	50 mg	tablet	YELLOW	20

(con't)

ADULT ED ACUTE AREA MEDICATION FLOOR STOCK PAR LEVEL LIST (con't)

Generic Name	Dose Strength	Dose Form	Pharmacovigilance Code	Quantity
metronidazole	500 mg/100 NaCl	premixed	GREEN	10
MVI for injection	5 mg/5 mL	injection	GREEN	10
Neutra-phos (take out)		packet	YELLOW	20
nitroglycerin	2%	ointment	YELLOW	20
nitroglycerin	50 mg/250 mL D5W	premixed	YELLOW	20
nitro-quick	0.4 mg	SL tablet	YELLOW	5
NovoLog	100 units/mL	10 mL vial	YELLOW	2
pancuronium	1 mg/mL	10 mL vial	RED	5
pantoprazole	40 mg	tablet	GREEN	25
phenytoin	250 mg/5 mL	vial	RED	12
potassium chloride	10 mEq/100 mL D5W	premixed	YELLOW	15
prednisone	5 mg	tablet	GREEN	10
prednisone	20 mg	tablet	GREEN	10
prednisone	50 mg	tablet	GREEN	10
procainamide	1 g/10 mL	vial	RED	2
prochlorperazine	5 mg	tablet	YELLOW	10
promethazine	25 mg/mL	vial	RED	10
sodium bicarbonate	44.6 mEq	50 mL brist.	RED	12
sodium chloride	0.9%	Inhalation solution	GREEN	20
sodium polystyrene sulfonate	15 g/60 mL	suspension	YELLOW	10
succinylcholine	20 mg/mL	20 mL vial	RED	10
tetanus/diphtheria toxoid		0.5 mL vial	RED	20
thiamine	100 mg/mL	2 mL vial	GREEN	10
vancomycin	500 mg	vial	YELLOW	10
vecuronium	1 mg/mL	10 mL	RED	10
Zemuron	10 mg/mL	5 mL vial	RED	2

MMC forms [Floor stock-ED acute – 7-07]

ACUTE CARE AREA MEDICATION FLOOR STOCK LIST FOR REFRIGERATED MEDICATIONS

Drug Name	Strength	Vial Size	Form	Pharmacovigilance Code	Par Level
acetaminophen	650 mg		suppository	GREEN	25
diltiazem	5 mg/mL	5 mL	injection	YELLOW	10
diltiazem	5 mg/mL	10 mL	Injection	YELLOW	10
famotidine	20 mg/2 mL	2 mL	Injection	GREEN	25
MVI for injection		5 mL/5 mL	Injection	GREEN	10
insulin regular	10 units/mL	10 mL	Injection	YELLOW	5
insulin NPH	10 units/mL	10 mL	Injection	YELLOW	5
pancuronium	1 mg/mL	10 mL	Injection	RED	5
succinylcholine	20 mg/mL	10 mL	Injection	RED	10
tetanus/diphtheria toxoid		0.5 mL	Injection	RED	20
vecuronium	1 mg/mL	10 mL	Injection	RED	10
NovoLog	100 units/mL	10 mL	Injection	YELLOW	2
Zemuron	10 mg/mL	5 mL	Injection	RED	2

Completed by Technician:

MMC forms: [ED-acute-Refrig Meds floor stock – 1/4/07]

ACUTE CARE AREA CONTROLLED DRUG FLOOR STOCK LIST

NURSING UNIT: <u>EMERGENCY DEPARTMENT – RESUSCITATION / TRAUMA ROOM</u>

FOR RAPID SEQUENCE INTUBATION

Approved by: **NURSING COORDINATOR / CHARGE NURSE:** _____
ASSOCIATE DIRECTOR OF PHARMACY: _____

These levels must be strictly adhered to and verified each shift as part of the narcotic inventory count. Any discrepancy in Par Level should be treated as a narcotic discrepancy and will require the immediate completion of the Controlled Drug Discrepancy Report Form. All requests for a permanent change in the Par Level should be made in writing and forwarded to the **Associate Director of Pharmacy**.

Item #	Controlled Drug	Number of Issues
1	diazepam (Valium) 5 mg/mL–2 mL injection	1 issue
2	fentanyl (Sublimaze) 50 mcg/mL–2 mL injection	1 issue
3	fentanyl (Sublimaze) 50 mcg/mL–5 mL injection	1 issue
4	ketamine (Ketalar) 10 mg/mL–20 mL injection	1 issue
5	lorazepam (Ativan) 2 mg/mL–1 mL injection	1 issue
6	methohexital Sodium (Brevital) 500 mg-injection	1 issue
7	midazolam (Versed) 1 mg/mL–5 mL injection	1 issue
8	midazolam (Versed) 5 mg/mL–10 mL injection	1 issue
9	morphine Sulfate 5 mg/mL–1 mL injection	1 issue
10	morphine Sulfate 10 mg/mL injection	1 issue
11	thiopental Sodium Injection (Pentothal) 400 mg 2% (20 mg/mL)–20 mL injection	1 issue
12	diazepam (Valium) 5 mg/mL–2 mL injection*	1 issue
13 a,b	*naloxone HCl (Narcan) 1 mg/mL–1 mL injection*	*2 issues*

*This issue of diazepam is for use in an emergency situation only. 9/14/06

RESUSCITATION CARE AREA MEDICATION FLOOR STOCK LIST

Generic Name	Dose Strength	Dose Form	Quantity
acetaminophen	650 mg	suppository	12
activated charcoal	50 g	solution	5
adenosine	6 mg/2 mL	vials	12
albuterol	0.083% 3 mL	Inhalation solution	30
amiodarone	50 mg/1 mL	vials	20
aspirin	.81 mg	Chewable tablet	30
atropine	0.1 mg/mL	10 mL brist.	10
atropine sulfate	0.4 mg/mL	vials	10
benzocaine	20%	spray	2
bumetanide	0.25 mg/mL	4 mL vials	4
bumetanide	0.25 mg/mL	10 mL vials	8
calcium chloride	10%	10 mL vials	8
calcium gluconate	10%	10 mL vials	8
dextrose	25 g/50 mL	Brist.	10
digoxin	500 mcg/2 mL	vials	10
diltiazem	5 mg/1 mL	5 mL vials	12
diltiazem	5 mg/1 mL	10 mL vials	12
dopamine	400 mg/250 D5W	Premixed	16
epinephrine	1:10,000	10 mL brist.	10

(con't)

RESUSCITATION CARE AREA MEDICATION FLOOR STOCK LIST (con't)

Generic Name	Dose Strength	Dose Form	Quantity
epinephrine	2 mg/mL	10 mL vials	10
epinephrine	1 mg/1 mL	vials	4
famotidine	20 mg	2 mL vials	20
furosemide	10 mg/mL	4 mL vials	20
furosemide	40 mg	Tablet	20
glucagon	1 mg	vials	8
haloperidol	5 mg/mL	vials	10
heparin	1,000 units/mL	10 mL vials	8
heparin	5,000 units/mL	10 mL vials	8
heparin	25,000 units/250 D5W	premixed	20
hydralazine	20 mg/mL	vials	5
insulin NPH	10 units/mL	10 mL vials	3
insulin regular	10 units/mL	10 mL vials	3
ipratropium	0.02% 3 mL	Inhalation solution	30
isoproterenol	0.2 mg/mL	5 mL vials	8
ketorolac	30 mg/mL	vials	20
labetalol	100 mg/mL	20 mL vials	5
lidocaine	1 g/250 D5W	premixed	10
lidocaine + epinephrine	1% - 10,000	20 mL vials	6
lidocaine HCl	1%	50 mL vials	5
lidocaine viscous	2%	15 mL UD solution	10
magnesium sulfate	0.5 g/mL	vials	10
mannitol	20% 500mL	premixed	2
mannitol	25% 50 mL	vials	5
methylprednisolone	125 mg/mL	vials	10
metoclopramide	10 mg/2 mL	vials	10
metoprolol	5 mg/5 mL	vials	10
MVI for injection h2	5 mL/5 mL	vials	10
neostigmine	10 mg/10 mL	vials	3
nitroglycerin	0.4 mg	SL tablet	5
nitroglycerin	2%	ointment	10
nitroglycerin	50 mg/250 mL D5W	premixed	16
nitroprusside	50 mg/5 mL	vials	3
norepinephrine	4 mg/4 mL	vials	10
NovoLog	100 units/mL	vials	2
pancuronium	1 mg/1 mL	10 mL vials	12
phenylephrine	10 mg/mL	vials	10
phenytoin	250 mg/5 mL	vials	15
prochlorperazine	5 mg/mL	2 mL vials	10
propofol	200 mg/20 mL	vials	10
propranolol	1 mg/1 mL	1 mL vials	5
Protonix	40 mg	vials	10
rocuronium	10 mg/mL	5 mL vials	4
sodium bicarbonate	7.5%	Brist.	12
succinylcholine	20 mg/mL	10 mL vial	10
tetanus/diphtheria toxoids		0.5 mL vials	20
vancomycin	500 mg	vials	10
vasopressin	20 units/mL	1 mL vial	10
vecuronium	1 mg/mL	10 mL vial	10
verapamil	5 mg/2 mL	vials	5

RESUSCITATION CARE AREA CONTROLLED DRUG FLOOR STOCK LIST

NURSING UNIT: Emergency Department

Approved by: NURSING COORDINATOR / CHARGE NURSE: _____
ASSOCIATE DIRECTOR OF PHARMACY: _____

These levels must be strictly adhered to and verified each shift as part of the narcotic inventory count. Any discrepancy in Par Level should be treated as a narcotic discrepancy and will require the immediate completion of the Controlled Drug Discrepancy Report Form. All requests for a permanent change in the Par Level should be made in writing and forwarded to the **Associate Director of Pharmacy**.

Item #	Controlled Drug	Number of Issues
1	alprazolam (Xanax) 0.25 mg tablet	1 issue
2	alprazolam (Xanax) 1 mg tablet	1 issue
3	chlordiazepoxide (Librium) 25 mg capsule	1 issue
4	clonazepam (Klonopin) 1 mg tablet	1 issue
5	diazepam (Valium) 5 mg/mL–2 mL injection	1 issue
6	diazepam (Valium) 5 mg tablet	1 issue
7	hydromorphone (Dilaudid) 2 mg/mL–1 mL ampule	1 issue
8	lorazepam (Ativan) 0.5 mg tablet	1 issue
9	lorazepam (Ativan) 2 mg tablets	1 issue
10	lorazepam (Ativan) 2 mg/mL–1 mL injection	1 issue
11	meperidine (Demerol) 50 mg/mL–1 mL injection	1 issue
12	methadone 10 mg tablet	1 issue
13	midazolam (Versed) 1 mg/mL–2 mL injection	1 issue
14	midazolam (Versed) 1 mg/mL–5 mL injection	1 issue
15	midazolam (Versed) 5 mg/mL–10 mL injection	1 issue
16 a,b	morphine Sulfate 5 mg/mL–1 mL injection	2 issues
17	morphine Sulfate 10 mg/mL–1 mL injection	1 issue
18	Percocet 5 mg/325 mg tablets	1 issue
19	phenobarbital 30 mg tablet	1 issue
20	phenobarbital 130 mg/mL–1 mL injection	1 issue
21	Tylenol and codeine #3 tablets	1 issue
22	zolpidem (Ambien) 5 mg tablet	1 issue
23	diazepam (Valium) 5 mg/mL–2 mL injection*	1 issue
24	HIV Kit	1 issue
25 a,b	flumazenil (Romazicon) 0.5 mg/5 mL injection	2 issues
26 a,b	naloxone HCl (Narcan) 1 mg/mL–2 mL injection	2 issues

*This issue of diazepam is for use in an emergency situation only.
6/6/07

PEDIATRIC ED CONTROLLED DRUG FLOOR STOCK LIST

CONTROLLED DRUG PAR LEVELS

NURSING UNIT: ____PEDIATRIC ED____   REVISED DATE: _____

Approved by: **NURSING COORDINATOR / CHARGE NURSE:** _____
        ASSOCIATE DIRECTOR OF PHARMACY: _____

These levels must be strictly adhered to and verified each shift as part of the narcotic inventory count. Any discrepancy in Par Level should be treated as a narcotic discrepancy and will require the immediate completion of the Controlled Drug Discrepancy Report Form. All requests for a permanent change in the Par Level should be made in writing and forwarded to the **Associate Director of Pharmacy**.

Item #	Controlled Drug	No. of Issues
1	acetaminophen 120 mg + codeine PO_4 12 mg (Tylenol + Codeine) 5 mL cups	1 issue
2	diazepam (Valium) 5 mg/mL–2 mL injection	1 issue
3	fentanyl (Sublimaze) 50 mcg/mL–2 mL injection	1 issue
4	ketamine (Ketalar) 10 mg/mL–20 mL injection	1 issue
5	ketamine (Ketalar) 50 mg/mL–10 mL injection	1 issue
6	lorazepam (Ativan) 2 mg/mL–1 mL injection	1 issue
7	midazolam (Versed) 1 mg/mL–2 mL injection	1 issue
8	midazolam (Versed) 1 mg/mL–5 mL injection	1 issue
9	midazolam (Versed) 2 mg/mL–118 mL syrup	1 issue
10	morphine Sulfate 5 mg/mL–1 mL injection	1 issue
11	pentobarbital Sodium (Nembutal) 50 mg/mL–20 mL injection	1 issue
12	phenobarbital 130 mg/mL–1 mL injection	1 issue
13	phenobarbital Elixir 20 mg/5 mL–5 mL cups	1 issue
14	thiopental sodium injection (Pentothal) 400 mg 2% (20 mg/mL)–20 mL injection	1 issue
15	diazepam (Valium) 5 mg/mL–2 mL injection*	1 issue
16	Rapid Intubation Kit	1 issue
17	flumazenil (Romazicon) 0.1 mg/mL–5mL injection	1 issue
18	naloxone (HCl) (Narcan) 1 mg/mL–2 mL injection	1 issue
19	naloxone HCl (Narcan) 0.4 mg/mL–1 mL injection	1 issue

*This issue of diazepam is for use in emergency situations only.

CLINICAL STEPS FOR SAFE ANTIDOTE ORDERING AND DELIVERY PROCESS IN THE ED

Key: P: Prescribing, T: Transcribing, D: Dispensing; A: Administer; M: Monitor; C: Continuity of Care

Medication[Ref.] Usual Dosage Concentration	40–50 kg	51–60 kg	61–70 kg	71–80 kg	81–90 kg	91–100 kg	Clinical Pearls Reference
Acetylcysteine Oral[11–17] 140 mg /kg 1st dose 70 mg/kg 2-17th dose 200 mg/mL (20%)	**28–35 mL** 14–18 mL	**36–42 mL** 18–21 mL	**43–49 mL** 21–25 mL	**50–56 mL** 25–28 mL	**57–63 mL** 28–32 mL	**64–70 mL** 32–35 mL	1. Mask taste with cola and ice 2. Use an enclosed container with a straw 3. Coaching may enhance adherence
Acetylcysteine[11–17] **Intravenous** 150 mg/kg in 200 mL D5W 1st dose 50 mg/kg in 500 mL D5W 2nd dose 100 mg/kg in 1000 mL D5W 3rd dose 200 mg/mL (20%)	**30–38 mL** 10–13 mL 20–25 mL	**38–45 mL** 13–15 mL 25–30 mL	**45–53 mL** 15–18 mL 30–35 mL	**53–60 mL** 18–20 mL 35–40 mL	**60–67 mL** 20–23 mL 40–45 mL	**68–75 mL** 23–25 mL 45–50 mL	1. Administer 1st dose over 60 minutes 2. Monitor for anaphylactoid reaction 3. Administer 2nd dose over 4 hours 4. Administer 3rd dose over 16 hours

Atropine[37]		
	P:	Indicated for nerve gas agent exposure repeat to resolution of wheezing and bronchorrhea
	P:	May need copious amount based on duration of nerve gas
	T:	1–2 mg IV push repeat every 10–30 minutes as needed
	A:	IV push over 1–2 minutes
	D:	Available as 0.1 mg/mL (5 and 10 mL), 0.4 mg/mL (20 mL)
	M:	Monitor for arrhythmia, hyperthermia, and sedation
	C:	Have 1500 mg on hand easily accessible to manage 50 patients up-to 30 mg for each
Calcium Chloride (Intravenous)[28–32]	P:	Use in cardiac arrest (PEA) associated with CCA toxicity; Preferred
	T:	1 gram (10 mL of a 10% solution) IV push q10–20 minutes ×3 doses
	A:	Bolus over 5 minutes; only increases ionized calcium for 5–10 minutes; start infusion
	A:	May be infused slowly over 20 min if intolerable to bolus dosing, dilute in 50 mL NS or D5W
	D:	Available as 100 mg/mL (10%); 270 mg elemental Ca/10 mL
	M:	Titrate infusion to goal blood pressure (MAP > 65 mm Hg) with other adjuvants
	M:	Monitor ionized Ca++ every 30 minutes initially then every 2 hours
	M:	Calciphylaxis is a risk with overzealous use of calcium
	C:	Extended release tablets of calcium channel blockers or beta blockers requires 24hr observation.
Calcium Gluconate (Intravenous)[28–32]	P:	CCA Overdose; Known or suspected
	P:	Many combination products contain CCA i.e. Tarka, Lotrel, Exforge
	T:	3 grams (30 ml of a 10% solution) of calcium gluconate bolus × 4 q10–20 minutes
	D:	100 mg/mL (10%); 90 mg elemental calcium /10 mL
	D:	If intolerable to bolus dosing, dilute dose indicated into 50 mL NS or D5W
	A:	IV push is recommended over 5 minutes
	A:	May be infused slowly over 20 minutes
	M:	Titrate infusion to goal blood pressure (MAP > 65 mm Hg) up to 5 grams[2] with other adjuvants
	M:	Monitor ionized Ca++ every 30 minutes initially then every 2 hours
	M:	Calciphylaxis is a risk with overzealous use of calcium
	C:	Extended release tablets of calcium channel blockers or beta blockers requires 24hr observation.

CLINICAL STEPS FOR SAFE ANTIDOTE ORDERING AND DELIVERY PROCESS IN THE ED (con't)

Key: P: Prescribing, T: Transcribing, D: Dispensing; A: Administer; M: Monitor; C: Continuity of Care

Deferoxamine (Desferal) (Intravenous Infusion)[3,4]	P:	Indicated for significant clinical signs of iron toxicity; metabolic acidosis, shock, profound lethargy, coma, iron level of >500 mcg/dL or pills on X-ray
	T:	Initial infusion of 1000 mg in 50 mL of NS, or D5W is administered at a rate of 15 mg/kg/hr; then 500 mg over 4 hours × 2 doses; and then based on clinical response
	D:	IM dose of 500 mg is reconstituted with 2 mL (210 mg/mL); 2 grams is reconstituted with 8 mL(230 mg/mL); should appear yellow but clear in color; for single use
	D:	IV preparation: Reconstitute 500 mg with sterile water 5 ml (95 mg/mL); or 2 grams reconstituted with 20 mL (95 mg/mL) add to NS or D5W
	A:	Assure adequate hydration at onset with deferoxamine due to rate related hypotension (adjust the infusion rate to 10 mg/hour or lower as tolerated)
	A:	15 mg/kg per hour not to exceed 1 gram/h over 6 hours in a 24 hour period (however higher doses have been used without incident)
	A:	IM is preferred when patient is not in shock.
	M:	Re-evaluate after initial infusion; Anaphylaxis; Infection; blood gas; perfusion; ALT/AST; ARDS with >24 hours of administration
	C:	Continue for 12 hours after patient is asymptomatic, serum iron level falls below 350 toward 150 mcg/dL; and urine turns to normal color
DIGIBIND/DigiFab Intravenous[3, 33–34]	P:	Avoid calcium salts in digoxin toxicity theoretical risk of cardiac asystole
	P:	Indicated in patient with potassium >5 mEq/L following acute ingestion; hemodynamic instability; potentially life threatening dysrhythmias
	P:	Phenytoin and lidocaine should be used for tachyarrhythmia,
	P:	Some ACLS measures may exacerbate the dysrhythmia i.e. class IA agents
	P:	Electrical cardioversion may induce ventricular fibrillation in dig toxicity (use as last resort at low 10–30 joules)
	P:	In Acute-on-chronic overdose calculate the dose: 40 mg of Fab (one vial) binds 0.6 mg of digoxin
	P:	(Usual dose (number of vials indicated) = {Serum digoxin level (ng/mL) × patient wt/100}
	P:	Usually - 2–3 vials is sufficient in acute on chronic overdose
	T:	In acute overdose unknown ingestion: DigiFab 40 mg vial; Infuse 5–10 vials(200–400 mg) in 100 ml NS over 30 minutes
	D:	Reconstitute Digifab/bind with 4 mL of sterile water for injection and add to 34 mL NS to make a 1 mg/ml concentration
	A:	Use an 0.22 micron in-line filter when infusing; infuse with a volumetric pump
	A:	May be administered in cardiac arrest as a bolus
	M:	Within 2 minutes life threatening dysrhythmia may resolve; within 30 minutes ventricular arrhythmia should settle
	M:	Within 6 hours 90% of patients have complete or partial response
	C:	Consult with cardiology as they will have to manage the patient inhospital care
	C:	Digifab does cross react with digoxin assay so levels will remain high for several days
Dimercaprol (BAL)	P:	Heavy metal poisoning; Lewisite exposure
	P:	Contains benzyl benzoate and peanut oil
	T:	4–5 mg/kg IM every 4 hours × 3–5 days
	D:	100 mg/mL (3 mL)
	A:	Inject deep into muscle
Ethanol solution for injection[32]		Methanol and ethylene glycol over dose
	P:	To estimate the plasma level Identify amount ingested by taking the percent in solution the total amount ingested, and weight of patient
	P:	Plasma level = (Amount ingested * percent solution * spec. grav.) / (Vd * weight); estimate body weight[2]
	P:	As part of risk assessment: Calculate Anion gap = Na − [HCO3 + Cl]; normal gap is 8–12 mEq/L
	P:	As part of risk assessment: Calculate Osmol gap: (Osmol gap increases because toxic alcohols contribute to osmolarity)
	P:	Osmol gap = measured − calculated; Calculated Osmol gap = 2(Na) + (glucose/18) + (BUN/2.8)
	P:	Normal Osmolarity = 275 mOsmol/L; Normal Osmol-gap = <10 mOsmol/L
	P:	Adjust ethanol dose based on whether initiating therapy or based on plasma level
	P:	Avoid if ethanol level is >130 mg/dL; goal is 100 mg/dl

(con't)

CLINICAL STEPS FOR SAFE ANTIDOTE ORDERING AND DELIVERY PROCESS IN THE ED (con't)

Key: P: Prescribing, T: Transcribing, D: Dispensing; A: Administer; M: Monitor; C: Continuity of Care

Ethanol solution for injection[32] *(continued)*	P:	Identify if drinker, nondrinker and adjust accordingly
	T:	Initiate loading dose with 10 mL/kg dose by continuous IV infusion over 1 hour; (70 kg = 700 mL over 1 hour)
	T:	Initiate maintenance 1.5 mL/kg/hr infusion then titrate based to achieve 100–150 mg/dl (70 kg = 105 mL/hr)
	D:	Ethyl alcohol 5% (50 mg/ml) in D5W or 10% (100 mg/ml) (V/V) are well tolerated
	M:	Identify if planning for hemodialysis as loading and maintenance dose needs to be adjusted
	M:	Identify current plasma level of ethanol to adjust maintenance dose
	M:	Monitor both blood glucose and ethanol levels (hypoglycemia may occur with ethanol administration)
	M:	Assure proper hydration
	C:	Folate should be administered at 50 mg IV every 4 hours
Flumazenil (Intravenous)[1, 3]	P:	Most appropriately used in reversal of benzodiazepine induced sedation during minor surgical procedures
	P:	May be effective in antihistamine overdose
	P:	Not to use for undifferentiated coma-reversal; may precipitate withdrawal; or seizures for those at risk
	P:	Not commonly used in the ED; Does not reliably reverse respiratory and cardiac depression
	T:	0.2 mg IV over 30 seconds; Repeat with 0.3 mg over 30 seconds if re-sedated;
	T:	After initial bolus administer 0.5 mg incremental doses at 1 minute intervals up-to a total dose of 3 mg or desired response
	D:	Should be made available in automated dispensing machines; available as a 0.1 mg/mL (5, 10 mL)
	A:	IV bolus over 30 seconds
	M:	Re-sedation does occur and re-dosing is needed
	C:	Assure that re-assessments is conducted
Fomepizole (Antizol)[3, 36]	P:	Suspected or confirmed ingestion and intoxication with ethylene glycol or methanol; see ethyl alcohol for important risk assessments
	T:	15 mg /kg 1st dose then; 10 mg/kg every 12 hours × 4 doses (48 hours); 15 mg/kg every 12 hours based on response
	D:	1 gram/mL (1.5 mL) Dilute in 100 mL NS or D5W (undiluted associated with phlebosclerosis)
	A:	Intravenously over 30 minutes
	M:	Increase dose frequency to every 4 hours if undergoing dialysis
	M:	Continue until ethylene glycol level is <20 mg/dl
	C:	Investigate and treat other coingestions
Glucagon (Intravenous)[28, 32]	P:	Used in Beta Blocker and Calcium Channel Antagonist Overdose
	P:	Very short duration of effect; after bolus start continuous infusion;
	P:	Use bolus dose as dose rate/hour that improved hemodynamic status
	T:	3–5 mg IV bolus; then start 1 mg/hr continuous infusion and titrate to desired blood pressure with other adjuvants[2]
	D:	Available as a 1 mg lyophilized powder; reconstitute with 1 mL sterile water for injection; Use a 0.22 filter needle;
	D:	For continuous infusion add to 50 ml of NS or D5W
	A:	Infuse bolus doses over 2–3 minutes; use inline filter for continuous infusion
	M:	Maintain airway as > 3 mg IV bolus is associated with rapid development of vomiting
	M:	Glucagon impact on heart rate blood pressure is inconsistent and requires other adjuvants, i.e. saline, pressors, calcium salts, HEIT
	C:	May have insufficient amount available; Notify pharmacy purchaser
	C:	Be sure to replenish infusion while in the ED if length of stay in the ED is longer than 6 hours
Hydroxocobalamin Cyanokit) Vitamin B12[6,35]	P:	Safe and effective for cyanide toxicity
	T:	50 mg/kg in 100 mL NS infused over 15 minutes; may repeat in 15 minutes to 1 hour based on response
	D:	Available as two 2.5 grams vials of lyophilized powder (5 grams)
	D:	Reconstitute with 100 mL of Normal Saline;
	D:	Gently invert vial to mix; solution is dark red and should not contain any praticles
	A:	Intravenously infuse over 15 minutes or 15 ml/minute
	M:	Patients will develop orange-red discoloration of skin and mucous membranes and urine
	M:	Should resolve in 24–8 hours
	M:	Hypertension, allergic reaction, rash

CLINICAL STEPS FOR SAFE ANTIDOTE ORDERING AND DELIVERY PROCESS IN THE ED (con't)

Key: P: Prescribing, T: Transcribing, D: Dispensing; A: Administer; M: Monitor; C: Continuity of Care

Methylene Blue (Urolene Blue)[32]	P:	Used empirically in patients with central cyanosis and chocolate brown blood as a sign of Methemoglobinemia
	P:	Many causes of methemeglobinemia such as nitrites from food, anesthetics, dyes
	T:	1–2 mg/kg IV push; and repeat in 1hour if needed
	A:	Administer IV undiluted over several minutes
	D:	10 mg/mL (1 and 10 mL); IV ampoules; Be sure to know location of storage
	D:	Procurement of dose is time consuming with 1 ml glass ampoules
	A:	Urine does turn blue upon administration
	A:	Use 0.22 micron filter to administer
	M:	Clinical resolution of cyanosis (color of face changes from blue or dusky to normal); MetHb level
	M:	Pulse oximetry may only increase slightly with administration
	C:	Contact purchaser as pharmacy may not stock sufficient amounts
	C:	Communicate with ICU as to the suspicion and doses given; too much methylene blue can induce methemglobinemia
Naloxone Hydrochloride[3]	P:	Used in comatose patients for therapeutic and diagnostic agent for opioid intoxication
	P:	May precipitate withdrawal symptoms
	T:	0.4 to 2 mg IV push, repeat every 5 minutes as needed
	D:	Available as 0.4 mg/mL (1 mL) or 1 mg/mL (2 mL)
	D:	Infusion prepared with (NS) or (D5W) to a concentration of 0.004 milligrams per milliliter (mg/mL) (2 mg in 500 mL)
	A:	Intravenous preferred; IM, Intraosseous SUBQ are viable options
	M:	Respiratory function restored; airway protected; mental status improved
	M:	Reasons for lack of response include: insufficient dose, absence of opioid, mixed exposure, medical or traumatic reason
	M:	If no response after 10 mg, reconsider diagnosis of opioid toxicity
Pralidoxime Chloride (Protopam vial), (Mark-1 autoinjector)[32]	P:	Nerve gas exposure with atropine
	T:	1–2 grams in 250 mL normal saline IV over 20–30 minutes
	D:	1 gram/20 mL (vial),
	D:	600 mg/2 mL (Autoinjector
	A:	If IV access is unobtainable use IM 1 gram in 3 mL diluents)
	M:	Repeat in 5 minutes if muscle weakness persists
	M:	Maximum dose 12 gram in 24 hours
Pyridoxine[32]	P:	Administer IV push in case of seizures, acidosis and coma due to Isoniazid or Gyrometria mushrooms[3]
	P:	Indicated in patients with overdose of > 80 mg/kg
	T:	1 gram for every 1 gram of INH consumed, to a maximum of 5 grams or 70 mg/kg; or 0.5 grams/minute until seizure stops
	D:	Available as 250 mg/5 mL or 100 mg/mL; Supply up-to 5–10 grams (50–100 vials) of pyridoxine for use at all times
	D:	Be sure to supply adequate amounts or create a rapid response to acquire sufficient amounts
	A:	Initially administer 5 grams over 30–60 minutes
	A:	Repeat if needed another 5 grams dilute in 50–100 mL of D5W and administer over the next 1–2 hours
	M:	Risk of neuropathies with high dose
Sodium Nitrite[35]	P:	Indicated in Cyanide toxicity
	T:	300 mg (10 mL) by IV over 5 minutes; May repeat 50% if response is inadequate
	D:	300 mg /10 mL as part of Cyanide Kit
	D:	Check expiration as not commonly used may be expired; check expiration monthly
	D:	Have at least two available in the ED
	A:	IV over 5 minutes
	M:	Goal is to produces 20–30% methemoglobin levels at 50 minutes after administration
	M:	Do not go over this level
	M:	Reduce dose rate if hypotension occurs or dilute in NS and give over 20 minutes
	M:	Patient may feel lightheaded, headache, abdominal pain, nausea and vomiting

(con't)

CLINICAL STEPS FOR SAFE ANTIDOTE ORDERING AND DELIVERY PROCESS IN THE ED (con't)

Key: P: Prescribing, T: Transcribing, D: Dispensing; A: Administer; M: Monitor; C: Continuity of Care

Sodium Thiosulfate	P:	Indicated in Cyanide toxicity; May be given empirically in case of fire
	P:	May be used for mustard gas as well
	T:	12.5 grams in 50 mL over 10 minutes
	D:	250 mg/mL (50 mL)
	A:	Give after sodium nitrite; unless empirically used
	M:	Repeat in 30 minutes with 50% of the dose

Note: This guide is based on experiences gained while managing toxicological emergencies within the ED combined with evidence-based pharmacotherapy literature.

References
1. Gora-Harper ML. The Injectable Drug Handbook. 140
2. Adler J, et al. NMS Clinical Manuals Emergency Medicine. Lippincott Williams & Wilkins, 1999.
3. Holstege CP, et al Critical Care Toxicology. Emerg Med Clin N Am. 2008; 25:715–739.
4. Chyka P. Clinical Toxicology. In: Pharmacotherapy: A Pathophysiological Approach. Sixth Edition. New York: McGraw-Hill, 2005.
5. Novartis Deferoxamine http://www.pharma.us.novartis.com/product/pi/pdf/desferal.pdf accessed January 2009
6. Dey Cyannokit http://www.cyanokit.com/pdf/cyanokit_pi.pdfaccessed January 2009

BIOTERRORISM MONTHLY INVENTORY LIST: ANTIDOTES FOR BIOLOGICAL AGENTS

Drug Name	Strength	Dosage Form	Location	Earliest Exp. Date	Target Qty	Qty In Stock	Total Qty
Activated charcoal	50 g	Oral Slurry	W MP ED		100	6 10	16
Cidofovir	75 mg/mL	Injectable	W MP ED		100	None found	
Ciprofloxacin	400 mg	Injectable	W MP ED	10/09 11/09	100	289 125	414
Ciprofloxacin	500 mg	Tablets	W MP ED		5000	None found	
Clindamycin	600 mg	Injectable	W MP ED	09/09 09/09	100	72 20 (+80 600 mg/ 4 mL)	92 (+80; 600 mg/ 4 mL)
Doxycycline (as the hyclate)	100 mg	Injectable	W MP ED	01/11 05/08	100	40 3	43
Doxycycline (as the hyclate)	100 mg	Tablets	W MP ED	06/09 10/08	5000	100 76	176
Gentamicin (as the sulfate)	10 mg/mL	Injectable	W MP ED	08/09	100	65	65
Gentamicin (as the sulfate)	40 mg/mL (20 ml Vials)	Injectable	W MP ED	07/09 04/09	100	50 55	105
Penicillin G (as the potassium)	20 million units	Injectable	W MP ED	10/09	100	4	
Rifampin	300 mg	Capsules	W MP ED	04/09 04/09	300	100 70	170
Streptomycin sulfate	1g	Injectable	W MP ED	07/10	100	10 vials	
Streptomycin (as the sulfate)	400 mg/mL	Injectable	W MP ED		100	None found	

ANTIDOTES FOR CHEMICAL AGENTS

Drug Name	Strength	Dosage Form	Location	Earliest Exp. Date	Target Qty	Qty In Stock	Total Qty
Amyl nitrite	0.3 mL	Crushable Ampul	W MP ED		50		
Atropine sulfate	1 mg/10 mL	Prefilled Syringes	W MP ED	10/09 08/09	300	250 130	380
Atropine sulfate	8 mg/20 mL	Multidose Injectable Vial	W MP ED		500	None found	
Calcium chloride	10 mg/10 mL	Injectable	W MP ED	10/10 10/09	150	2800 400	3200
Calcium gluconate	10%, 10 mg/100 mL	Injectable	W MP ED	03/10 01/10	150	200 52	252
Diazepam	5 mg/mL,	Injectable	W MP ED		100	Controlled Substance	
Dimercaprol	100 mg/mL,	Injectable	W MP ED	07/08 07/08	250	40 (3 mL vials) 10	50
Diphenhydramine hydrochloride	50 mg/mL,	Injectable	W MP ED	10/08 01/10	250	975 100	1075
Methylene Blue	1%, 10 mg/mL (10 mL)	Injectable	W MP ED	02/10 03/09	50	90 10	100
Pralidoxime chloride	1 g/20 mL	Injectable	W MP ED	08/11	150	6	6
Pyridostigmine bromide	60 mg	Tablets	W MP ED	02/09	300	120	120
Pyridoxine hydrochloride	3 g/30 mL	Injectable	W MP ED	12/08	100	250	
Sodium nitrite	300 mg/mL	Injectable	W MP ED		300		
Sodium thiosulfate	12.5 mg/50 mL (12.5 g/50 mL)	Injectable	W MP ED	05/09	50	3	3

RADIOLOGIC AND NUCLEAR ANTIDOTES MONTHLY INVENTORY LIST

Drug Name	Strength	Dosage Form	Location	Earliest Exp. Date	Target Qty	Qty In Stock	Total Qty
Aluminum hydroxide	240 mL	Suspension	W MP ED		50	None Found	
Calcium carbonate	1 g 1.25 g	Tablets	W MP ED	09/09 09/09	300	200 320	520
Chlorthalidone	100 mg	Tablets	W MP ED	03/10 06/08	100	150 (50 mg), 165 (25 mg)	150 (50 mg), 165 (25 mg)
Deferoxamine mesylate	1 g	Injectable	W MP ED	11/09 05/08	100	16 (500 mg) 12 (500 mg	28 (500 mg)
Edetic acid	200 mg/mL	Injectable	W MP ED		100	None found	
Furosemide	100 mg/ 10 mL	Injectable	W MP ED	12/08	100	25 33	58
Magnesium sulfate	25 g/50 mL		W MP ED	04/09	100		
Magnesium oxide			W MP ED			None found	
Penicillamine	250 mg	Tablets	W MP ED	04/09		65	
Potassium iodide	130 mg	Tablets	W MP ED		5000	None found	
Prussian blue			W MP ED		50	None found	
Sodium iodide	130 mg	Tablets	W MP ED		5000	None found	
Trisodium calcium diethylenetriamine-pentaacetate	1 g	Injectable	W MP ED		50	None found	
Trisodium zinc diethylenetriamine-pentaacetate	1 g	Injectable	W MP ED		50	None found	

Drugs for Treating Acute Radiation Syndrome

Drug Name	Strength	Dosage Form	Location	Earliest Exp. Date	Target Qty	Qty In Stock	Total Qty
Acyclovir (as the sodium)	25 mg/mL	Injectable	W MP ED	04/09	100	40 (500 mg/10 mL) 8 (500 mg/10 mL)	48(500 mg/ 10 mL)
Acyclovir	400 mg	Tablets	W MP ED		100	None found	
Antidiarrheal			W MP ED		100		
Cefepime hydrochloride	1 g	Injectable	W MP ED	10/09 04/25/2008	100	420 90	510
Filgrastim	300 µg/mL	Injectable	W MP ED		100		
Fluconazole,	200 mg/mL	Tablets	W MP ED		100		
Ganciclovir,	250–500 mg	Capsules	W MP ED		100	None found	
Ganciclovir (as the sodium)	500 mg/mL	Injectable	W MP ED		100	None found	
Granisetron (as the hydrochloride)	1 mg/mL	Injectable	W MP ED	06/10	100	62	62
Granisetron (as the hydrochloride)	1 mg	Tablets	W MP ED		100	None found	
Ondansetron (as the hydrochloride)	2 mg/mL	Injectable	W MP ED	11/10 11/10	100	33 70	103
Pegfilgrastim	6 mg	Injectable	W MP ED		100		
Trimethoprim & sulfamethoxazole	160 mg/800 mg	Tablets	W MP ED	10/09 10/09	100	300 100	400
Trimethoprim & sulfamethoxazole	80 mg/5 mL (80 mg/mL, 10 mL vials)	Injectable	W MP ED	04/09 04/10	100	130 51	181

PANDEMIC INFLUENZA PREPAREDNESS

Drug Name	Strength	Dosage Form	Location	Earliest Exp. Date	Target Qty	Qty In Stock	Total Qty
Antivirals							
Tamiflu			W				
			MP				
			ED				
Relenza			W				
			MP				
			ED				
Symmetrel			W				
			MP				
			ED				
Flumadine			W				
			MP				
			ED				
Analgesics							
Ibuprofen			W				
			MP				
			ED				
Naproxen			W				
			MP				
			ED				
Acetaminophen			W				
			MP				
			ED				
Aspirin			W				
			MP				
			ED				
Morphine oral			W				
			MP				
			ED				
Morphine IV			W				
			MP				
			ED				
Acetaminophen with codeine			W				
			MP				
			ED				
Acetaminophen with oxycodone			W				
			MP				
			ED				
Decongestants							
Sudafed			W				
			MP				
			ED				
Allegra D			W				
			MP				
			ED				

PANDEMIC INFLUENZA PREPAREDNESS (con't)

Drug Name	Strength	Dosage Form	Location	Earliest Exp. Date	Target Qty	Qty In Stock	Total Qty
Decongestants							
Claritin D			W				
			MP				
			ED				
Coricidin HBP			W				
			MP				
			ED				
Phenylephrine			W				
			MP				
			ED				
Antihistamines							
Claritin			W				
Allegra			MP				
Benadryl			ED				
Antidiarrheals							
Imodium AD			W				
			MP				
			ED				
Pepto Bismol			W				
			MP				
			ED				
Lomotil			W				
			MP				
			ED				
Antinausea							
Emetrol			W				
Meclizine			MP				
Phenergan			ED				
Topical Decongestants							
Phenylephrine			W				
			MP				
			ED				
Oxymetazoline			W				
			MP				
			ED				
Naphazoline			W				
			MP				
			ED				
Short-acting beta agonists							
Albuterol			W				
			MP				
			ED				
Ipratropium			W				
			MP				
			ED				

CHRONIC CARE MEDICATIONS FOR NATURAL DISASTERS

Drug Name	Strength	Dosage Form	Location	Earliest Exp. Date	Target Qty	Qty In Stock	Total Qty
Albuterol		Inhaler	W MP ED				
Alprazolam	0.5 mg	Tablets	W MP ED				
Amoxicillin	500 mg	Capsule	W MP ED				
Atenolol	25 mg	Tablets	W MP ED				
Atenolol	50 mg	Tablets	W MP ED				
Ambien	10 mg	Tablets	W MP ED				
Advair	250/50 mcg	Diskus	W MP ED				
Carisoprodol	350 mg	Tablet	W MP ED				
Cephalexin	500 mg	Capsule	W MP ED				
Ciprofloxacin	500 mg	Tablet	W MP ED				
Combivent		Inhaler	W MP ED				
Cyclobenzaprine	10 mg	Tablet	W MP ED				
Furosemide	40 mg	Tablet	W MP ED				
Flonase		Nasal spray	W MP ED				
Hydrochlorothiazide	12.5 mg 25 mg	Tablet	W MP ED				

(con't)

CHRONIC CARE MEDICATIONS FOR NATURAL DISASTERS (con't)

Drug Name	Strength	Dosage Form	Location	Earliest Exp. Date	Target Qty	Qty In Stock	Total Qty
Hydrocodone with APAP	5 mg/500 mg	Tablet	W MP ED				
Hydrocodone with APAP	7.5 mg/750 mg	Tablet	W MP ED				
Hydrocodone with APAP	10 mg/500 mg	Tablet	W MP ED				
Hydrocodone with APAP	7.5 mg/500 mg	Tablet	W MP ED				
Ibuprofen	800 mg	Tablet	W MP ED				
Lantus	U-100	10 ml	W MP ED				
Lipitor	10 mg	Tablet	W MP ED				
Lipitor	20 mg	Tablet	W MP ED				
Lipitor	40 mg	Tablet	W MP ED				
Lisinopril	10 mg	Tablet	W MP ED				
Lisinopril	20 mg	Tablet	W MP ED				
Lexapro	10 mg	Tablet	W MP ED				
Metformin	500 mg	Tablet	W MP ED				
Metformin	1000 mg	Tablet	W MP ED				
Metoprolol	50 mg	Tablet	W MP ED				
Nexium	40 mg	Capsule	W MP ED				

CHRONIC CARE MEDICATIONS FOR NATURAL DISASTERS (con't)

Drug Name	Strength	Dosage Form	Location	Earliest Exp. Date	Target Qty	Qty In Stock	Total Qty
Norvasc	5 mg	Tablet	W MP ED				
Norvasc	10 mg	Tablet	W MP ED				
Plavix	75 mg	Tablet	W MP ED				
Potassium chloride	20 mEq	ER tablet	W MP ED				
Prevacid	30 mg	Capsule	W MP ED				
Propoxyphene-N 100 with APAP		Tablet	W MP ED				
Protonix	40 mg	Tablet	W MP ED				
Promethazine	25 mg	Tablet	W MP ED				
Singulair	10 mg	Tablet	W MP ED				
Sulfamethoxazole/ Trimethoprim	800/160 mg	Tablet	W MP ED				
Triamterene/ Hydrochlorothiazide	37.5 mg	Tablet	W MP ED				
Tramadol	50 mg	Tablet	W MP ED				
Toprol XL	50 mg	Tablet	W MP ED				
Zithromax	250 mg	Tablet	W MP ED				
Zocor	40 mg	Tablet	W MP ED				

EMERGENCY MEDICINE PHARMACOTHERAPIST GENERAL PRINCIPLES AND GUIDE FOR MANAGING CRITICAL CARE INFUSIONS

Prescribing (Recommending/Verifying)
1. This situation requires you to multi-task.
2. Try to anticipate need for infusion before hemodynamic compromise.
3. Assess whether infusion is permitted based on the location the patient is to be admitted.
4. Estimate patient weight and identify if renal, hepatic or other cause for exacerbating effects, i.e. CHF or on BB requires a dose adjustment.
5. Assure the order is in the system or on paper and recompose if needed.
6. Cognitively verify patient allergies and medication history.

Procuring
1. Know the location of all resuscitation medications IV bags, and pumps in the ED.
2. Confirm the reason for the infusion as you prepare as well (you have time after to assure it makes sense).
3. Decide whether to prepare the infusion or request it from central pharmacy immediately.

Dispensing
1. Prepare a label include drug name, concentration, rate of infusion, diluents, and who prepared it, and date of preparation, and provide a date of expiration.
2. Set the pump on an IV pole (verify the patient name tag).
3. Set the pump using pre-existing profiles or directly entering the rate of infusion (be sure to re-check the rate).

Administration
2. Spike the infusion bag with a volumetric pump-line, and prime the infusion line to remove any air bubbles.
3. Calculate the rate in mL/hour and re-check if that rate corresponds to recommended dose rate in mg/min or mcg/min or mcg/kg/min or mg/kg/min.
4. Have the nurse connect the drip and check for occlusions in the line.

Monitoring
1. Set the cardiac monitor to assess BP and MAP (Goal[3]: MAP > 65 mm Hg but no higher) every 5–10 minutes initially and titrate using this titration guide to desired endpoint.
2. Noninvasive measures may be affected by volume status and cardiac function).
3. Use arterial line for titration of vasopressor or vasodilator[3].
4. Titration is guided by best clinical response: minimize myocardial ischemia (ECG and HR); Renal (Dec GFR and/or Urine output); Splanchnic/gastric (Low pHi bowel ischemia); peripheral (cold extremities) hypoperfusion (PaO2 and PAOP)[5].

Continuity
1. Investigate other pharmacotherapy needs as you monitor.
2. Plan for continuity of care and assure sufficient amount of infusion is available while in the ED.
3. Continue therapy until stable clinically.
3. Discontinuation should be executed slowly.

Drug / Std Conc Recommended Dose rate	Onset/Offset Titration Management	Routinely Monitored in the Emergency Department				Not routinely monitored in the Emergency Department			
		HR beats/min	SBP(%) mmHg	DBP mmHg	MAP mmHg	PCWP mmHg	CO L/min	SVR Dynes-sec-9 *cm −5	ICP
Amiodarone 900 mg in 500 mL D5W 0.5-1 mg/min	Administer at a rate of 1 mg/min (33.3 mL/hr) for 6 hours, and then 0.5 mg/min (16.6 mL/hr) for 18 hours[4]	↓	↔ to ↓	↔ to ↓	↔ to ↓	↔ to ↓	↓	↓	N/A
Clevidipine butyrate (Cleviprex)[1] 25 mg/50 mL or 50 mg/100 mL (Emulsion) 0.5 mg/mL 1-2 mg/hr (2-4 mL/hr) initially	2-4 min/ 5-15 min Double dose every 90 seconds until blood pressure achieves goal	↔ (↑ with too rapid upward titration)	↓(15%)	↓	↓	↔ to ↓ (In heart failure patients- may exacerbate heart failure)	↔ to ↓ (In heart failure patients- may exacerbate heart failure)	↓	N/A

Drug	Dosing	Effects
Diltiazem 125 mg in 125 mL NS or D5w 5–15 mg/hr	2–5 min/ Initially, administer IV bolus 0.25 mg/kg, then repeat with 0.35mg/kg 5 mg/hr up to 15 mg/hr to a stable HR	↔ to ↓ · ↓ · ↓ · ↓ · ↔ · ↔ to ↑ · ↔ to ↓ · ↑
Dobutamine 250 or 500 mg/250 mL NS or D5W 2.5–15 mcg/kg/min	2.5 mcg/kg/min every 2–10 minutes up to 20 mcg/kg/min	↑ · ↑ · ↑ · ↑ · → · ↑ · N/A · N/A
Dopamine 400 or 800 mg/250 mL NS or D5W	5–10 mcg/kg/min[5] Titrate up every 5-15 min Up to max of 20 mcg/kg/min Higher doses-tachycardia[5] Hypovolemic patients more susceptible[5] Lower dose –not recommended for renal failure[5] May reduce splanchnic circulation at high doses	↑↑ · ↑ · ↑↑ · ↑ · ↔ · ↑ · ↓ · ↓ · ↑ · ↑ (35%) ↑ Risk of Pulmonary edema · ↑ · N/A
Epinephrine 4 or 8 mg/250 mL NS or D5W 0.05–2 mcg/kg/min	Start at 0.05 mcg/minute (low dose) titrate every 5 minutes by 0.2 mcg/kg/minute 2 mcg/kg/minute (considered a large dose) Last line in septic shock; with other pressors[5] Reduces splanchnic circulation at high doses in sever septic shock patients[5]	↑ · ↑ · ↑ · ↑ · ↑ · ↑ · → ↑ · N/A
Esmolol 2500 mg/250 mL NS Bolus 250–500 mcg/kg over 1 min Maintenance 50–200 mcg/kg/min	Start at 25 mcg/kg/min Titrate by 25–50 mcg/kg/min every 10–20 min until desired response and max if 300 mcg/kg/min	→ · → · → · → · ↔ to ↑ · → · ↔ to ↑ · ↔

EMERGENCY MEDICINE PHARMACOTHERAPIST GENERAL PRINCIPLES AND GUIDE FOR MANAGING CRITICAL CARE INFUSIONS (continued)

Drug / Dosing	Titration							
Isoproterenol 1 mg/250 mL or 2 mg/500 mL NS or D5W 0.5–20 mcg/min	Start with 2 mcg/min (1.25 mL/min), and titrate by 2–4 mcg/min every 5 min until asymptomatic heart rate is achieved to 10–20 mcg/min until HR is 60 BPM No more than 10 mcg/min are needed in most cases RARELY USED IN THE ED	↑	↓	↔ to ↓	↓	↑	↑	↓	N/A
Labetalol 200 mg/200 ml NS or D5W (withdraw 40 mL of diluent to make a 0.1 mg/mL concentration) 0.5–3 mg /min	5–10 minutes/6 hours Start infusion with 2 mg/min and titrate upward; Elderly may requires lower doses;	↓	↓	↓	↔ to ↓	↔ to ↓	↔ to ↓	↓	↔
Lidocaine 1 or 2 g/250 mL NS or D5W 20–50 mcg/kg/min	Titrate to 15–30 mcg/kg/minute or 2–4 mg/minute Usually Premixed	↔ to ↑	↔	↔	N/A	N/A	N/A	N/A	N/A
Nicardipine 25 mg/250 mL D5W or NS (withdraw 10 mL of diluent to make a 0.1 mg/mL concentration) 1–15 mg/hr	Start at 5 mg/hour and titrate every 5 minutes to a maximum of 15 mg/hour	↔ (↑ with too rapid upward titration)	↓	↓	↓	↔ to ↓	↔ to ↓	↓	N/A
Nitroglycerin 50 or 100 mg/250 mL (premix bottle) 5–200 mcg/min	2–5 min/15–30 min Start at 5 mcg/min and titrate every 3–5 minutes For PE Start at 10 mcg/minute and titrate upward 10–20 mcg/min upward 10–20 mcg/min every 10 minutes	↔ to ↑	↓	↓	↓	↑	↑	↓	↑
Nitroprusside 50 or 100 mg/250 mL D5W 0.25–10 mcg/kg/min 0.3–10 mcg/kg/min	1 min/1–2 min Start at 0.1 mcg/kg/min and titrate at 0.05 mcg/kg/min every 5–10 min until desired blood pressure is reached; most respond to 0.5–3 mcg/kg/min; max 10 mcg/kg/min	↔ to ↑	↓	↓	↓	↑	↑	↓	↑

Drug	Concentration / Dose	Comments	HR	SBP	DBP	MAP	PCWP	CO	SVR	ICP
Norepinephrine	4 or 8 mg /250 mL D5W 0.01–3 mcg /kg/min (2–20 mcg/min)*	Routinely started first in septic shock Start at 0.01 mcg/kg/min and titrate at a rate of 0.02 mcg/kg/min every 5–10 min up to a max of 3 mcg/kg/min based on MAP = 65 mmHg	↔ to ↑	↑	↑	↑	↔	↔ to ↓	↑	N/A
Phenylephrine	100 mg /250 mL NS 0.5–0.9 mcg / kg/min	Start at a rate of 0.5 mcg/kg/ per minute and titrated quickly to hemodynamic response up to a max of 9 mcg/kg/min Beneficial in those who cannot tolerate tachycardia	↔	↑	↑	↑	↔	↔	↑	N/A
Procainamide	240 mL D5W (withdraw 10 mL of diluent to make a 4–8 mg/mL concentration)	15–18 mg/kg over 25–30 min Administer typically 1 gram over 45–60 min Maintenance at a rate of 1–4 mg/min	↔ to ↑	↔ to ↓	↔ to ↓	↔ to ↓	N/A	↔ to ↓	N/A	N/A

* Assuming normal lung function.

HR – Heart Rate, SBP – Systolic Blood Pressure, DBP – Diastolic Blood Pressure, MAP – Mean Arterial Pressure, PCWP – Pulmonary Capillary Wedge Pressure, CO – Cardiac Output, SVR – Systemic Vascular Resistance, ICP – Intracranial Pressure

Key:
↓ Decrease. ↑ Increase, ↔ No Change, N/A Information not available

References

1. Cleviprex http://www.cleviprex.com/files/pdf1/ClevidipinePI1.pdf Accessed December 2008.
2. Gora-Harper ML. The Injectable Drug Reference. Bioscientific Resources, Inc., 1998.
3. Winters ME et al., Monitoring the Critically Ill Emergency Department Patient. Emerg Med Clin N Am. 2008;26:741–757.
4. Berk WA. Detroit Receiving Hospital Emergency Medicine Handbook. Fifth Edition. 2005
5. Rudis M, Dasta JF. Vasopressors and Inotropes in the Pharmacotherapy of Shock. Dipiro JT. Pharmacotherapy A Pathophysiologic Approach. 6th Edition. 2005

Appendix C
Educational Outcomes, Goals, and Objectives for Emergency Medicine

EDUCATIONAL OUTCOMES, GOALS, AND OBJECTIVES FOR POSTGRADUATE YEAR TWO (PGY2) PHARMACY RESIDENCIES IN EMERGENCY MEDICINE

OVERVIEW OF PGY2 PHARMACY RESIDENCY IN EMERGENCY CARE

The PGY2 residency in Emergency medicine pharmacotherapy is designed to transition PGY1 residency graduates from generalist practice to specialized practice that meets the needs of emergency medicine patients. PGY2 residency graduates exit equipped to be fully integrated members of the interdisciplinary emergency care team, able to make complex pharmacotherapy recommendations in this fast-paced environment. Training focuses on developing resident capability to deal with the range of diseases and disorders that occur in the emergency medicine setting. Special emphasis is placed on the complexities of emergent care in the face of minimal information and the breadth of diseases that may be experienced and how to lead a safe medication use system and enhance quality in this unique environment. Furthermore, emphasis is placed on acutely stabilizing multiple organ system failure and the difficulties imposed on care when patients require life-sustaining equipment.

Graduates of the Emergency medicine pharmacotherapy residency are experienced in short-term research in the emergency care environment and excel in their ability to teach other health professionals and those in training to be health professionals. They also acquire the experience necessary to exercise leadership for emergency care practice in the health system.

EXPLANATION OF THE CONTENTS OF THIS DOCUMENT

Each of the document's objectives has been classified according to educational taxonomy (cognitive, affective, or psychomotor) and level of learning. An explanation of the taxonomies is available elsewhere.[1]

The order in which the required educational outcomes are presented in this document does not suggest relative importance of the outcome, amount of time that should be devoted to teaching the outcome, or sequence for teaching.

The educational outcomes, goals, and objectives are divided into those that are required and those that are elective. The required outcomes, including all of the goals and objectives falling under them, must be included in the design of all programs. The elective outcomes are provided for those programs that wish to add to the required outcomes. Programs selecting an elective outcome are not required to include all of the goals and objectives falling under that outcome. In addition to the potential elective outcomes contained in this document, programs are free to create their own elective outcomes with associated goals and objectives. Other sources of elective outcomes may include elective educational outcomes in the list provided for PGY1 pharmacy residencies and educational outcomes for training in other PGY2 areas. Each of the goals falling under the program's selection of program outcomes (required and elective) must be evaluated at least once during the resident's year.

Educational Outcomes (Outcome): Educational outcomes are statements of broad categories of the residency graduates' capabilities.

Educational Goals (Goal): Educational goals listed under each educational outcome are broad sweeping statements of abilities.

Educational Objectives (OBJ): Resident achievement of educational goals is determined by assessment of the resident's ability to perform the associated educational objectives below each educational goal.

---

[1] Nimmo, CM. Developing training materials and programs: creating educational objectives and assessing their attainment. In: Nimmo CM, Guerrero R, Greene SA, Taylor JT, eds. Staff development for pharmacy practice. Bethesda, MD: ASHP; 2000.

Instructional Objectives (IO): Instructional objectives are the result of a learning analysis of each of the educational objectives. They are offered as a resource for preceptors encountering difficulty in helping residents achieve a particular educational objective. The instructional objectives falling below the educational objectives suggest knowledge and skills required for successful performance of the educational objective that the resident may not possess upon entering the residency year. Instructional objectives are teaching tools only. They are not required in any way nor are they meant to be evaluated.

Outcome EM1: Demonstrate th e knowledge of the emergency medicine specialty

Goal EM1.1   Describe the Emergency Medicine Specialty

Objective EM 1.1.1:   Define Emergency Medicine Specialty

Objective EM 1.1.2:   Trace back the history of the Emergency Medicine Specialty

Objective EM 1.1.3:   Describe the Emergency Physicians Approach to the Patient
  IO: Describe the management vs. diagnosis approach

Objective EM 1.1.4:   Describe how emergency medicine physicians are trained to think
  IO: Describe the various decision models and errors that occur due to them

Objective EM 1.1.5:   Describe strategies for reducing cognitive errors

Objective EM 1.1.6:   Describe the current ED overcrowding crisis
  *IO: Describe the current trends in ED epidemiology
  Describe the current demands and reduced supply*

Goal EM 1.2:   Demonstrate an mastery of the current internal challenges facing Emergency medicine including the Institute of Medicine's National Aims and the The Joint Commission's Medication Management Standards

Objective EM 1.2.1:   Describe the public's concern for safety

Objective EM 1.2.2:   Describe the incidence and cost of medical injury
  IO: Explain the tip of the iceberg model

Objective EM 1.2.3:   Define medical error, where they occur, and how they are classified
  IO: Explain and define Latent vs. active errors

Objective EM 1.2.4:   Elaborate on the Emergency Department as a high risk environment

Objective EM 1.2.5:   Define the healthcare quality chasm

Objective EM 1.2.6:   List the IOMs national aims for healthcare improvement
  IO: Describe examples of how to apply these aims to medication safety in the ED

Objective EM 1.2.7:   Describe the Joint Commission's Medication Management Standards

Outcome EM2: Demonstrates the unique nature of the emergency department and how this may impact the establishment of clinical pharmacy services.

Goal EM 2.1:   Describe the alignment of principles of pharmacotherapy and that of the clinical practice of emergency medicine.

Objective EM 2.1.1:   Describe divergent principles of pharmacotherapy and emergency medicine.

Objective EM 2.1.2:   List and define aligning principles of pharmacotherapy and emergency medicine.

Objective EM 2.1.3:   Describe divergent principles of pharmacotherapy and emergency medicine.

Objective EM 2.1.4:   Describe the role of the emergency medicine pharmacists in filling the gaps where there is misalignment in principles.

Objective EM 2.1.5:   Describe Emergency Care Pharmacotherapy Principles and continue to synthesize new principles.

Goal EM 2.2:   Define the emergency medicine clinical pharmacist.

Objective EM 2.2.1:   Provide a historical perspective of published account of the pharmacists providing services to the emergency department.
  IO: Quote the evidence based pharmacotherapy on the descriptions of pharmacy services to the emergency department.

Objective EM 2.2.2:   Provide a quantitative discussion on the impact of clinical pharmacy services in the emergency department.
  IO: Quote the evidence based pharmacotherapy on the numerical value of the pharmacist in the emergency department.

Objective EM 2.2.2:   Describe the outcome data describing the value of the clinical pharmacist in the emergency department and its current limitations of such data.
  IO: Quote the evidence based pharmacotherapy on the

economic, humanistic, and clinical value of the pharmacist in the emergency department.

IO: *Identify current limitations of evidence based pharmacotherapy as it pertains to outcome data.*

Goal EM 2.3: Describe the unique characteristics of the emergency department that requires a unique specialized emergency department pharmacist to manage.

Objective EM 2.3.1: Explain the impact of physical constraints of the ED and how this may impact provision of pharmaceutical care.

Objective EM 2.3.2: Describe the impact of time and volume issues of the emergency department setting and how that modifies the role of the traditional pharmacist.

Objective EM 2.3.3: List the variety of conditions that may be observed in the emergency department setting and its implication on the pharmacists' knowledge and specialization.

Objective EM 2.3.4: Identify the role of pharmacotherapy in the emergency department as a temporizing measure.

Objective EM 2.3.5: Demonstrate the team approach required to acutely stabilize the emergency department patients.

Objective EM 2.3.6: Discuss the paucity of information available in the emergency department and how this impact emergency pharmacotherapy care.

Objective EM 2.3.7: Compare and contrast the unique challenges for discharge counseling in the emergency department as compared to other sites, i.e. community, inpatient.

Outcome EM3: Establish an Academic Based Emergency Medicine Clinical Pharmacy Service, through implementation of "the PharmER pyramid model," a management approach.

Goal EM 3.1: Describe the elements needed to establish an Academic based emergency medicine clinical pharmacy service.

Objective EM 3.1.1: Identify common characteristics of metropolitan emergency departments

IO: *Describe affiliations, frequency of patient's visits, and number of admissions, and it's most intense hours of operations.*

IO: *Illustrate the layout of a metropolitan emergency department, and training*

level of the emergency care staff.

Objective EM 3.1.2: Identify clinical operations associated with use of pharmaceuticals within the emergency department.

IO: *Describe the central pharmacy's role in distribution of medications to the emergency department.*

Objective EM 3.1.3: Describe the role of the clinical pharmacist in the emergency department as a generalist and subspecialist in emergency medicine.

IO: *Describe the training and education conducive to achieving this role.*

IO: *Describe certification that may assist in managing the breadth of conditions observed.*

IO: *Describe ED clinical pharmacist approach in medical emergencies and resuscitative events.*

Objective EM 3.1.4: Introduce "the PharmER pyramid model" as a management strategy to a safe medication use system in the emergency department that also assures that patient's medication needs are being met.

IO: *Describe the PharmER pyramid and its symbolism.*

IO: *Describe the elements of the PharmER pyramid.*

IO: *Define, characterize, assure, and sustain a safe medication use system in the emergency department.*

Outcome EM4: Establish clinical pharmacy presence and leadership in the emergency department.

Goal EM 4.1: Describe the leadership elements needed to establish an Academic based emergency medicine clinical pharmacy service.

Objective EM 4.1.1: Describe leadership and quality of life tools to facilitate establishing an ED clinical pharmacy service.

IO: *Define the mnemonic TEAM.*

IO: *Describe the importance of sharpening the saw and peak performance.*

IO: *Demonstrate "Win-Win" relationships with emergency nursing and medicine staff*

Objective EM 4.1.2:   Describe an FMEA (Failure Mode Effect Analysis)

     IO: *Apply an FMEA to Emergency Care Pharmacotherapy.*

     IO: *Describe the conceptual model of gaps in oversight in ED medication use.*

Objective EM 4.1.3:   Explain how to use existing hospital infrastructure to facilitate clinical pharmacy services in the ED.

Objective EM 4.1.4:   Establish a pharmacy administrative presence in the ED.

     IO: *Describe knowledge translation gap and the pharmacist role in filling these gaps.*

     IO: *List the Joint Commission standards and annual national patient safety goals and the ED clinical pharmacy services role to assure compliance.*

Outcome EM5: Establish a clinical pharmacy presence and leadership in the emergency department in information technology.

Goal EM 5.1:   Describe the elements of information technology that contribute to a safe medication use system.

Objective EM 5.1.1:   Explain the benefits and failures of computerized physician order entry (CPOE) for medication ordering in the emergency department.

     IO: *List outcome benefits of associated with use of CPOE.*

     IO: *List failures associated with CPOE implementation*

Objective EM 5.1.2:   Describe the various types of emergency department information systems that exist and their advantages and disadvantages.

Objective EM 5.1.3:   Characterize the recommendations for preferred implementation CPOE and clinical decision support system.

Objective EM 5.1.4:   Describe medication management standards that CPOE systems help comply with.

     IO: *Describe MM3.20. 1.10, 4.10 and how CPOE may facilitate compliance with these standards.*

Objective EM 5.1.5:   Describe CPOE tools to facilitate implementation of pharmaceutical care.

     IO: *Explain preformed order sets to streamline order verification, and transcription errors.*

     IO: *Illustrate the use of clinical alert icons*

     IO: *Define the tracking board*

     IO: *Describe the integration of preformed order sets with Smart pump technology*

Outcome EM6: Design an optimal medication use process for the emergency department.

Goal EM 6.1:   Contribute to expediting safe and effective pharmaceutical care in the emergency department.

Objective EM 6.1.1:   List and describe medication management standards 2.10, 2.20, 2.40 and how they apply to the emergency department.

Objective EM 6.1.2:   Design a unit of use formulary for the emergency department.

     IO: *Identify common medication used in the emergency department*

     IO: *List medications that should not be used in the emergency department.*

     IO: *Provide updated list of medications floor stock specific to each region of the ED, acute, resuscitation, refrigerated, controlled substances, pediatrics that includes their par levels with the route, dosage strength in a table format.*

     IO: *Provide case illustration of the cost avoidance advantage of a unit of use formulary in the emergency department.*

Objective EM 6.1.2:   Design a unit dose distribution system for the emergency department.

     IO: *Provide a work flow diagram of a unit dose distribution system for the emergency department.*

     IO: *Write a policy and procedures for unit dose distribution for boarded patients.*

     IO: *Describe pitfalls associated with unit dose distribution in the emergency department*

Objective EM 6.1.3:   Compare and contrast advantages and disadvantages of various methods of securing medications in the emergency department.

Goal EM 6.2:   Conduct prospective review of medication order in the emergency department.

Objective EM 6.2.1:   Compare and contrast the traditional role of prospective review of medication orders and other strategies that may be used.

IO: Describe the Joint Commissions MM4.10 standard.

IO: Compare and contrast the emergency medicine and pharmacy society's position on prospective review of medication orders.

IO: Describe alternative approaches and compromises to MM4.10.

Objective EM 6.2.2:   Design a policy and procedure for compliance of MM4.10 in the emergency department taking into consideration the limitations described.

IO: Update or illustrate a policy and procedure for MM4.10

Objective EM 6.2.3:   Report findings of prospective review of medication orders in the emergency department using the PharmER model.

IO: Explain in graphs and tabular format the interventions and problem medication orders identified and resolved.

IO: Using various software applications document interventions onto a PDA to assure documentation of activities.

Outcome EM7: Optimize the quality of emergency care pharmacotherapy.

Goal EM 7.1:   Optimize antimicrobial pharmacotherapy in the emergency department for variety of infectious diseases.

Objective EM 7.1.1:   Describe pay for performance incentives for the emergency department management of Community Acquired Pneumonia and the surviving sepsis campaign and its impact on appropriate antimicrobial use in the ED.

IO: Describe PN5B.

IO: Describe the surviving sepsis campaign

Objective EM 7.1.2:   Initiate a modified antimicrobial stewardship in the emergency department.

IO: Describe the antimicrobial stewardship.

IO: Describe the economic outcomes benefits of an antimicrobial stewardship in the ED.

Objective EM 7.1.3:   Describe tools that emergency department clinical pharmacist may implement to prevent overuse and underuse of antimicrobials.

IO: Describe an Infectious Disease Clinical pathway.

IO: Describe an empiric antimicrobial request form

IO: Describe the use of the emergency department information System and embedding of a clinical decision support algorithm that assures optimal use of antimicrobials.

Objective EM 7.1.4:   List the responsibilities and duties of the emergency department-infectious disease clinical pharmacy services.

Objective EM 7.1.5:   Develop an infectious disease clinical pathway and empiric antimicrobial request form for the emergency department as part of a larger antimicrobial control program.

IO: Describe the contents of the infectious disease guideline

IO: Explain the rationale for the use of the empiric antimicrobial request form.

IO: Describe the goals of a hospital wide antimicrobial restricted pathway.

Objective EM 7.1.6:   Develop and design and empiric antimicrobial guideline, alternative choices, and oral conversion s for common infectious diseases such as Pneumonia, Soft Tissue Infections, Pyelonephritis, Bacterial Meningitis, Biliary Tract Infections, Bowel Related Infections, Surgical Wound Infections, Neutropenic sepsis.

Goal EM 7.2:   Detect, anticipate, recommend, tailor, dose, prepare, and procure antimicrobials for a variety of infectious diseases to expedite emergency care pharmacotherapy.

Goal EM 8.1:   Optimize antidotal pharmacotherapy in the emergency department for variety of Toxicological emergencies

Objective EM 8.1.1:   Describe the risks associated with antidote use and rationale for increases vigilance with their use

IO: Describe the EDTA associated deaths

IO: Describe the errors associated with Intravenous NAC

Objective EM 8.1.2: Review the evidence on the role of pharmacists in management of toxicological emergencies

IO: Describe Czajka's account

IO: Describe Levy and Barrone's description

Objective EM 8.1.2: Assuring safe and effective use of antidotes in the ED

IO: Describe the national problem of under-stocking antidotes in the ED

IO: Describe the consensus on minimal quantities and costs of antidotes

IO: Describe the monthly inventory check list used to assure appropriate quantities and stocking of antidotes

IO: Compare and contrast antidotes that should be stored in the ED and those that should not, and describe procedures that enable improved use of antidotes without delay.

IO: Apply toxicokinetics and toxicodynamics to predict extent of toxicity, observation period and disposition.

IO: Describe what activities, knowledge and skills the ED pharmacist must acquire to respond to toxicological emergencies

IO: Describe the optimal references and resources to acquire the knowledge and skills needed for managing toxicological emergencies

IO: Illustrate errors in diagnosis associated with toxicological emergencies - Interpretation of the acetaminophen level

IO: Describe cognitive tasks conducted by the ED Pharmacist to screen for error of antidote use

IO: List considerations needed to be made with safe and effective use of NAC

IO: Compare and contrast oral and intravenous use of NAC and which is the preferred route

IO: Prescribe, procure, dispense and monitor NAC use

IO: Describe the cognitive tasks needed to assure safe and effective use of calcium during CCA overdose

IO: Compare and contrast dosage forms of calcium - Gluconate versus chloride

IO: List toxicity of calcium and describe protocol orders to prevent

Goal EM 9.1: Optimize emergency care and critical care pharmacotherapy in the emergency department for a variety of medical emergencies

Objective EM 9.1.1: Identify the role of emergency care of the critical care patient in the ED

Objective EM 9.1.2: Describe the importance of early treatment to improve outcomes in the critically ill

IO: Describe the impact of early goal directed therapy for sepsis

Objective EM 9.1.3: List levels of management of the critically ill patient and the risk inherent in each level

Objective EM 9.1.4: Describe the importance of the Critical Care pharmacist and the gap in management while in the ED

IO: Review current evidence based pharmacotherapy of the impact of the Critical Care Pharmacist

Objective EM 9.1.5: Identify the role of the ED Pharmacist the initial management of the critical care patient in the ED

Objective EM 9.1.6: Use tools to expedite emergency care of the critical care patient.

IO: Rapidly identify the dose concentration, titration range procurement guide and expected effects of dopamine, dobutamine, norepinephrine, phenylephrine, epinephrine

IO: Rapidly identify the dose concentration, titration range procurement guide and expected effects of amiodarone, diltiazem, esmolol, isoproterenol, labetalol, milrinone, nitroglycerin, nitroprusside, procainamide

Objective EM 9.1.7: List the activities of the ED Pharmacist during the dispensing, administering and monitoring stage of the medication use process during resuscitation of the critical care patient

Objective EM 9.1.8: Describe the role of the ED Pharmacist in assisting with procedures

Objective EM 9.1.9: Describe the Emergency Physician's approach to responding to medical emergencies.

IO: Describe the primary survey.

IO: List the early evaluation and management of resuscitation

Goal EM 9.2: *Describe emergency care pharmacotherapy used during acute respiratory failure and when intubation is indicated*

Objective EM 9.2.1: Describe the pretreatments represented by the nemonic LOAD used during rapid sequence intubation.

Objective EM 9.2.2: Differentiate amongst the most commonly used sedative and paralytic used to facilitate rapid endotracheal intubation.

IO: Describe the dose regimen, procurement, product available method of administration and monitoring for etomidate, midazolam, methohexital, thiopental, propofol and ketamine.

IO: Describe the dose regimen, procurement,, product available method of administration and monitoring for succinylcholine vecuronium, pancuronium, rocuronium

IO: describe the order of administration of sedation and paralysis and its importance.

IO: Describe the differences amongst paralytics in onset, and Duration of action of each paralytic

IO: Describe the difference between depolarizing and Non-depolarizing agents

IO: Describe how to monitor for effectiveness of paralysis

IO: Describe safety precautions used to prevent look-alike and sound-alike errors with paralytics

IO: Describe the side effect profile of paralytics

IO: describe the clinical relevance of hyperkalemia with paralytics

IO: Describe contraindications of raised ICP associated with succinylcholine

Objective EM 9.2.3: Describe maneuvers used by the pharmacist to assist in during rapid endotracheal intubation.

IO: Describe the Sellick's maneuver and why it's used

IO: Describe the BURP maneuver and why it is used

IO: Identify the methods used to assure correct placement of the ETT

IO: Describe the colorimetric end-tidal CO2 detector

Objective EM 9.2.4: Describe post intubation complications.

Objective EM 9.2.5: Describe a therapeutic plan for long term sedation and paralysis

IO: Describe the use of the Ramsey scale for sedation

IO: Describe the need for analgesia and the medication used for it

IO: Recall the doses of morphine and fentanyl

Goal EM 9.3.0: *Describe emergency care pharmacotherapy for circulation management*

Objective EM 9.3.1: Describe the importance of CPR in survival of cardiac arrest

Objective EM 9.3.2: Identify ominous but treatable cardiac rhythms

IO: Differentiate Asystole, Pulseless electrical activity and ventricular fibrillation, tachycardia

Objective EM 9.3.3: List the medications to have on hand for pulseless ventricular fibrillation or tachycardia

IO: Describe the dose regimen, procurement, product available, method of administration and monitoring for epinephrine, vasopressin, amiodarone, lidocaine, magnesium, and procainamide

IO: Describe mechanism of effects, side effects of epinephrine, vasopressin, amiodarone, lidocaine, magnesium, and procainamide and the evidence based pharmacotherapy supporting their use

Objective EM 9.3.4: List the medications to have on hand for bradycardia leading to Asystole

Objective EM 9.3.5: Describe the reasons for persistent asystole

Objective EM 9.3.6: Recall the etiologies for Pulseless Electrical Activity

IO: Describe the 5 H's and 5 T's of PEA

Objective EM 9.3.7: Describe the emergency care pharmacotherapy of 5 H's and 5 T's

IO: Describe the dose regimen, procurement, product available, method of administration and monitoring for saline, sodium bicarbonate, potassium chloride, glucose and insulin, calcium chloride/gluconate, Dextrose 50% and thiamine

IO: Describe mechanism of effects, side effects of saline, sodium bicarbonate, potassium chloride, glucose and insulin, calcium chloride/gluconate, Dextrose 50% and thiamine and the evidence based pharmacotherapy supporting their use

Goal EM 10.1: Optimize emergency medicine pharmacotherapy for special populations: Geriatric, Pediatric and Pregnancy and Lactation

Goal EM 11.1: Implement a multidisciplinary medication reconciliation process in the ED

INDEX

Page numbers followed by "f" denote figures; those followed by "t" denote tables

A

AAEM. *See* American Academy of Emergency Medicine
ACEP. *See* American College of Emergency Physicians
Acetaminophen overdose, 122–123
Acetylcysteine, 120–123
Activated partial thromboplastin time, 165
Acuity levels, 70, 70t
Acute meningitis, 102–103
Adenosine, 179t
Administration of medications, 63, 69
Advanced cardiovascular life support, 143
Advanced hazardous material life support training, 131
Adverse drug events, 83
Adverse outcomes, 46f–47f
Airway management, 141
Albuterol, 147
Alcohol abuse screening, 215
Alteplase, 150
American Academy of Emergency Medicine, 83, 168
American College of Emergency Physicians, 83–84, 168
American Society of Health-System Pharmacists, 84, 191–192, 212f
Amiodarone, 145
Analgesic therapy, 16
Anchoring, 5
Anthrax, 129
Antiarrhythmic drugs, 145
Antibiotic surveillance committee, 96
Antibiotics
    acute meningitis treated with, 102–103
    community-acquired methicillin-resistant *Staphylococcus aureus,* 103–104
    early use of, 99
    empiric, 98t, 99, 101, 105, 160f
    pharmacist's role in expediting, 95, 96t
    pneumonia treated with, 104–105
    during pregnancy, 184t
    request form for, 96f, 97
    sepsis treated with, 100–102
    timing of, 100
    urinary tract infections treated with, 104
Antidote(s)
    calcium salts as, 123–124
    cyanide, 125–126
    Digibind, 125
    DigiFab, 125
    effective use of, 118–119
    flumazenil, 127
    fomepizole, 126–127
    glucagon as, 124–125

high-dose insulin–euglycemia, 123, 128
intravenous ethanol solution, 126–127
methylene blue, 127–128
monthly inventory verification record for, 119f
N-acetylcysteine, 120–123
naloxone hydrochloride, 128
risk associated with, 117–118
types of, 118t
Antimicrobial stewardship
    definition of, 95
    procedures for, 96–97
    programs for, 95
Assessing Care of Vulnerable Elders, 175, 176t
Asymptomatic bacteriuria, 104
Asystole, 145–146
Atropine, 145, 179t
Australian College of Emergency Medicine, 3
Automated dispensing machines for medications, 76f, 77t, 77–78
Automated medication management systems, 70
Availability heuristic, 6

B

Bacterial meningitis, 97, 98t, 100
Bacteriuria, asymptomatic, 104
Basic life support, 143
Benzodiazepine overdose, 127
Beta lactams, 102
Biases, 5–6
Bicarbonate, 180t
Bioterrorism, 134, 135f
Blood transfusion, 152
Bounded rationality, 5
Bradycardia, 145
Breathing management, 141
Brief intervention, 113
BURP, 142

C

Calcium channel blocker overdose, 123–124
Calcium chloride, 179t
Calcium salts, 123–124
Cardiac arrest, 148, 150
Cardiac rhythms, 143
Cardiogenic shock, 151
Cardiopulmonary resuscitation
    of critically ill patients, 141, 141t, 145
    description of, 143
    form for, 144f
    for pediatric emergencies, 177–178, 179t–181
CDSS. *See* Clinical decision support system
Certifications, 39
Change, 51
Change practitioner, 215

Ciprofloxacin, 104
Circulation management, 143
Clinical decision support system
    definition of, 57, 155
    deployment of, 156, 156t
    implementation of, 58–67, 155–162
    infectious disease guide incorporated into, 97–99
    protocol orders, 157f–162f, 162–165
    quality achieved through, 165
Clinical pharmacy services. *See* Emergency care pharmacy services
Cognitive biases, 5
Colorimetric end tidal carbon dioxide detection, 142
Community-acquired methicillin-resistant *Staphylococcus aureus,* 103–104
Community-acquired pneumonia, 97, 98t, 104–106
Computerized physician order entry
    advantages of, 57, 166
    continuity of care, 97
    definition of, 57
    disadvantages of, 58
    errors associated with, 156
    formulary compliance and, 70, 75, 175
    implementation of, 58–67, 155–157
    infectious disease guide incorporated into, 97–99
    medication error reduction through, 57–58
    pharmacist's role in, 58–67, 67
Confirmation bias, 5
Conjunction fallacy, 5
Continuity of care, 78–79, 97, 125, 175
Coronary thrombosis, 150
Covey, Stephen, 51
CPOE. *See* Computerized physician order entry
Critical care, 139
Critical care pharmacist, 140
Critical patient, 192
Critically ill patients
    airway management, 141
    asystole, 145–146
    breathing management, 141
    cardiac arrest, 148, 150
    circulation management in, 143
    emergency care for, 140t
    emergency department's role in treating, 139
    high-risk areas for, 139–140
    hypercalcemia, 147
    hyperkalemia in, 146–147
    hypermagnesemia, 147
    hypokalemia in, 146
    hypomagnesemia, 147
    intubation of, 141–142
    management of, 140
    peri-infusion complications, 150

Critically ill patients *(continued)*
  primary survey of, 141
  pulmonary embolism, 148
  pulseless electrical activity, 146–147
  resuscitation of, 141, 141t, 145
  shock, 150–152
  tamponade, 147–148
  tension pneumothorax, 147–148
  thrombolysis, 148–150, 149f
  thrombosis, 148, 150
Cyanide antidote, 125–126

D
Decision making
  approaches to, 4–5
  by doctor-nurse team, 84
  errors in, 5–7
Decision threshold, 4
Dextrose, 179t
Diagnosis
  decision making approach to, 4–5
  emergency physician's approach to, 4
  errors in, 7
  time from emergency department entry
    until, 32
Digibind, 125
DigiFab, 125
Disaster preparedness, 129–135
Discharge counseling, 33
Dispensing of medications, 63, 69–70
Distributive shock, 151–152
Dobutamine, 152
Doctor-nurse team, 84
Documentation systems, 58, 58t
Dopamine, 152
Drug Abuse Warning Network, 110, 111f,
  213–214, 214t
Drug administration, 17–20, 63, 69
Drug interactions
  barriers to prevention of, 114–115
  brief intervention, 113
  challenges associated with, 109
  high-risk medications for, 113
  incidence of, 115
  multimodal approach to, 110
  oral formulations and, 120, 122
  pharmacist's role, 110–111
  prevention of, 110, 114–115
  safe medication use practices for, 113–114
  screening for, 109, 112–114
Drug order and delivery. *See also* Formulary;
    Medication order(s)
  for boarded patients, 78
  computerized physician order entry for. *See*
    Computerized physician order entry
  stages of, 6f, 6–7, 47f

E
Early goal-directed therapy, 139
Edetate disodium, 117
Elderly
  continuity of care for, 175
  discharge planning for, 211
  emergency care for, 173–174
  geriatric emergency care pharmacotherapeu-
    tic interventions, 175, 176t
  geriatric emergency department interven-
    tions, 174t, 174–175
  less-than-optimal quality care for, 174
Electrocardiogram, 146–147
Electronic medical records, 59, 60f–61f, 162
Electronic medication administration records,
  67, 89f
Emergency care pharmacotherapist, 15

Emergency care pharmacy services. *See also*
    Pharmacist
  discharge counseling, 33
  elements of performance, 130t
  epidemiology of, 22
  future of, 211–216
  historical perspective of, 21–22
  limited therapeutic options, 32
  nursing staff and, 52
  physical constraint effects on, 31
  prioritization in, 32
  requirements of, 31
  systematic review of, 22–25, 26t–28t, 28–29
  time pressures, 31–32
  variety of patients, 32
  volume pressures, 31–32
Emergency department
  boarding of patients, 78–81, 80f
  closure of, 11
  crisis for, 10–12
  errors in, 4
  increased usage of, 9–10
  at Maimonides Medical Center, 35–39
  overcrowding in, 11, 31, 131
  pharmacy verification in, 85–86
  physical constraints of, 31
  quality of care in, 10
  regulatory challenges for, 11
  statistics regarding, 10
  temporizing treatments offered in, 33
  variety of patients in, 32
Emergency Department Information Systems,
  155
Emergency department pharmacist
  academic-based, 35, 39
  advanced hazardous material life support
    training for, 131
  certifications, 39
  clinical decision support system implementa-
    tion and, 58–67
  computerized physician order entry imple-
    mentation and, 58–67
  cost-related benefits of, 25, 27t
  discharge counseling by, 33
  drug interaction screening, 110–111
  education of, 39
  emergency physicians and, collaboration
    between, 52, 54
  future of, 215
  historical perspective of, 21–22
  impact of, 25, 27t
  information gathering by, 33
  job responsibilities of, 24–25
  knowledge-transition facilitated by, 54
  limited therapeutic options for, 33
  management tools for, 49–51
  medication order review by, 165
  nursing staff and, 52
  pediatric care, 177, 178t
  prioritization by, 32
  public health initiatives and, 215–216
  public health role of, 129–131
  responsibilities of, 140
  resuscitative care by, 39
  role of, 21–22, 24–25, 140t, 215
  systematic review of, 22–25, 26t–28t, 28–29
  as team member, 33
  time and volume pressures on, 31–32
  toxicologic emergencies and, 118–119
  training of, 39
  variety of patients experienced by, 32
Emergency Medical Treatment and Active
    Labor Act (EMTALA), 11
Emergency medicine
  administrative components of, 193
  definition of, 3

  documentation systems, 58, 58t
  history of, 3–4
  pharmacotherapy principles and, 15–20
  practice model for, 191–192
  public health and, 129
  verification of, 85
Emergency medicine undergraduate clerkship
  advantages of, 202, 203t
  assessment tools and outcomes, 203,
    204f–205f
  challenges associated with, 202–203
  course objectives, 195, 196t
  course session description, 195, 200
  hands-on learning, 200
  instructional methods and content, 195
Emergency Nursing Association, 83–84, 168
Emergency operations center, 132
Emergency physician
  approach used for patients, 4
  challenges for, 6
  decision making by, 4–5
  mistakes by, 85
  pharmacist and, collaboration between,
    52, 54
  temporizing treatments by, 33
Emergent illness, 192
Empiric antibiotic therapy, 98t, 99, 101,
  105, 160f
ENA. *See* Emergency Nursing Association
Endotracheal intubation, 141–142
Enoxaparin, 16
Epinephrine, 143, 145, 150, 179t
Errors. *See also* Medication errors
  in children, 175, 177
  computerized physician order entry, 156
  costs of, 9
  decision making, 5–7
  diagnostic, 7
  drug order and delivery, 7
  in emergency department, 4
  pediatric, 175, 177
  prevention of, 6, 177
  resuscitation, 145
  system-related causes for, 6–7
Ethylene glycol poisoning, 126–127
Etomidate, 179t
Event-driven decision making, 5
Evidence-based medicine, 4, 120,
  214–215

F
Failure mode effect analysis, 49–51, 50f, 52t
Fentanyl, 179t
Flumazenil, 127
Focused reconciliation, 168–169, 171f
Fomepizole, 126–127
Formulary
  barriers for restricting, 69
  computerized physician order entry effects on
    compliance with, 70, 75, 175
  Joint Commission for the Accreditation of
    Healthcare Organization standards, 69
  sample, 71t–74t
  unit of use, 70
Full reconciliation, 169
Furosemide, 179t

G
Gentamicin, 104
Geriatric emergency care pharmacotherapeutic
  interventions, 175, 176t
Geriatric emergency department interventions,
  174t, 174–175
Glucagon, 124–125

H

Hazardous exposures, 134
Healthcare
   equity of, 12
   national goals for, 12, 12t
   timeliness of, 12
Healthcare quality
   in emergency department, 10
   enhancing of, 94
Healthcare-acquired pneumonia, 97,
      98t, 105
Healthcare-associated medication errors, 123
HEICS. *See* Hospital emergency incident
      command systems
Heparin weight-based nomogram, 163f, 165
Herbal–drug interactions, 109
Herman-Miller carts, 75, 77f
Heuristics thinking, 5
High-dose insulin–euglycemia, 123, 128
High-risk discharge assessment instrument,
      211–212
Hindsight bias, 6
Hospital emergency incident command systems,
      131–132
Hospital-acquired pneumonia, 97, 98t
HRDAI. *See* High-risk discharge assessment
      instrument
Hydralazine, 183t
Hydroxocobalamin, 126
Hypercalcemia, 147
Hyperkalemia, 141–142, 146–147
Hypermagnesemia, 147
Hypokalemia, 146
Hypomagnesemia, 147
Hypothetico-deductive method of decision
      making, 4
Hypovolemic shock, 151

I

Iceberg model, of medical errors, 9, 10f
Index of suspicion, 4
Infectious disease guidelines, 97–99, 101
Intern. *See* Pharmacy intern
Intracranial pressure, 142
Intravenous ethanol solution, 126–127
Intubation
   of critically ill patients, 141–142
   rapid sequence, 178, 182t
Ischemic chest pain order set, 158f–159f,
      162–165

J

Joint Commission for the Accreditation of
      Healthcare Organization (JCAHO)
   description of, 11, 21
   emergency management standards, 132
   formulary standards, 69
   mock survey, 53f
   National Patient Safety Goals, 54

K

Ketamine, 180t
Ketorolac, 17
KLAS, 58
Knowledge base inadequacies, 59
Knowledge-transition, 54, 155

L

Labetalol, 16, 183t
Lactation, 182, 184
Leadership, 49
Lidocaine, 145, 180t

M

Magnesium, 145, 183t
Maimonides Medical Center, 35–39, 85–86,
      165
Manufacture-associated medication errors,
      123–125
Mean arterial blood pressure, 151
Medical decision making, 4–5
Medical errors. *See* Errors
Medical injury, 9
Medication(s). *See also* Formulary
   acuity levels and, 70, 70t
   administration of, 63, 69
   automated dispensing machines for, 76f, 77t,
      77–78
   automated management systems, 70
   case study of, 18–20
   dispensing of, 63, 69–70
   high-risk, identification of, 64f–65f
   in lactation, 182, 184, 184t
   newly approved, 17
   in pregnancy, 182, 184, 184t
   principles for, 15–20
   prospective review of, 115
   storage of, 75–77, 76f
   timing of administration, 17
Medication errors. *See also* Errors
   computerized physician order entry for
      reduction of, 57–58
   continuity-related, 123
   cost containment and, 123
   deaths caused by, 11
   economic costs associated with, 11
   healthcare-associated, 123
   knowledge base inadequacies as cause of, 59
   manufacture-associated, 123–125
   national goals for, 12
   pharmacist's role in reducing, 22, 25, 27t
   prevalence of, 110
   procurement-related, 125
   transcription-related, 57
Medication history, 113, 113f, 211
Medication management technician, 207
Medication order(s)
   boarded, 78
   pharmacist's role in reviewing, 165
   preformed, 61, 62f
   prescribing of, 57
   problem, 86
   prospective review of, 61, 63, 89f–91f,
      115, 165
   transcribing of, 57
   verification of, 85
Medication order review, 32
Medication reconciliation
   barriers to, 168
   definition of, 167
   flowchart for, 168f
   focused, 168–169, 171f
   form for, 170f
   full, 169
   levels of, 168–169
   at Maimonides, 169–172
   multidisciplinary process for, 168
   resistance to, 167–168
   screening, 168–169
Medication therapy management services,
      211–214, 214t
Meningitis, 97, 98t, 100, 102–103
Methanol poisoning, 126–127
Methemoglobinemia, 127–128
Methicillin-resistant *Staphylococcus aureus*,
      103–104
Methotrexate, 181, 183t
Methylene blue, 127–128
Midazolam, 180t

Mitigation strategies, 51
Mixed soft tissue infection, 97, 98t
MM4.10, 25, 52, 84
Morphine, 180t

N

N-acetylcysteine, 120–123
Naloxone, 180t
Naloxone hydrochloride, 128
National Patient Safety Goals, 54
Naturalistic decision making, 5
Necrotizing pneumonia, 104
Neurogenic shock, 151–152
Neutropenic sepsis, 97, 98t
Nicardipine, 183t
Norepinephrine, 152
Nursing staff, 52

O

Obstetrical emergency care, 181–184
Obstructive shock, 151–152
Older adults. *See* Elderly
"Out of sight, out of mind" failure mode, 6
Outcomes, 84
Oxytocin, 183t

P

Pancuronium, 142
Paracetamol, 118
Paralysis, 142
Paralytics, 141
Patient safety
   enhancing of, 94
   goals for improving, 12
   public concern of, 9
   training curriculum for, 199t
Pay for performance, 99–100
Pediatrics
   cardiopulmonary resuscitation in, 177–178,
      179t–181
   emergency department pharmacists' role,
      177, 178t
   medical errors, 175, 177
Peth, Howard A., 6
PGY-1
   mastery of goals and objectives by, 190
   role and activities of, 189–191
PGY-2
   credentialing book, 190
   emergency medicine model and, 191–193
   goals and objectives for, 190, 192
   procedural pharmacotherapy, 192
   role and activities of, 190–191
   standards for, 191
Pharmaceutical care, 129–131, 130f, 215
Pharmacist
   critical care, 140
   emergency department. *See* Emergency
      department pharmacist
Pharmacotherapists, 15, 39, 120, 122
Pharmacotherapy principles
   automation effects, 67
   case study of, 18–20
   emergency medicine and, 15–20
   list of, 16t
Pharmacotherapy screening, 87f
Pharmacy emergency response team, 132, 134,
      135f
Pharmacy intern
   activities for, 200
   personal attributes of, 200, 202
   undergraduate clerkship for. *See* Emergency
      medicine undergraduate clerkship

Pharmacy services. *See* Emergency care
    pharmacy services
Pharmacy technician, 207–209
PharmER pyramid model, 39–41, 45–48,
    85, 187
Phenylephrine, 152
Physician. *See* Emergency physician
Piperacillin–tazobactam, 104
PN-5b, 100
Pneumonia, 97, 98t, 104–106
Post-graduate year one residency. *See* PGY-1
Post-graduate year two residency. *See* PGY-2
Preformed medication orders, 61, 62f
Pregnancy, 181–184
Prevalence bias, 6
Problem medication order, 86
Procainamide, 145
Procedural pharmacotherapy, 192
Process, 84
Procurement-related medication errors, 125
Propofol, 180t
Prospective review, 61, 63, 83–84, 89f–91f,
    114f, 165
Protocol orders, 157, 157f–162f, 162–165
Public health emergencies, 129–135
Public health initiatives, 215–216
Pulmonary embolism, 148
Pulseless electrical activity, 146–147
Pyelonephritis, 97, 98t, 104

Q

Quality
    clinical decision support system and, 165
    enhancing of, 94
Quality indicators, 84t, 101

R

RACQITO, 6
Ramsay scale, 142

Rapid sequence intubation, 178, 182t
Representative bias, 6
Resuscitation
    of critically ill patients, 141,
        141t, 145
    description of, 39, 143
    form for, 144f
    for pediatric emergencies, 177–178,
        179t–181
RhoGAM, 181, 183t
Rocuronium, 141, 180t

S

Safe medication use system, 45–49,
    113–114
Safety. *See* Patient safety
SATO effect/phenomenon, 6, 85
Screening reconciliation, 168–169
Search satisficing, 5
Sedation, 142
Selection bias, 28
Sellick's maneuver, 142
Sepsis, 100–102, 139
Serotonin syndrome, 111
Shock, 150–152
Society for Academic Emergency Medicine,
    191
Soft tissue infection, 97, 98t
Speed over accuracy tradeoff effect, 85
Stat medications, 79
Status epilepticus, 123
Storage of medications, 75–77, 76f
Streptokinase, 150
Structure, 84
Succinylcholine, 141–142, 180t
Sumatriptan, 18–20, 110
Surgical wound infections, 97, 98t
Sutton's law, 5
Swiss cheese model of adverse outcomes,
    46f–47f

System change, 51
Systems thinking, 45

T

Tamponade, 147–148
Taniguchi, Theodore, 3–4, 21
TEAM, 49
Technology-enabled knowledge transition, 155
Tension pneumothorax, 147–148
Thiopental, 180t
Thrombolysis, 148–150, 149f
Thrombosis, 148, 150
Timeliness, 12
Toxic shock syndrome, 103
Toxicologic emergencies
    antidotes for. *See* Antidote(s)
    case studies of, 117–118
    pharmacists' role in, 118–119
Transfusion, 152
Triage, 169

U

Undergraduate clerkship. *See* Emergency
    medicine undergraduate clerkship
Unit dose distribution system, 78–81
Unit of use formulary, 70
Urinary tract infections, 104

V

Vasopressin, 143, 145
Vecuronium, 142, 180t–181t
Ventilator associated pneumonia, 97
Ventricular fibrillation, 143
Ventricular tachycardia, 143

W

Win-win relationships, 51–52